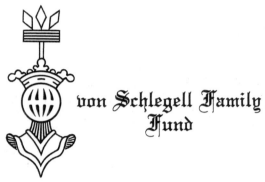

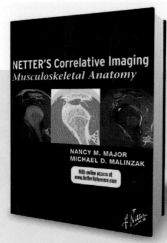 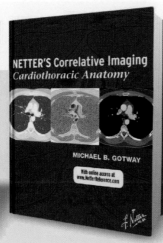 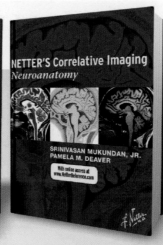 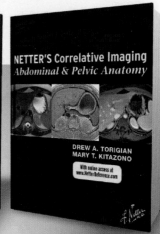
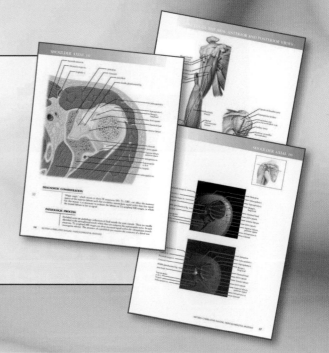

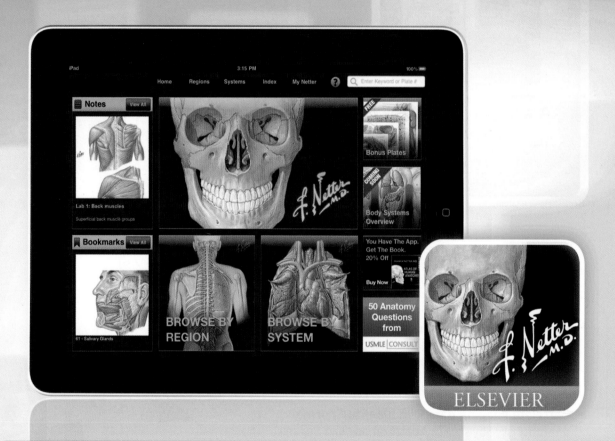
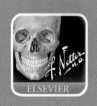

NETTER'S
Correlative Imaging: Neuroanatomy

Volume Editors
THOMAS C. LEE, MD
Assistant Section Head
Neuroradiology
Instructor
Harvard Medical School
Boston, Massachusetts

SRINIVASAN MUKUNDAN, JR., MD, PhD
Neuroradiology Network Chief
Brigham and Women's Hospital
Associate Professor of Radiology
Harvard University
Boston, Massachusetts

Series Editor
NANCY M. MAJOR, MD
Director of Diagnostic Imaging
Orthopaedic Associates of Allentown
Allentown, Pennsylvania

Illustrations by
Frank H. Netter, MD

Contributing Illustrators
Tiffany Slaybaugh DaVanzo, MA, CMI
Carlos Machado, MD

ELSEVIER
SAUNDERS

ELSEVIER
SAUNDERS

1600 John F. Kennedy Blvd.
Ste 1800
Philadelphia, PA 19103-2899

NETTER'S CORRELATIVE IMAGING: NEUROANATOMY   ISBN: 978-1-4377-0415-0
Copyright © 2015 by Saunders, an imprint of Elsevier Inc.

Notices

Knowledge and best practice in this field are constantly changing. As new research and experience broaden our understanding, changes in research methods, professional practices, or medical treatment may become necessary.

Practitioners and researchers must always rely on their own experience and knowledge in evaluating and using any information, methods, compounds, or experiments described herein. In using such information or methods they should be mindful of their own safety and the safety of others, including parties for whom they have a professional responsibility.

With respect to any drug or pharmaceutical products identified, readers are advised to check the most current information provided (i) on procedures featured or (ii) by the manufacturer of each product to be administered, to verify the recommended dose or formula, the method and duration of administration, and contraindications. It is the responsibility of practitioners, relying on their own experience and knowledge of their patients, to make diagnoses, to determine dosages and the best treatment for each individual patient, and to take all appropriate safety precautions.

To the fullest extent of the law, neither the Publisher nor the authors, contributors, or editors, assume any liability for any injury and/or damage to persons or property as a matter of products liability, negligence or otherwise, or from any use or operation of any methods, products, instructions, or ideas contained in the material herein.

Library of Congress Cataloging-in-Publication Data
Netter's correlative imaging. Neuroanatomy / volume editors, Thomas C. Lee,
Srinivasan Mukundan, Jr. ; illustrations by Frank H. Netter, contributing
illustrators, Tiffany Slaybaugh DaVanzo, Carlos Machado.
        p. ; cm. -- (Netter clinical science)
  Correlative imaging: neuroanatomy
  Neuroanatomy
  Includes bibliographical references and index.
  ISBN 978-1-4377-0415-0 (hardcover: alk. paper)
  I. Lee, Thomas C., editor. II. Mukundan, Srinivasan, Jr., editor. III.
Netter, Frank H. (Frank Henry), 1906-1991, illustrator. IV. Title:
Correlative imaging: neuroanatomy. V. Title: Neuroanatomy. VI. Series:
Netter clinical science.
  [DNLM: 1. Nervous System--anatomy & histology--Atlases. 2. Magnetic
Resonance Imaging--Atlases. WL 17]
  QM451
  611.8022'2--dc23   2014001295

Senior Content Strategist: Elyse O'Grady
Senior Content Development Editor: Marybeth Thiel
Publishing Services Manager: Patricia Tannian
Project Manager: Kate Mannix
Design Direction: Louis Forgione

Printed in China

Last digit is the print number: 9 8 7 6 5 4 3 2 1

To my wonderful parents, Wendy and Doug,
for their unwavering support and encouragement
To my siblings, Ashley, Hillary, MacGregor, and Alex,
who have been permanent sources of love and inspiration
McKinley D. Nickerson, Project Coordinator

To my inspirational parents, Sun Hyee and Chang Whan Lee,
who provided my foundation
To my sister and brother-in-law, Jane and Richard, and their son,
Alexander, for bringing bright hope for the future
To my supportive wife, Ji In, who is my one and only soulmate
Thomas C. Lee

To my wife, Nancy, and our sons, TJ and Dev
To my parents, teachers, and mentors
To students past, present, and future, who,
through their study and dedication, validate this effort
Srinivasan Mukundan

About the Artists

FRANK H. NETTER, MD

Frank H. Netter was born in 1906 in New York City. He studied art at the Art Students League and the National Academy of Design before entering medical school at New York University, where he received his MD in 1931. During his student years, Dr. Netter's notebook sketches attracted the attention of the medical faculty and other physicians, allowing him to augment his income by illustrating articles and textbooks. He continued illustrating on the side after establishing a surgical practice in 1933, but he ultimately opted to give up his practice in favor of a full-time commitment to art. After service in the United States Army during World War II, Dr. Netter began his long collaboration with the CIBA Pharmaceutical Company (now Novartis Pharmaceuticals). This 45-year partnership resulted in the production of the extraordinary collection of medical art so familiar to physicians and other medical professionals worldwide.

In 2005, Elsevier, Inc., purchased the Netter Collection and all publications from Icon Learning Systems. There are now more than 50 publications featuring the art of Dr. Netter available through Elsevier, Inc. (in the US: www.us.elsevierhealth.com/Netter; outside the US: www.elsevierhealth.com).

Dr. Netter's works are among the finest examples of the use of illustration in the teaching of medical concepts. The 13-book *Netter Collection of Medical Illustrations*, which includes the greater part of the more than 20,000 paintings created by Dr. Netter, became and remains one of the most famous medical works ever published. *The Netter Atlas of Human Anatomy*, first published in 1989, presents the anatomical paintings from the Netter Collection. Now translated into 16 languages, it is the anatomy atlas of choice among medical and health professions students the world over.

The Netter illustrations are appreciated not only for their aesthetic qualities, but, more important, for their intellectual content. As Dr. Netter wrote in 1949, ". . . clarification of a subject is the aim and goal of illustration. No matter how beautifully painted, how delicately and subtly rendered a subject may be, it is of little value as a *medical illustration* if it does not serve to make clear some medical point." Dr. Netter's planning, conception, point of view, and approach are what inform his paintings and what make them so intellectually valuable.

Frank H. Netter, MD, physician and artist, died in 1991.

Learn more about the physician-artist whose work has inspired the Netter Reference collection: http://www.netterimages.com/artist/netter.htm

CARLOS MACHADO, MD

Carlos Machado was chosen by Novartis to be Dr. Netter's successor. He continues to be the main artist who contributes to the *Netter Collection of Medical Illustrations*.

Self-taught in medical illustration, cardiologist Carlos Machado has contributed meticulous updates to some of Dr. Netter's original plates and has created many paintings of his own in the style of Netter as an extension of the Netter Collection. Dr. Machado's photorealistic expertise and his keen insight into the physician/patient relationship inform his vivid and unforgettable visual style. His dedication to researching each topic and subject he paints places him among the premier medical illustrators at work today.

Learn more about his background and see more of his art at: http://www.netterimages.com/artist/machado.htm

TIFFANY SLAYBAUGH DAVANZO, MA, CMI

Tiffany Slaybaugh DaVanzo is a Certified Medical Illustrator and graduate of the Johns Hopkins University School of Medicine's Art as Applied to Medicine master's degree program. She has been a self-employed medical illustrator since 2006, and her work has received numerous awards. She specializes in art for medical publications, education, and the medical legal field.

The first medical text Tiffany owned was Netter's *Atlas of Human Anatomy*. It currently sits on her desk tattered and littered with Post-It notes from years of hard use, but is a tribute to Dr. Netter's influence on her art. She considers it a career highlight to be creating new artwork for the Netter collection. Tiffany lives in Tennessee with her husband and two young daughters.

About the Editors

Thomas C. Lee, MD, grew up in Toronto, Ontario. He attended Harvard College and earned an AB degree with honors in biochemical studies. He graduated from medical school at McGill University in Montreal before returning to his hometown, where he completed a residency in diagnostic radiology, followed by a fellowship in neuroradiology, at the University of Toronto.

While a student at Harvard, he attended Addenbrooke's Hospital at Cambridge University, United Kingdom, as a Weissman Awardee. As a medical student, he won the BiochemPharma Award for McGill medical student research of highest scientific merit, and as a resident, he won the Radiological Society of North America Award for research excellence. He has co-authored several peer-reviewed manuscripts and book chapters. He has lectured at many local, national, and international meetings with a focus on head, neck, and spine imaging and intervention, most recently on MRI-guided cryoablation of nerves and tumors of the head, neck, and spine.

Dr. Lee is currently an instructor of radiology at Harvard Medical School, as well as assistant section head of neuroradiology at Brigham and Women's Hospital, and is a premedical advisor for Quincy House of Harvard College.

Srinivasan Mukundan, Jr., MD, PhD, grew up in Atlanta, Georgia, where he attended Emory University to study chemistry, earning his BS, MS, and PhD degrees. He then entered Emory University School of Medicine, earning his MD and completing a postdoctoral fellowship in cardiac MRI, a residency in diagnostic radiology, and a clinical fellowship in neuroradiology.

Dr. Mukundan has won research awards as a graduate student, medical student, and resident. He also received the Berlex-Neuroradiology Education Research Foundation Scholar Award from the American Society of Neuroradiology and the Scholar Award from the American Roentgen Ray Society. He has co-authored more than 80 peer-reviewed manuscripts, as well as 10 book chapters and one textbook. In addition, he is a frequent speaker both nationally and internationally on a variety of topics related to neuroradiology, MRI, and preclinical imaging.

Dr. Mukundan is currently an associate professor of radiology at Harvard Medical School and the section head of neuroradiology at Brigham and Women's Hospital. In addition, he holds several other administrative positions at Brigham and Women's Hospital, including neuroradiology network director, co-director of the Clinical Functional MRI Program, and chair of the Contrast Agent Safety Committee. He is also the first director of the Brigham and Women's Hospital Small Animal Imaging Laboratory.

Acknowledgments

From our perspective, this project began several years ago with a phone call from Dr. Nancy Major, a dear colleague and friend. Nancy has served as the driving force behind the Netter's Correlative Imaging series, finding the authors and helping define the unique format of this project. In our specific project, she provided support and guidance at several key stages of the project.

The Elsevier publishing team is led by Elyse O'Grady, Senior Content Strategist, and Marybeth Thiel, Senior Content Development Editor. They practice their craft according to the finest traditions of book editing and publishing that have evolved from the time of the first presses. This is particularly admirable given that many of these traditions are challenged in our modern world. Mostly, Marybeth and Elyse are recognized for their patience and their passion in seeing this project through to its conclusion.

Several colleagues and friends have played significant roles during the evolution of this project. We extend heartfelt gratitude to these individuals:

Dr. Pamela Deaver

Dr. Leahthan Domeshak

Dr. Gerald Grant

Dr. Jeffrey Marcus

Dr. Karli Spetzler

Special thanks go to Frank H. Netter, MD, often considered the "Michelangelo of Medicine," who created and perfected this genre. Our artist, Tiffany DaVanzo, immersed herself in creating illustrations that are of high artistic quality, and then spent countless hours in conferences reviewing the fine details of the artwork on a plate-by-plate basis to ensure anatomic accuracy. Tiffany is recognized for her stewardship of the Netter tradition to which we are all committed.

Finally, **McKinley Nickerson** served as our project coordinator. Her myriad contributions have ranged from scheduling and coordination to assistance with image segmentation and digital proofs. Simply stated, this project would never have been completed without McKinley's participation.

Preface

The study of anatomy, by its very nature, exposes the student to both the forms and the functions responsible for the inner workings of the human body—one of the most elegant demonstrations of the synthesis of art and science. This statement is never truer than when reviewing the works of Frank H. Netter, MD (1906-1991). His monumental works of art have educated countless generations of physicians and will continue to do so for many years to come.

The evolution of cross-sectional imaging technologies, including computed tomography (CT) and magnetic resonance imaging (MRI), has allowed physicians and aspiring physicians the ability to peer into the human body in many ways previously impossible. This, in turn, has forced the review of anatomy in a manner that was not contemplated when Dr. Netter began rendering his artwork more than three-quarters of a century ago. Limited spatial and temporal resolution, tissue parameters, image contrast, and partial volume averaging are all issues that confound the interpretation of MRI and CT images and are not part of conventional anatomic teaching in the dissection laboratory.

Despite the changing nature of the anatomy education problem, Dr. Netter's approach still provides the template for how to teach modern medical imaging. By directly correlating cross-sectional medical images with "Netter art" that is voxel matched, the student is provided with the key to unlock the anatomy hidden within.

Many existing textbooks with radiology images and clarifying illustrations focus on showing 3D renderings for better understanding of the entire course of a particular structure, such as a cranial nerve. Our goal, however, is to provide a more rigorous "slice-by-slice" reference guide for both the cross-sectional medical image and the corresponding illustration. For instance, someone may understand the general course of the facial nerve, yet still have difficulty identifying the fractional component of this structure on a single axial image. Conversely, individuals may need help identifying an unknown structure on a given image, particularly in the coronal or sagittal planes. Finally, the imaging characteristics on CT versus different sequences of MRI, such as T1- or T2-weighted imaging, can often be confusing and will hopefully be partially clarified through this book.

This volume remains true to the goals of the *Netter's Correlative Imaging* series. There is high-quality imaging, allowing the demonstration of important anatomic structures, including structures not always included in other sources. The book also serves as a user-friendly anatomy reference for commonly employed imaging techniques of the brain, head, neck, and spine. As with the other volumes in the series, the text is not inclusive of pathology. In addition, normal variant anatomy and clinical pearls are presented.

Structures are labeled using the most common terms and should be acceptable to radiologists, neurosurgeons, and neurologists.

It is our hope that this volume will serve as a primary source of knowledge to the novice and as a reference text for the seasoned veteran. In either case, we hope that it will be useful on a daily basis.

Contents

CONTENTS

PART 3 SPINE

PART 1 BRAIN

Chapter 1 OVERVIEW OF BRAIN

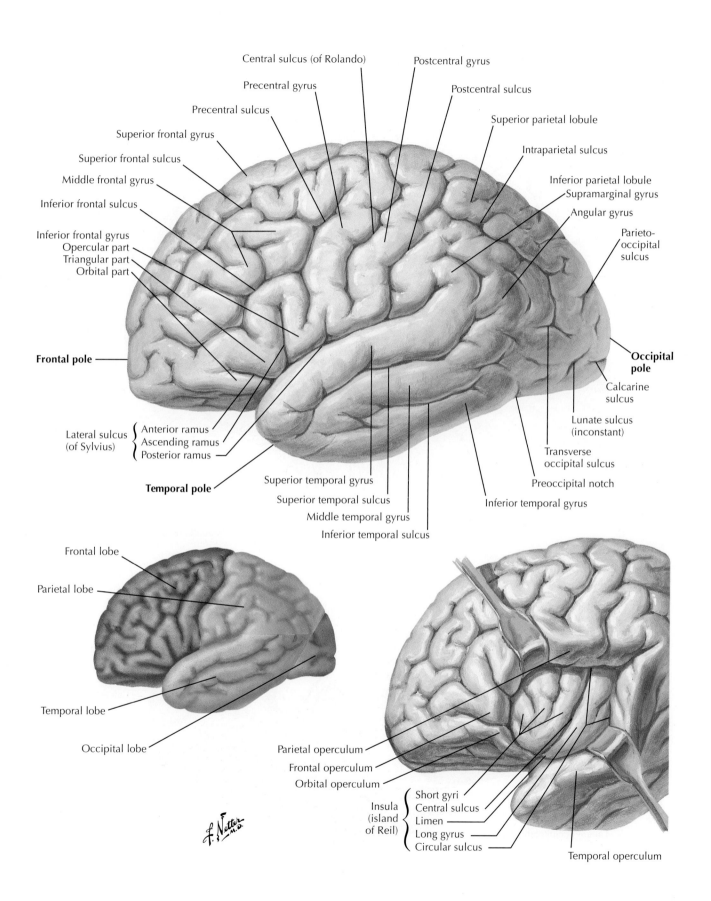

Central sulcus (of Rolando)

Precentral gyrus

Precentral sulcus

Superior frontal gyrus

Superior frontal sulcus

Middle frontal gyrus

Inferior frontal sulcus

Inferior frontal gyrus
Opercular part
Triangular part
Orbital part

Frontal pole

Lateral sulcus
(of Sylvius)
{ Anterior ramus
Ascending ramus
Posterior ramus

Temporal pole

Superior temporal gyrus

Superior temporal sulcus

Middle temporal gyrus

Inferior temporal sulcus

Postcentral gyrus

Postcentral sulcus

Superior parietal lobule

Intraparietal sulcus

Inferior parietal lobule
Supramarginal gyrus

Angular gyrus

Parieto-
occipital
sulcus

**Occipital
pole**

Calcarine
sulcus

Lunate sulcus
(inconstant)

Transverse
occipital sulcus

Preoccipital notch

Inferior temporal gyrus

Frontal lobe

Parietal lobe

Temporal lobe

Occipital lobe

Parietal operculum

Frontal operculum

Orbital operculum

Insula
(island
of Reil)
{ Short gyri
Central sulcus
Limen
Long gyrus
Circular sulcus

Temporal operculum

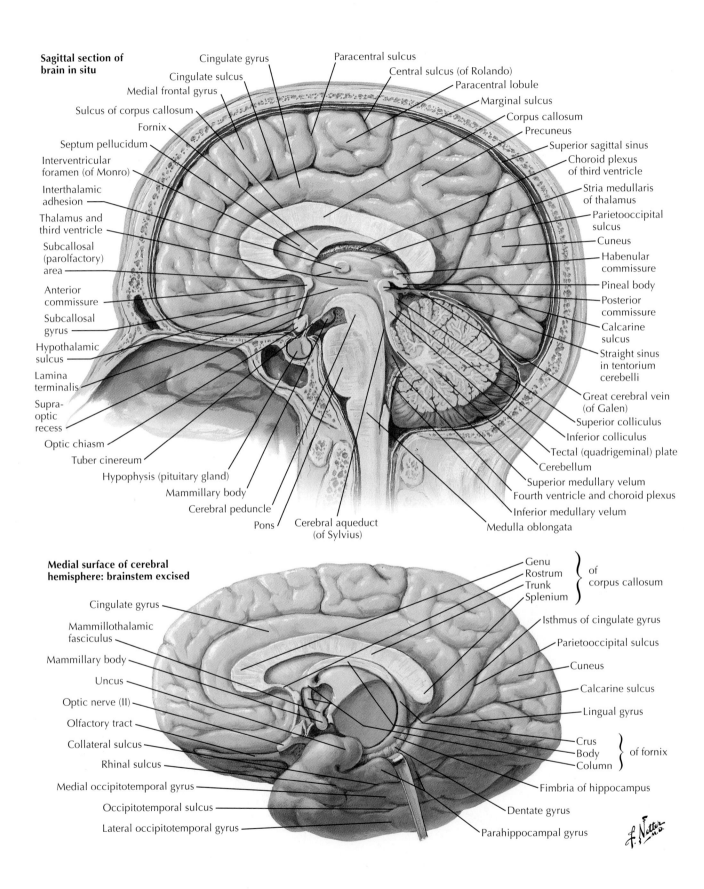

Sagittal section of brain in situ

Cingulate gyrus
Paracentral sulcus
Central sulcus (of Rolando)
Cingulate sulcus
Paracentral lobule
Medial frontal gyrus
Marginal sulcus
Sulcus of corpus callosum
Corpus callosum
Fornix
Precuneus
Septum pellucidum
Superior sagittal sinus
Interventricular foramen (of Monro)
Choroid plexus of third ventricle
Interthalamic adhesion
Stria medullaris of thalamus
Thalamus and third ventricle
Parietooccipital sulcus
Subcallosal (parolfactory) area
Cuneus
Habenular commissure
Anterior commissure
Pineal body
Subcallosal gyrus
Posterior commissure
Hypothalamic sulcus
Calcarine sulcus
Lamina terminalis
Straight sinus in tentorium cerebelli
Supra-optic recess
Great cerebral vein (of Galen)
Optic chiasm
Superior colliculus
Tuber cinereum
Inferior colliculus
Tectal (quadrigeminal) plate
Hypophysis (pituitary gland)
Cerebellum
Mammillary body
Superior medullary velum
Cerebral peduncle
Fourth ventricle and choroid plexus
Pons
Cerebral aqueduct (of Sylvius)
Inferior medullary velum
Medulla oblongata

Medial surface of cerebral hemisphere: brainstem excised

Genu
Rostrum
Trunk
Splenium
of corpus callosum
Cingulate gyrus
Isthmus of cingulate gyrus
Mammillothalamic fasciculus
Parietooccipital sulcus
Mammillary body
Cuneus
Uncus
Calcarine sulcus
Optic nerve (II)
Lingual gyrus
Olfactory tract
Crus
Body
Column
of fornix
Collateral sulcus
Rhinal sulcus
Fimbria of hippocampus
Medial occipitotemporal gyrus
Dentate gyrus
Occipitotemporal sulcus
Lateral occipitotemporal gyrus
Parahippocampal gyrus

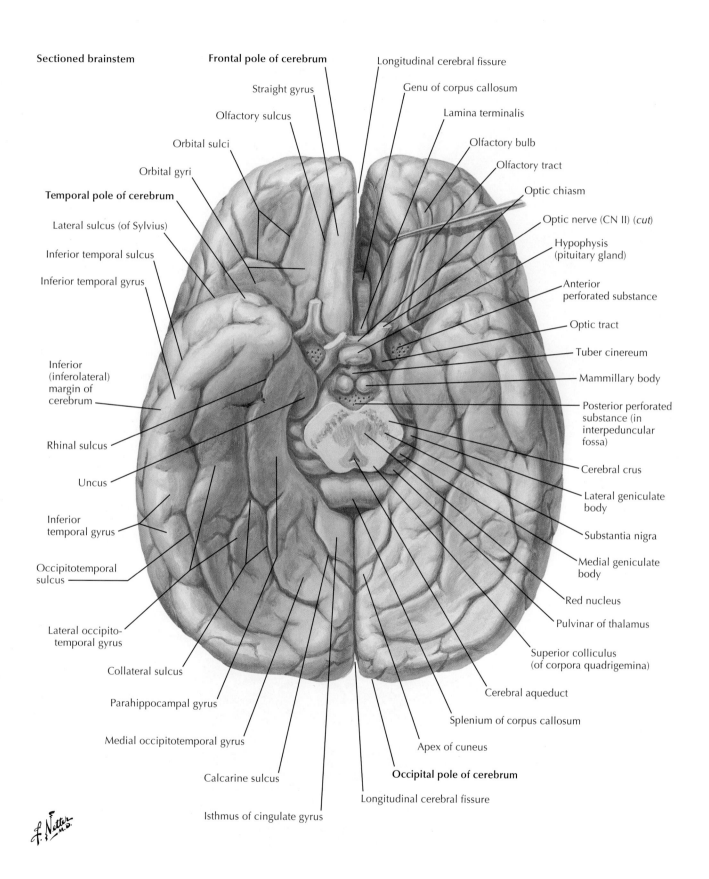

Sectioned brainstem

Frontal pole of cerebrum

Longitudinal cerebral fissure

Straight gyrus

Genu of corpus callosum

Olfactory sulcus

Lamina terminalis

Orbital sulci

Olfactory bulb

Orbital gyri

Olfactory tract

Temporal pole of cerebrum

Optic chiasm

Lateral sulcus (of Sylvius)

Optic nerve (CN II) (cut)

Inferior temporal sulcus

Hypophysis (pituitary gland)

Inferior temporal gyrus

Anterior perforated substance

Optic tract

Inferior (inferolateral) margin of cerebrum

Tuber cinereum

Mammillary body

Posterior perforated substance (in interpeduncular fossa)

Rhinal sulcus

Uncus

Cerebral crus

Lateral geniculate body

Inferior temporal gyrus

Substantia nigra

Occipitotemporal sulcus

Medial geniculate body

Red nucleus

Lateral occipito-temporal gyrus

Pulvinar of thalamus

Superior colliculus (of corpora quadrigemina)

Collateral sulcus

Parahippocampal gyrus

Cerebral aqueduct

Medial occipitotemporal gyrus

Splenium of corpus callosum

Calcarine sulcus

Apex of cuneus

Occipital pole of cerebrum

Longitudinal cerebral fissure

Isthmus of cingulate gyrus

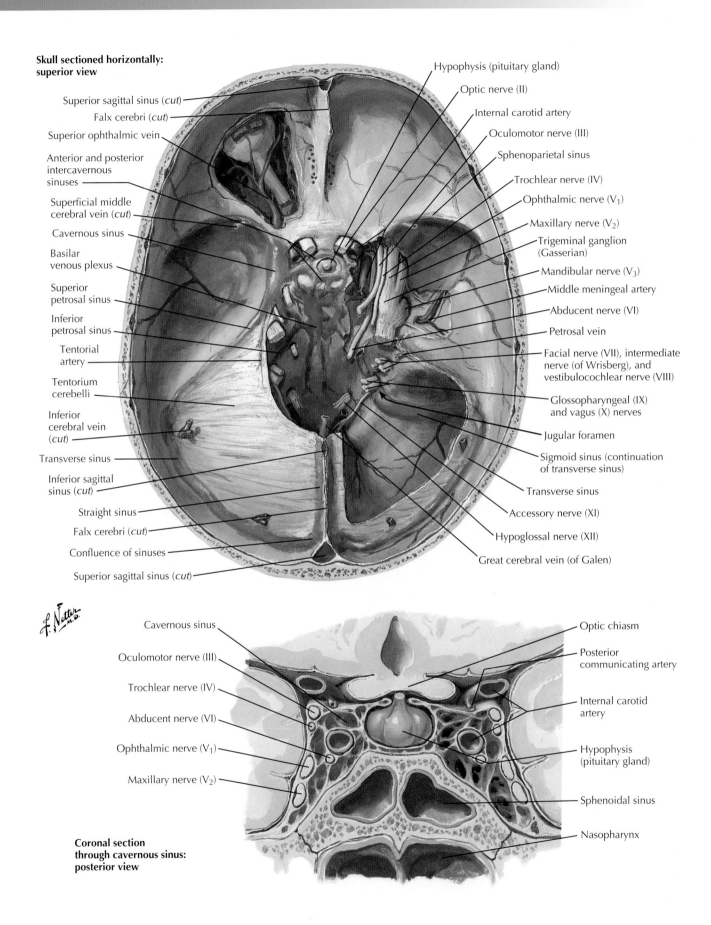

Skull sectioned horizontally: superior view

Superior sagittal sinus (*cut*)

Falx cerebri (*cut*)

Superior ophthalmic vein

Anterior and posterior intercavernous sinuses

Superficial middle cerebral vein (*cut*)

Cavernous sinus

Basilar venous plexus

Superior petrosal sinus

Inferior petrosal sinus

Tentorial artery

Tentorium cerebelli

Inferior cerebral vein (*cut*)

Transverse sinus

Inferior sagittal sinus (*cut*)

Straight sinus

Falx cerebri (*cut*)

Confluence of sinuses

Superior sagittal sinus (*cut*)

Hypophysis (pituitary gland)

Optic nerve (II)

Internal carotid artery

Oculomotor nerve (III)

Sphenoparietal sinus

Trochlear nerve (IV)

Ophthalmic nerve (V$_1$)

Maxillary nerve (V$_2$)

Trigeminal ganglion (Gasserian)

Mandibular nerve (V$_3$)

Middle meningeal artery

Abducent nerve (VI)

Petrosal vein

Facial nerve (VII), intermediate nerve (of Wrisberg), and vestibulocochlear nerve (VIII)

Glossopharyngeal (IX) and vagus (X) nerves

Jugular foramen

Sigmoid sinus (continuation of transverse sinus)

Transverse sinus

Accessory nerve (XI)

Hypoglossal nerve (XII)

Great cerebral vein (of Galen)

Cavernous sinus

Oculomotor nerve (III)

Trochlear nerve (IV)

Abducent nerve (VI)

Ophthalmic nerve (V$_1$)

Maxillary nerve (V$_2$)

Coronal section through cavernous sinus: posterior view

Optic chiasm

Posterior communicating artery

Internal carotid artery

Hypophysis (pituitary gland)

Sphenoidal sinus

Nasopharynx

Sagittal section

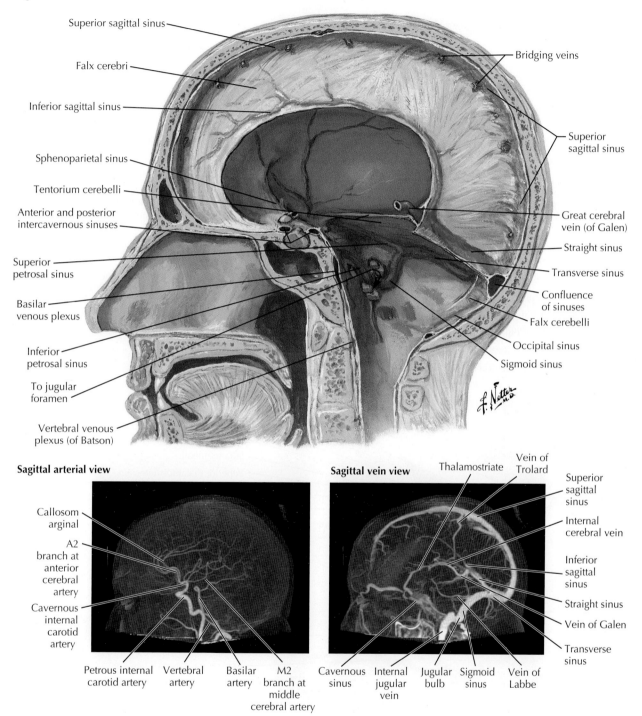

Superior sagittal sinus

Falx cerebri

Inferior sagittal sinus

Sphenoparietal sinus

Tentorium cerebelli

Anterior and posterior intercavernous sinuses

Superior petrosal sinus

Basilar venous plexus

Inferior petrosal sinus

To jugular foramen

Vertebral venous plexus (of Batson)

Bridging veins

Superior sagittal sinus

Great cerebral vein (of Galen)

Straight sinus

Transverse sinus

Confluence of sinuses

Falx cerebelli

Occipital sinus

Sigmoid sinus

Sagittal arterial view

Callosom arginal

A2 branch at anterior cerebral artery

Cavernous internal carotid artery

Petrous internal carotid artery

Vertebral artery

Basilar artery

M2 branch at middle cerebral artery

Sagittal vein view

Thalamostriate

Vein of Trolard

Superior sagittal sinus

Internal cerebral vein

Inferior sagittal sinus

Straight sinus

Vein of Galen

Transverse sinus

Cavernous sinus

Internal jugular vein

Jugular bulb

Sigmoid sinus

Vein of Labbe

Left lateral phantom view

Right lateral ventricle

Frontal (anterior) horn

Central part

Temporal (inferior) horn

Occipital (posterior) horn

Left lateral ventricle

Cerebral aqueduct (of Sylvius)

Fourth ventricle

Left lateral aperture (foramen of Luschka)

Left lateral recess

Median aperture (foramen of Magendie)

Left interventricular foramen (of Monro)

Third ventricle

Supraoptic recess

Interthalamic adhesion

Infundibular recess

Pineal recess

Suprapineal recess

Central canal of spinal cord

Corpus callosum

Septum pellucidum

Lateral ventricle

Caudate nucleus (body)

Choroid plexus of lateral ventricle

Stria terminalis

Superior thalamostriate vein

Body of fornix

Internal cerebral vein

Tela choroidea of third ventricle

Choroid plexus of third ventricle

Thalamus

Putamen

Globus pallidus

Lentiform nucleus

Internal capsule

Third ventricle and interthalamic adhesion

Hypothalamus

Caudate nucleus (tail)

Optic tract

Choroid plexus of lateral ventricle

Temporal (inferior) horn of lateral ventricle

Fimbria of hippocampus

Hippocampus

Dentate gyrus

Mammillary body

Parahippocampal gyrus

White arrow in left interventricular foramen (of Monro)

Ependyma

Pia mater

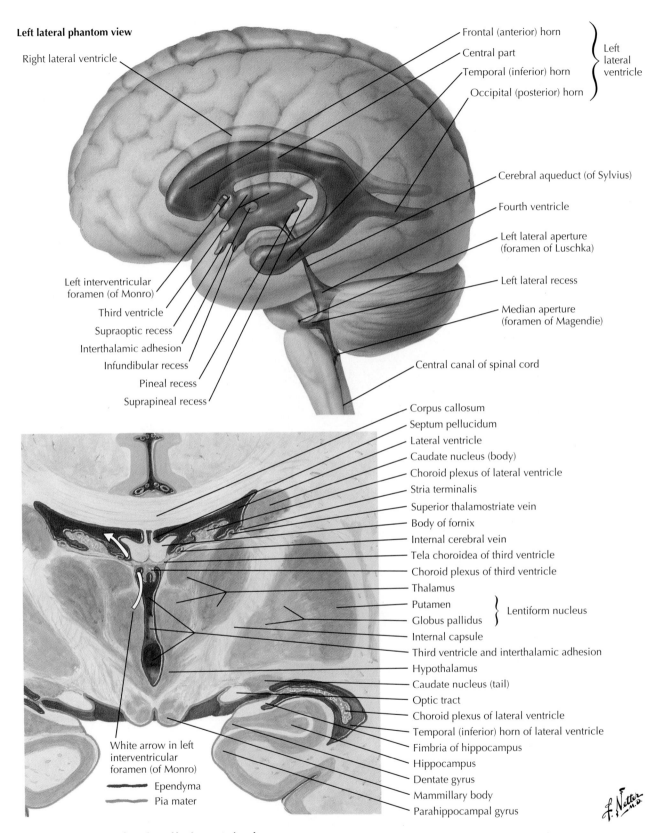

Coronal section of brain: posterior view

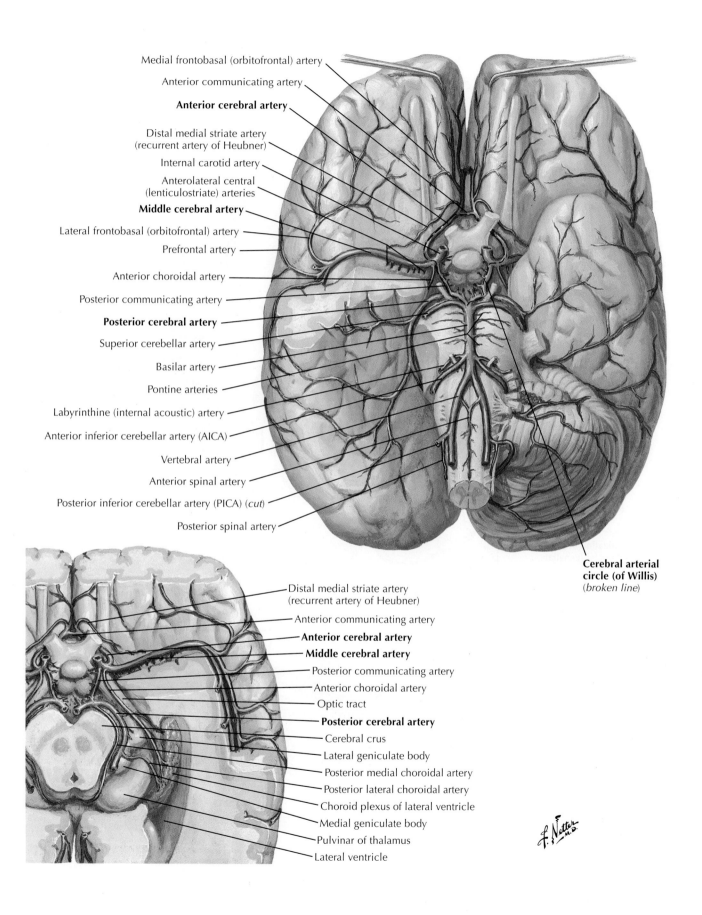

Medial frontobasal (orbitofrontal) artery

Anterior communicating artery

Anterior cerebral artery

Distal medial striate artery (recurrent artery of Heubner)

Internal carotid artery

Anterolateral central (lenticulostriate) arteries

Middle cerebral artery

Lateral frontobasal (orbitofrontal) artery

Prefrontal artery

Anterior choroidal artery

Posterior communicating artery

Posterior cerebral artery

Superior cerebellar artery

Basilar artery

Pontine arteries

Labyrinthine (internal acoustic) artery

Anterior inferior cerebellar artery (AICA)

Vertebral artery

Anterior spinal artery

Posterior inferior cerebellar artery (PICA) (*cut*)

Posterior spinal artery

Cerebral arterial circle (of Willis) (*broken line*)

Distal medial striate artery (recurrent artery of Heubner)

Anterior communicating artery

Anterior cerebral artery

Middle cerebral artery

Posterior communicating artery

Anterior choroidal artery

Optic tract

Posterior cerebral artery

Cerebral crus

Lateral geniculate body

Posterior medial choroidal artery

Posterior lateral choroidal artery

Choroid plexus of lateral ventricle

Medial geniculate body

Pulvinar of thalamus

Lateral ventricle

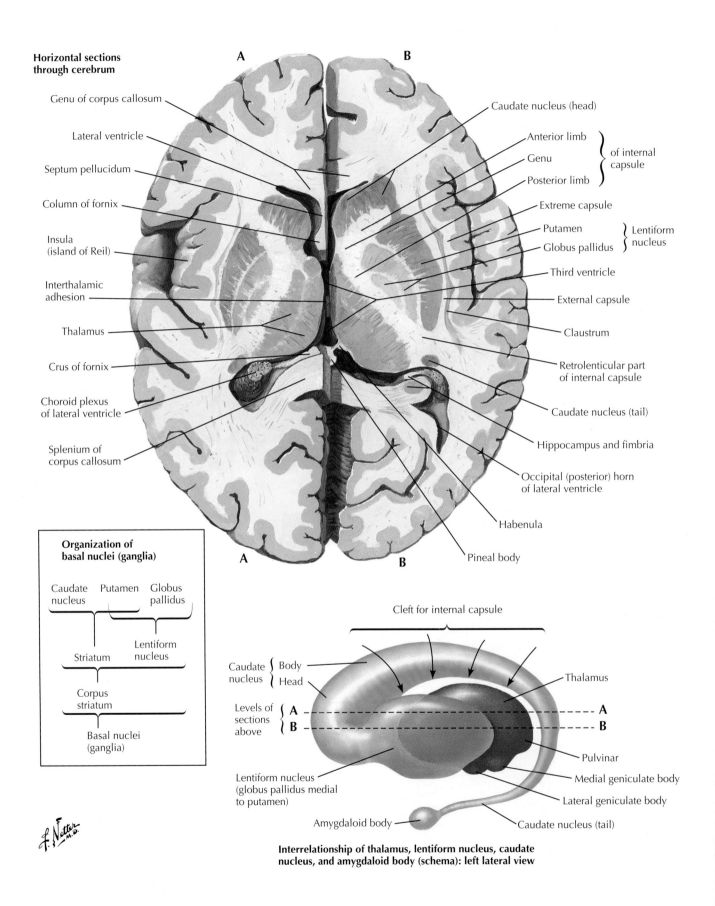

Horizontal sections through cerebrum

A   B

Genu of corpus callosum

Lateral ventricle

Septum pellucidum

Column of fornix

Insula (island of Reil)

Interthalamic adhesion

Thalamus

Crus of fornix

Choroid plexus of lateral ventricle

Splenium of corpus callosum

A   B

Caudate nucleus (head)

Anterior limb

Genu } of internal capsule

Posterior limb

Extreme capsule

Putamen } Lentiform nucleus

Globus pallidus

Third ventricle

External capsule

Claustrum

Retrolenticular part of internal capsule

Caudate nucleus (tail)

Hippocampus and fimbria

Occipital (posterior) horn of lateral ventricle

Habenula

Pineal body

Organization of basal nuclei (ganglia)

Caudate nucleus   Putamen   Globus pallidus

Striatum

Lentiform nucleus

Corpus striatum

Basal nuclei (ganglia)

Cleft for internal capsule

Caudate nucleus { Body Head

Levels of sections above { A B

Lentiform nucleus (globus pallidus medial to putamen)

Amygdaloid body

Thalamus

A
B

Pulvinar

Medial geniculate body

Lateral geniculate body

Caudate nucleus (tail)

Interrelationship of thalamus, lentiform nucleus, caudate nucleus, and amygdaloid body (schema): left lateral view

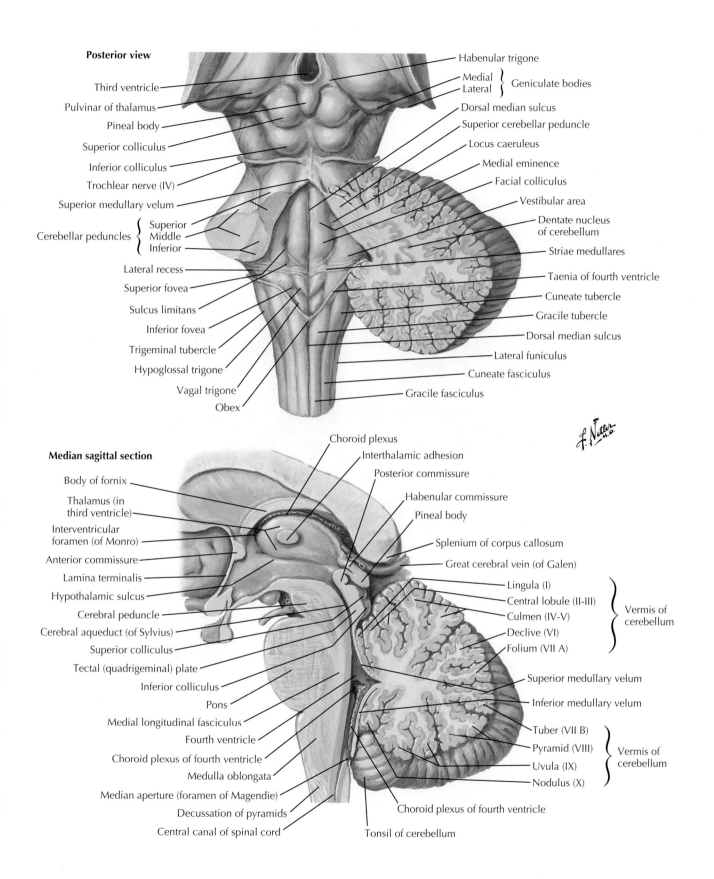

Posterior view

Third ventricle
Pulvinar of thalamus
Pineal body
Superior colliculus
Inferior colliculus
Trochlear nerve (IV)
Superior medullary velum

Cerebellar peduncles
  Superior
  Middle
  Inferior

Lateral recess
Superior fovea
Sulcus limitans
Inferior fovea
Trigeminal tubercle
Hypoglossal trigone
Vagal trigone
Obex

Habenular trigone
Medial
Lateral } Geniculate bodies
Dorsal median sulcus
Superior cerebellar peduncle
Locus caeruleus
Medial eminence
Facial colliculus
Vestibular area
Dentate nucleus of cerebellum
Striae medullares
Taenia of fourth ventricle
Cuneate tubercle
Gracile tubercle
Dorsal median sulcus
Lateral funiculus
Cuneate fasciculus
Gracile fasciculus

Median sagittal section

Choroid plexus
Interthalamic adhesion
Posterior commissure
Habenular commissure
Pineal body

Body of fornix
Thalamus (in third ventricle)
Interventricular foramen (of Monro)
Anterior commissure
Lamina terminalis
Hypothalamic sulcus
Cerebral peduncle
Cerebral aqueduct (of Sylvius)
Superior colliculus
Tectal (quadrigeminal) plate
Inferior colliculus
Pons
Medial longitudinal fasciculus
Fourth ventricle
Choroid plexus of fourth ventricle
Medulla oblongata
Median aperture (foramen of Magendie)
Decussation of pyramids
Central canal of spinal cord

Splenium of corpus callosum
Great cerebral vein (of Galen)
Lingula (I)
Central lobule (II-III)
Culmen (IV-V)
Declive (VI)
Folium (VII A)
} Vermis of cerebellum
Superior medullary velum
Inferior medullary velum
Tuber (VII B)
Pyramid (VIII)
Uvula (IX)
Nodulus (X)
} Vermis of cerebellum
Choroid plexus of fourth ventricle
Tonsil of cerebellum

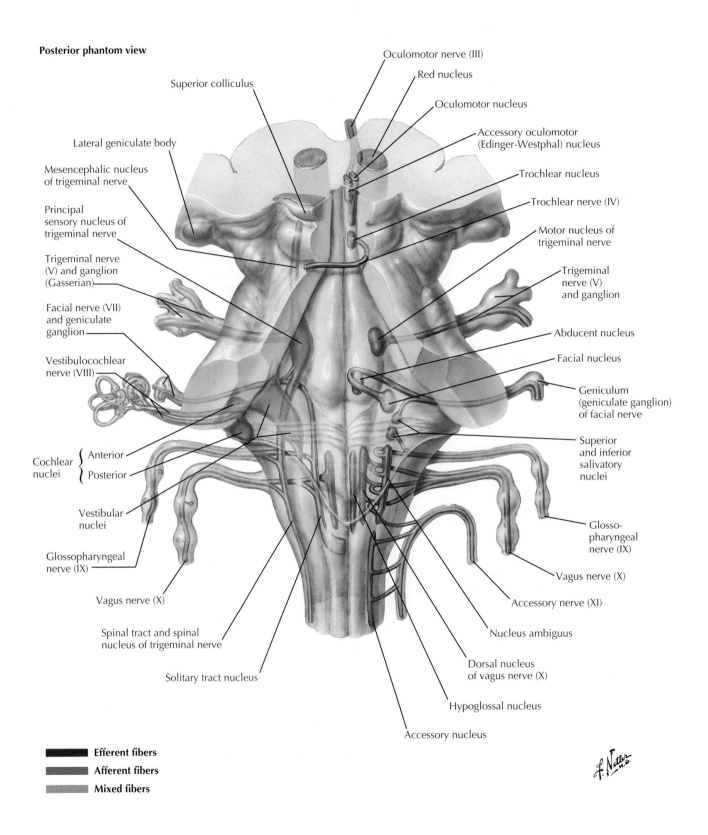

Posterior phantom view

Oculomotor nerve (III)

Superior colliculus

Red nucleus

Oculomotor nucleus

Lateral geniculate body

Accessory oculomotor
(Edinger-Westphal) nucleus

Mesencephalic nucleus
of trigeminal nerve

Trochlear nucleus

Principal
sensory nucleus of
trigeminal nerve

Trochlear nerve (IV)

Motor nucleus of
trigeminal nerve

Trigeminal nerve
(V) and ganglion
(Gasserian)

Trigeminal
nerve (V)
and ganglion

Facial nerve (VII)
and geniculate
ganglion

Abducent nucleus

Facial nucleus

Vestibulocochlear
nerve (VIII)

Geniculum
(geniculate ganglion)
of facial nerve

Cochlear { Anterior
nuclei { Posterior

Superior
and inferior
salivatory
nuclei

Vestibular
nuclei

Glosso-
pharyngeal
nerve (IX)

Glossopharyngeal
nerve (IX)

Vagus nerve (X)

Vagus nerve (X)

Accessory nerve (XI)

Spinal tract and spinal
nucleus of trigeminal nerve

Nucleus ambiguus

Dorsal nucleus
of vagus nerve (X)

Solitary tract nucleus

Hypoglossal nucleus

Accessory nucleus

■■■ **Efferent fibers**
■■■ **Afferent fibers**
■■■ **Mixed fibers**

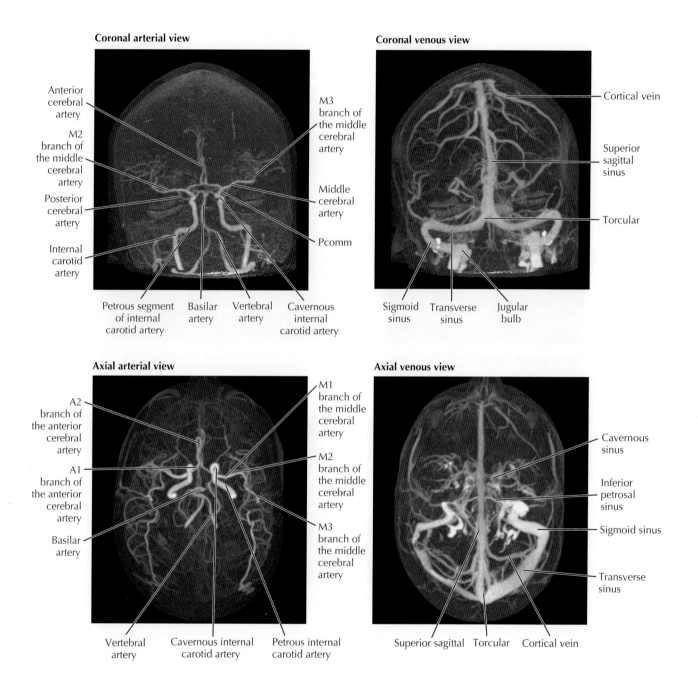

Coronal arterial view

Anterior cerebral artery

M2 branch of the middle cerebral artery

Posterior cerebral artery

Internal carotid artery

M3 branch of the middle cerebral artery

Middle cerebral artery

Pcomm

Petrous segment of internal carotid artery

Basilar artery

Vertebral artery

Cavernous internal carotid artery

Coronal venous view

Cortical vein

Superior sagittal sinus

Torcular

Sigmoid sinus

Transverse sinus

Jugular bulb

Axial arterial view

A2 branch of the anterior cerebral artery

A1 branch of the anterior cerebral artery

Basilar artery

M1 branch of the middle cerebral artery

M2 branch of the middle cerebral artery

M3 branch of the middle cerebral artery

Vertebral artery

Cavernous internal carotid artery

Petrous internal carotid artery

Axial venous view

Cavernous sinus

Inferior petrosal sinus

Sigmoid sinus

Transverse sinus

Superior sagittal

Torcular

Cortical vein

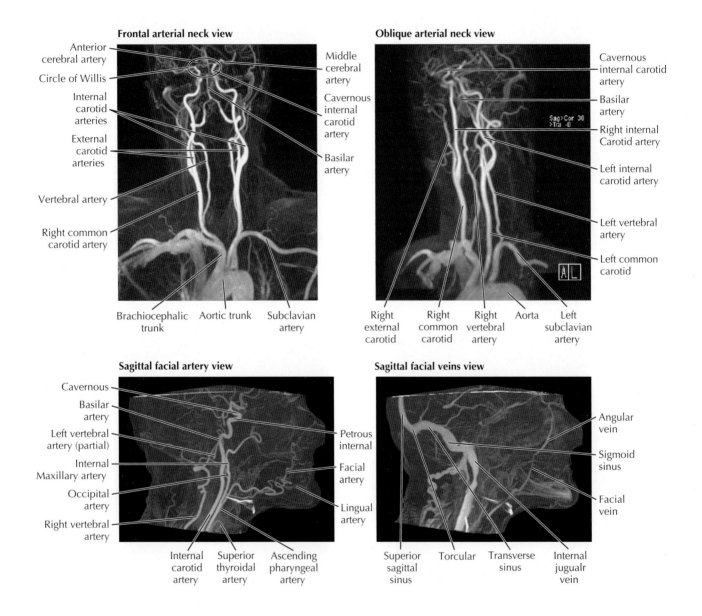

Frontal arterial neck view

Anterior cerebral artery
Circle of Willis
Internal carotid arteries
External carotid arteries
Vertebral artery
Right common carotid artery

Middle cerebral artery
Cavernous internal carotid artery
Basilar artery

Brachiocephalic trunk
Aortic trunk
Subclavian artery

Oblique arterial neck view

Cavernous internal carotid artery
Basilar artery
Right internal Carotid artery
Left internal carotid artery
Left vertebral artery
Left common carotid

Sag>Cor 38
>Tra -0

A L

Right external carotid
Right common carotid
Right vertebral artery
Aorta
Left subclavian artery

Sagittal facial artery view

Cavernous
Basilar artery
Left vertebral artery (partial)
Internal Maxillary artery
Occipital artery
Right vertebral artery

Petrous internal
Facial artery
Lingual artery

Internal carotid artery
Superior thyroidal artery
Ascending pharyngeal artery

Sagittal facial veins view

Angular vein
Sigmoid sinus
Facial vein

Superior sagittal sinus
Torcular
Transverse sinus
Internal jugualr vein

Chapter 2 BRAIN

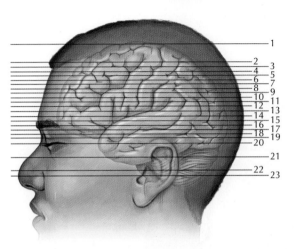

AXIAL   16

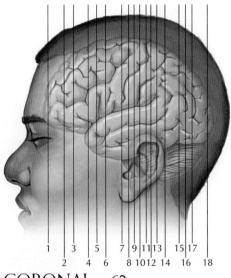

CORONAL   62

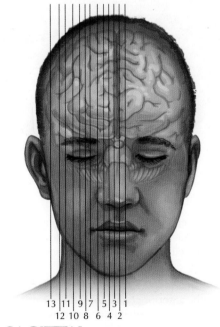

SAGITTAL   98

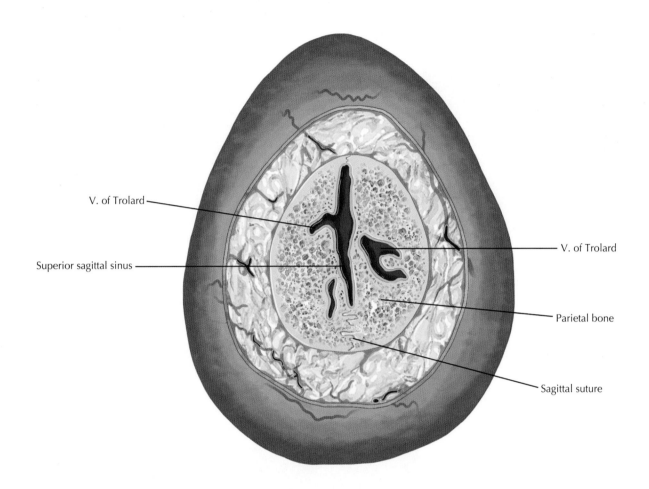

V. of Trolard

Superior sagittal sinus

V. of Trolard

Parietal bone

Sagittal suture

NORMAL ANATOMY

Named after the French anatomist Paulin Trolard (1842–1910) and also known as the superior anastomotic vein, the vein of Trolard is the largest cortical vein at the convexity (see also Brain Coronal 15). The vein of Trolard anastomoses with the middle cerebral vein and the superior sagittal sinus.

Note the first cranial nerves, the olfactory nerves, in the olfactory grooves along the medial inferior floor of the anterior cranial fossa. Please note there is volume averaging of cortical veins with the top of the calvaria such that the veins artifactually appear to be within the bone rather than within the cranial vault (see Brain Coronal 2).

DIAGNOSTIC CONSIDERATION

A lesion, such as a metastatic lesion in the marrow, can often be missed at the vertex (vertex cranii). Diffusion-weighted magnetic resonance imaging (MRI) is often useful in identifying such lesions, not because the lesion is diffusion restricted, but because all the other structures are often low in signal, making the lesion conspicuously bright. The same principle holds for the base of the skull, where the presence of many structures can make pathologic lesions easy to overlook.

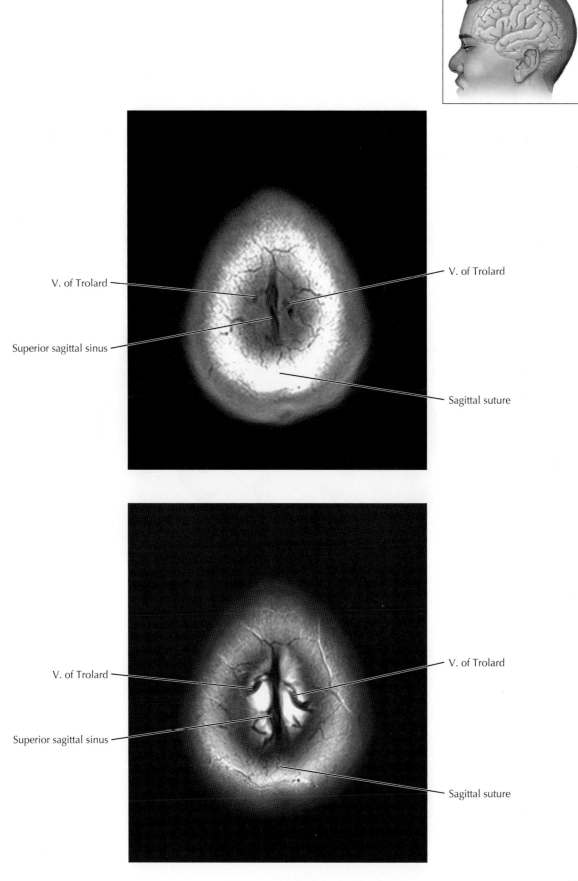

V. of Trolard

V. of Trolard

Superior sagittal sinus

Sagittal suture

V. of Trolard

V. of Trolard

Superior sagittal sinus

Sagittal suture

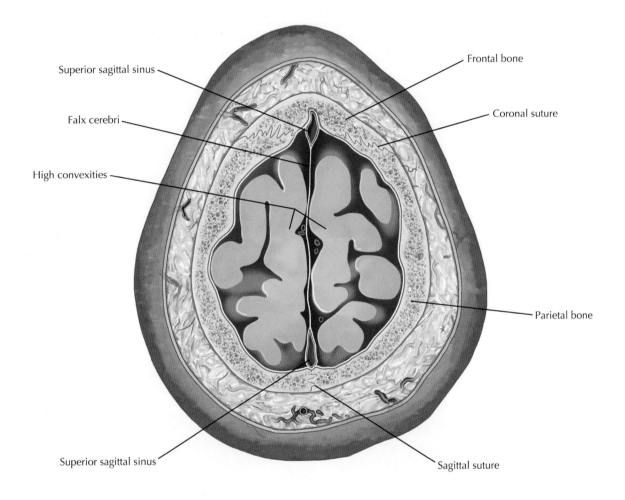

Superior sagittal sinus

Falx cerebri

High convexities

Frontal bone

Coronal suture

Parietal bone

Superior sagittal sinus

Sagittal suture

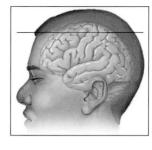

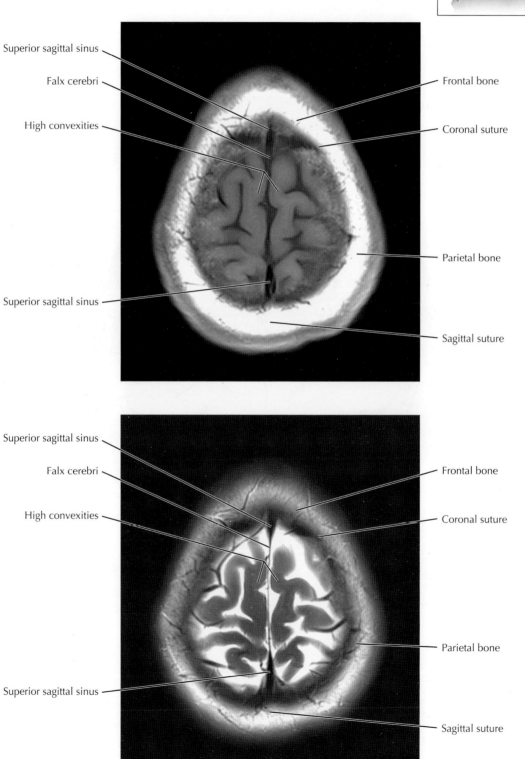

Superior sagittal sinus

Falx cerebri

High convexities

Superior sagittal sinus

Frontal bone

Coronal suture

Parietal bone

Sagittal suture

Superior sagittal sinus

Falx cerebri

High convexities

Superior sagittal sinus

Frontal bone

Coronal suture

Parietal bone

Sagittal suture

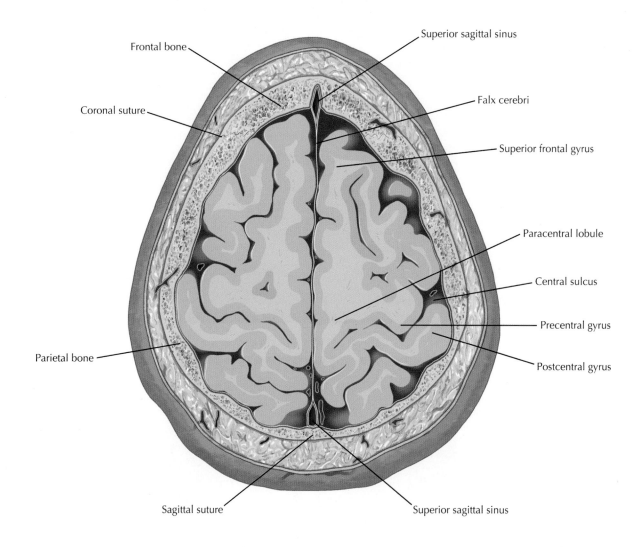

Frontal bone

Coronal suture

Superior sagittal sinus

Falx cerebri

Superior frontal gyrus

Paracentral lobule

Central sulcus

Precentral gyrus

Parietal bone

Postcentral gyrus

Sagittal suture

Superior sagittal sinus

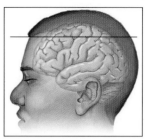

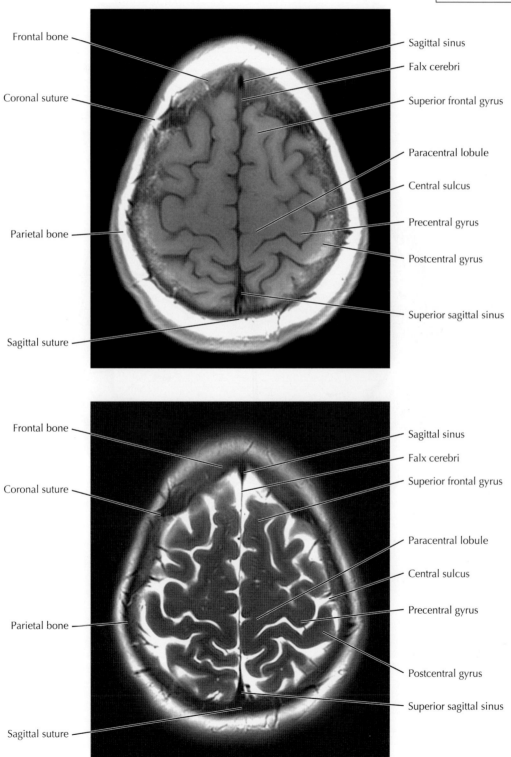

Frontal bone

Coronal suture

Parietal bone

Sagittal suture

Sagittal sinus

Falx cerebri

Superior frontal gyrus

Paracentral lobule

Central sulcus

Precentral gyrus

Postcentral gyrus

Superior sagittal sinus

Frontal bone

Coronal suture

Parietal bone

Sagittal suture

Sagittal sinus

Falx cerebri

Superior frontal gyrus

Paracentral lobule

Central sulcus

Precentral gyrus

Postcentral gyrus

Superior sagittal sinus

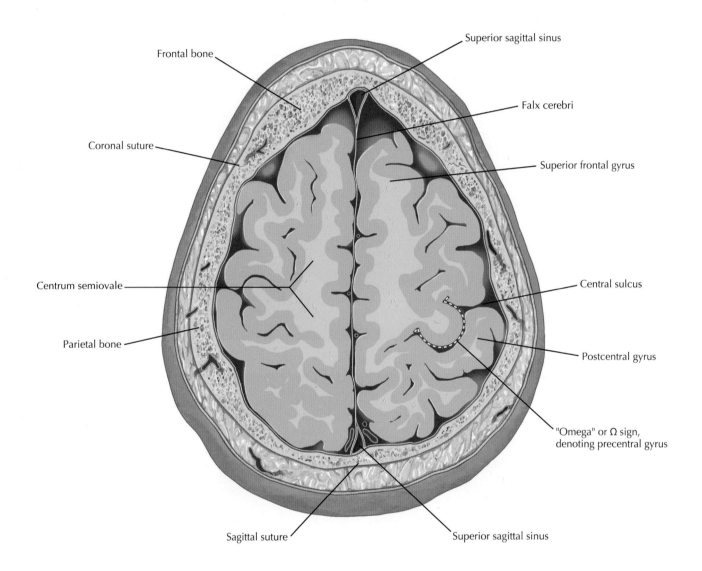

Frontal bone

Superior sagittal sinus

Falx cerebri

Coronal suture

Superior frontal gyrus

Centrum semiovale

Central sulcus

Parietal bone

Postcentral gyrus

"Omega" or Ω sign,
denoting precentral gyrus

Sagittal suture

Superior sagittal sinus

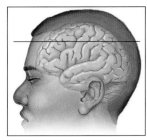

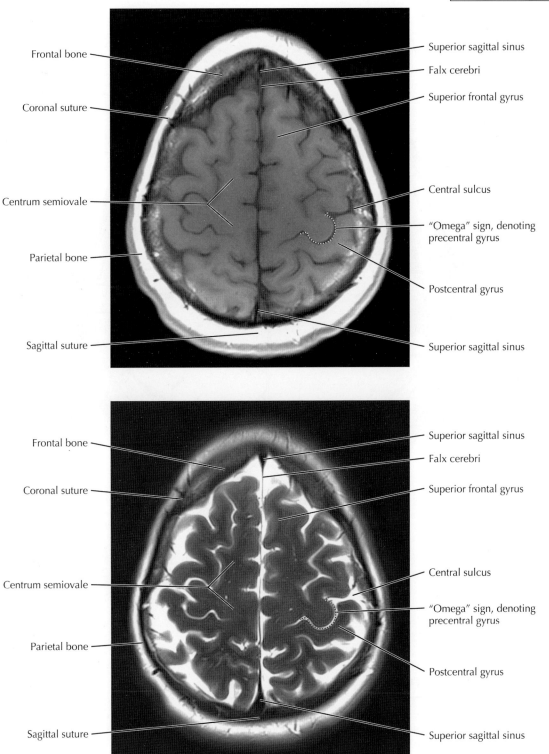

Frontal bone

Coronal suture

Centrum semiovale

Parietal bone

Sagittal suture

Superior sagittal sinus

Falx cerebri

Superior frontal gyrus

Central sulcus

"Omega" sign, denoting precentral gyrus

Postcentral gyrus

Superior sagittal sinus

Frontal bone

Coronal suture

Centrum semiovale

Parietal bone

Sagittal suture

Superior sagittal sinus

Falx cerebri

Superior frontal gyrus

Central sulcus

"Omega" sign, denoting precentral gyrus

Postcentral gyrus

Superior sagittal sinus

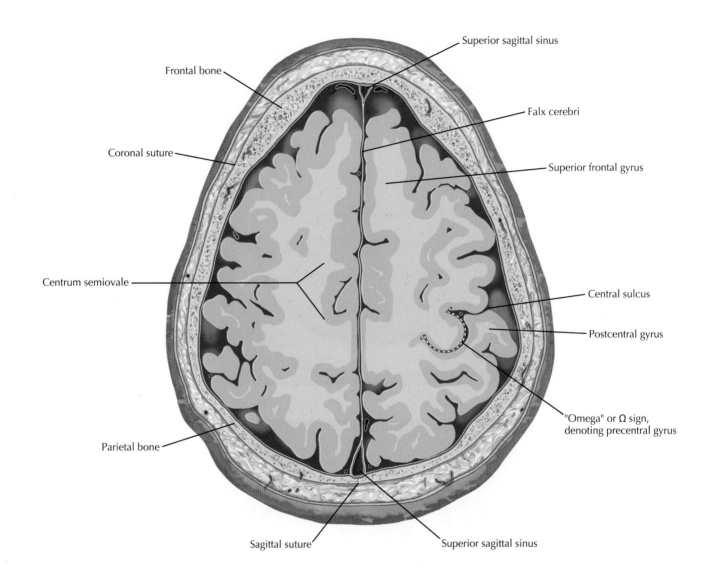

Superior sagittal sinus

Frontal bone

Falx cerebri

Coronal suture

Superior frontal gyrus

Centrum semiovale

Central sulcus

Postcentral gyrus

"Omega" or Ω sign, denoting precentral gyrus

Parietal bone

Sagittal suture

Superior sagittal sinus

NORMAL ANATOMY

The "omega sign" denotes a sulcal configuration similar to the Greek letter Ω and is one sign of the central sulcus separating the motor strip anteriorly and the sensory cortex posteriorly. The omega sign also demarcates the frontal lobe from the parietal lobe. Note that the two sulci in the midline immediately posterior to the medial ends of the central sulci should resemble a smile.

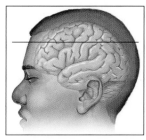

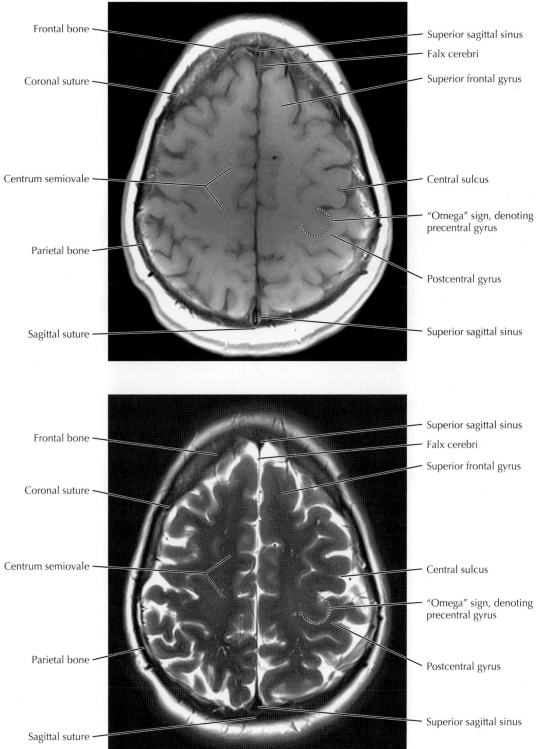

Frontal bone

Coronal suture

Centrum semiovale

Parietal bone

Sagittal suture

Superior sagittal sinus

Falx cerebri

Superior frontal gyrus

Central sulcus

"Omega" sign, denoting precentral gyrus

Postcentral gyrus

Superior sagittal sinus

Frontal bone

Coronal suture

Centrum semiovale

Parietal bone

Sagittal suture

Superior sagittal sinus

Falx cerebri

Superior frontal gyrus

Central sulcus

"Omega" sign, denoting precentral gyrus

Postcentral gyrus

Superior sagittal sinus

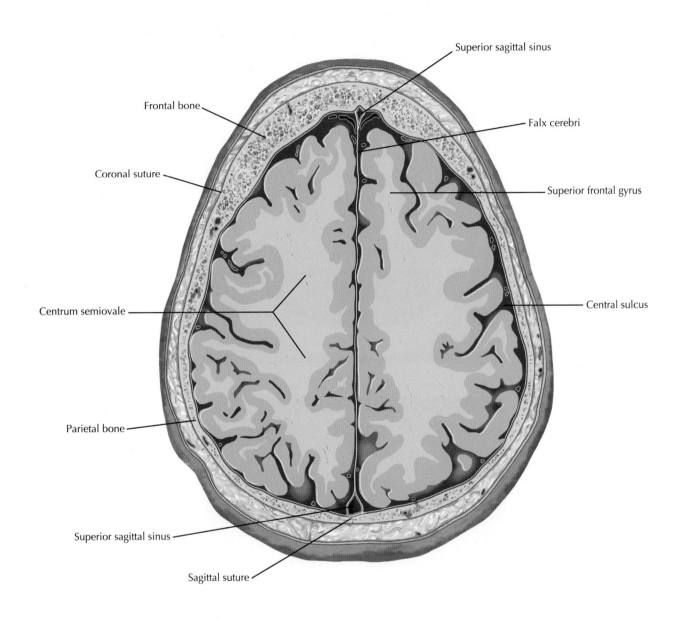

Superior sagittal sinus

Frontal bone

Falx cerebri

Coronal suture

Superior frontal gyrus

Centrum semiovale

Central sulcus

Parietal bone

Superior sagittal sinus

Sagittal suture

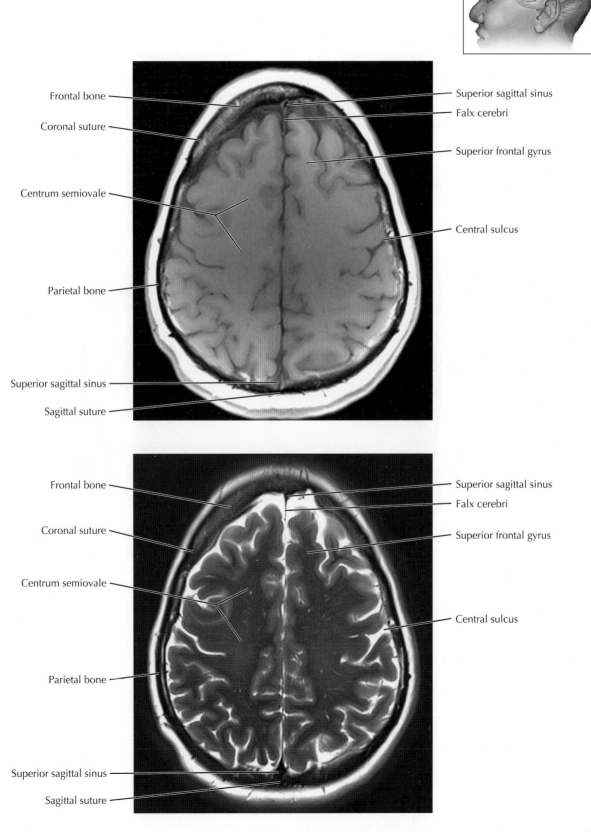

Frontal bone

Coronal suture

Centrum semiovale

Parietal bone

Superior sagittal sinus

Sagittal suture

Superior sagittal sinus

Falx cerebri

Superior frontal gyrus

Central sulcus

Frontal bone

Coronal suture

Centrum semiovale

Parietal bone

Superior sagittal sinus

Sagittal suture

Superior sagittal sinus

Falx cerebri

Superior frontal gyrus

Central sulcus

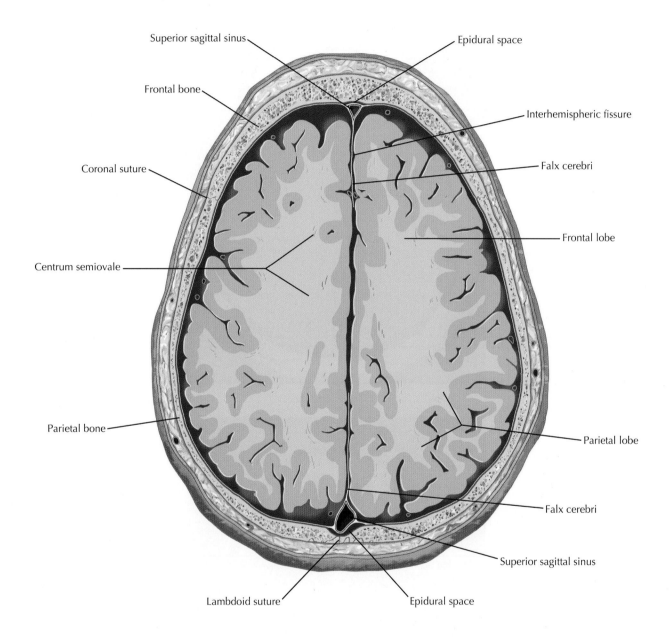

Superior sagittal sinus

Frontal bone

Coronal suture

Centrum semiovale

Parietal bone

Lambdoid suture

Epidural space

Interhemispheric fissure

Falx cerebri

Frontal lobe

Parietal lobe

Falx cerebri

Superior sagittal sinus

Epidural space

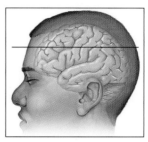

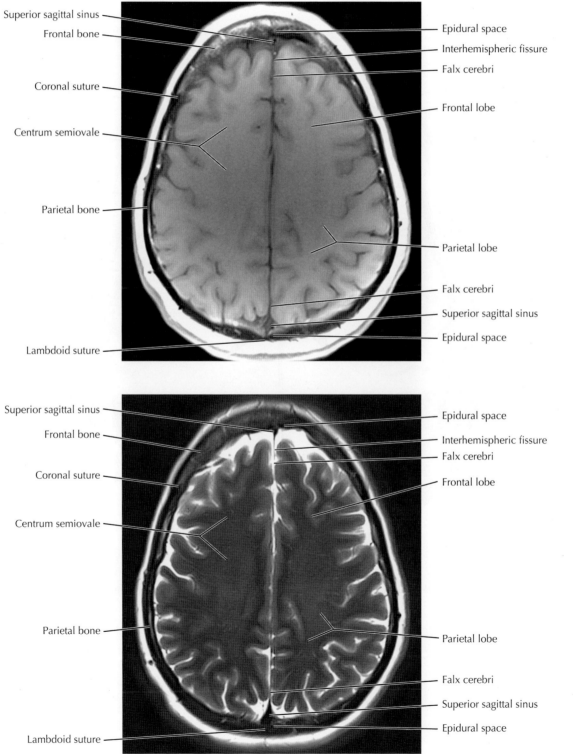

Superior sagittal sinus

Frontal bone

Coronal suture

Centrum semiovale

Parietal bone

Lambdoid suture

Epidural space

Interhemispheric fissure

Falx cerebri

Frontal lobe

Parietal lobe

Falx cerebri

Superior sagittal sinus

Epidural space

Superior sagittal sinus

Frontal bone

Coronal suture

Centrum semiovale

Parietal bone

Lambdoid suture

Epidural space

Interhemispheric fissure

Falx cerebri

Frontal lobe

Parietal lobe

Falx cerebri

Superior sagittal sinus

Epidural space

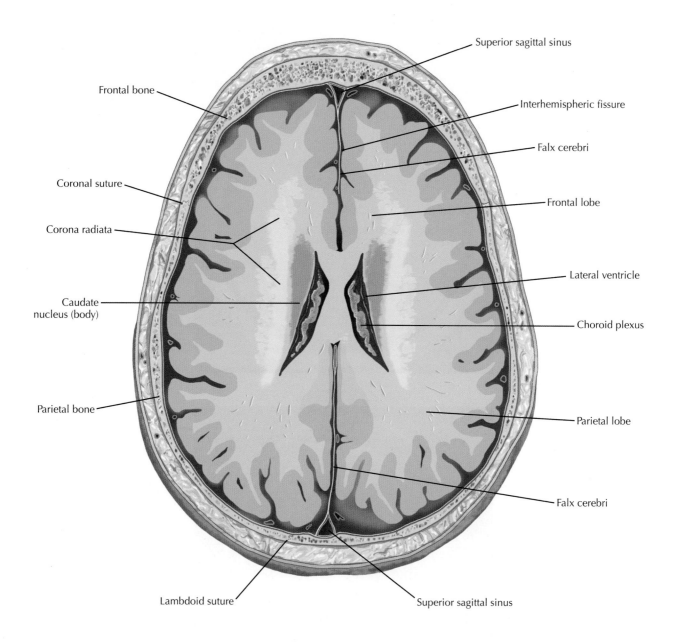

Superior sagittal sinus

Frontal bone

Interhemispheric fissure

Falx cerebri

Coronal suture

Frontal lobe

Corona radiata

Lateral ventricle

Caudate nucleus (body)

Choroid plexus

Parietal bone

Parietal lobe

Falx cerebri

Lambdoid suture

Superior sagittal sinus

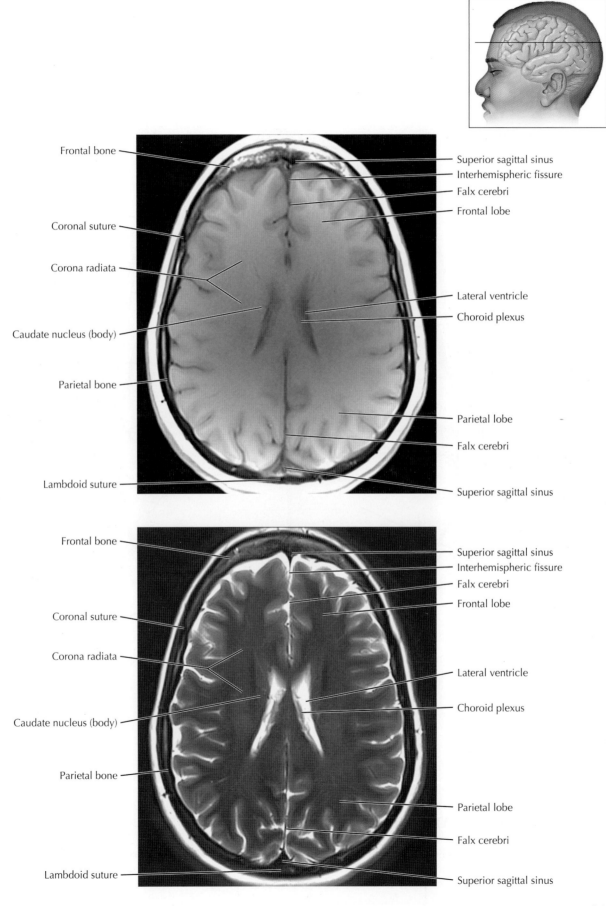

Frontal bone

Coronal suture

Corona radiata

Caudate nucleus (body)

Parietal bone

Lambdoid suture

Superior sagittal sinus
Interhemispheric fissure
Falx cerebri
Frontal lobe

Lateral ventricle
Choroid plexus

Parietal lobe

Falx cerebri

Superior sagittal sinus

Frontal bone

Coronal suture

Corona radiata

Caudate nucleus (body)

Parietal bone

Lambdoid suture

Superior sagittal sinus
Interhemispheric fissure
Falx cerebri
Frontal lobe

Lateral ventricle

Choroid plexus

Parietal lobe

Falx cerebri

Superior sagittal sinus

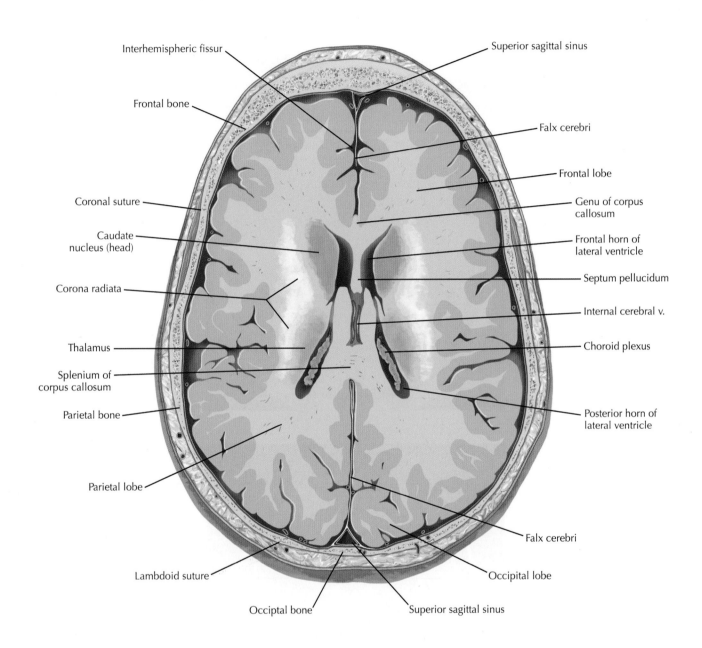

Interhemispheric fissur

Frontal bone

Coronal suture

Caudate nucleus (head)

Corona radiata

Thalamus

Splenium of corpus callosum

Parietal bone

Parietal lobe

Lambdoid suture

Occiptal bone

Superior sagittal sinus

Falx cerebri

Frontal lobe

Genu of corpus callosum

Frontal horn of lateral ventricle

Septum pellucidum

Internal cerebral v.

Choroid plexus

Posterior horn of lateral ventricle

Falx cerebri

Occipital lobe

Superior sagittal sinus

NORMAL ANATOMY

The white matter fibers at the level of the basal ganglia known as *internal capsule* (Axials 10 and 11) are known as *corona radiata* (Axials 8 and 9) more superiorly along the lateral margins of the ventricles, and as the centrum semiovale superior to the ventricles (Axial 7).

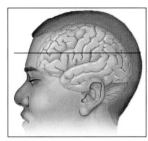

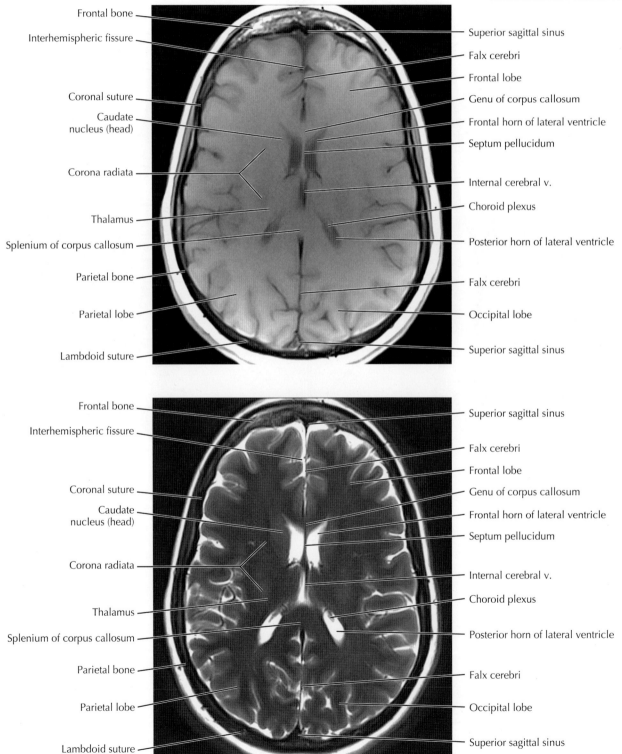

Frontal bone

Interhemispheric fissure

Coronal suture

Caudate nucleus (head)

Corona radiata

Thalamus

Splenium of corpus callosum

Parietal bone

Parietal lobe

Lambdoid suture

Superior sagittal sinus

Falx cerebri

Frontal lobe

Genu of corpus callosum

Frontal horn of lateral ventricle

Septum pellucidum

Internal cerebral v.

Choroid plexus

Posterior horn of lateral ventricle

Falx cerebri

Occipital lobe

Superior sagittal sinus

Frontal bone

Interhemispheric fissure

Coronal suture

Caudate nucleus (head)

Corona radiata

Thalamus

Splenium of corpus callosum

Parietal bone

Parietal lobe

Lambdoid suture

Superior sagittal sinus

Falx cerebri

Frontal lobe

Genu of corpus callosum

Frontal horn of lateral ventricle

Septum pellucidum

Internal cerebral v.

Choroid plexus

Posterior horn of lateral ventricle

Falx cerebri

Occipital lobe

Superior sagittal sinus

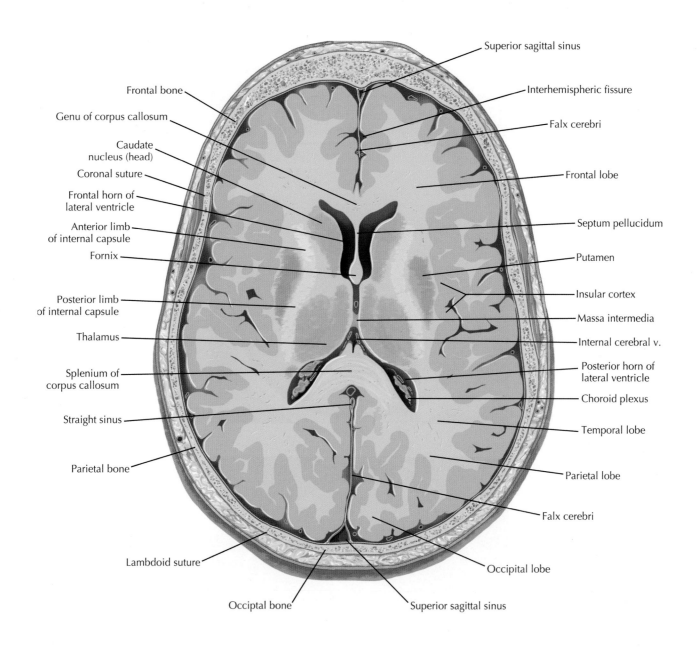

Superior sagittal sinus

Frontal bone

Genu of corpus callosum

Caudate nucleus (head)

Coronal suture

Frontal horn of lateral ventricle

Anterior limb of internal capsule

Fornix

Posterior limb of internal capsule

Thalamus

Splenium of corpus callosum

Straight sinus

Parietal bone

Lambdoid suture

Occiptal bone

Interhemispheric fissure

Falx cerebri

Frontal lobe

Septum pellucidum

Putamen

Insular cortex

Massa intermedia

Internal cerebral v.

Posterior horn of lateral ventricle

Choroid plexus

Temporal lobe

Parietal lobe

Falx cerebri

Occipital lobe

Superior sagittal sinus

NORMAL ANATOMY

Note how the signal of the basal ganglia is not ideal on this MR sequence tailored to capture the entire brain. For better delineation, see Chapter 3.

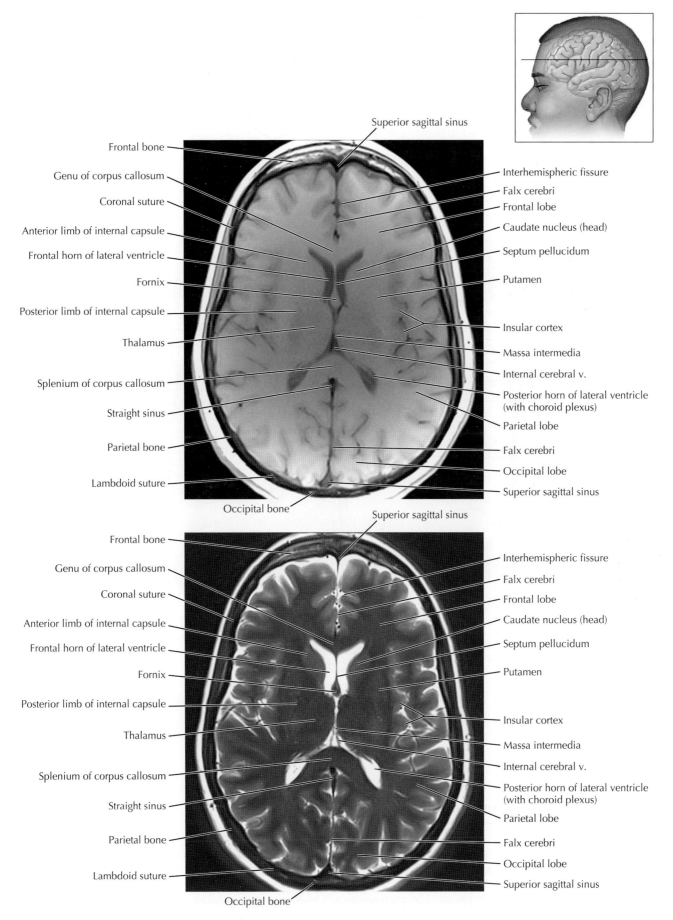

Superior sagittal sinus

Frontal bone

Genu of corpus callosum

Coronal suture

Anterior limb of internal capsule

Frontal horn of lateral ventricle

Fornix

Posterior limb of internal capsule

Thalamus

Splenium of corpus callosum

Straight sinus

Parietal bone

Lambdoid suture

Occipital bone

Interhemispheric fissure

Falx cerebri

Frontal lobe

Caudate nucleus (head)

Septum pellucidum

Putamen

Insular cortex

Massa intermedia

Internal cerebral v.

Posterior horn of lateral ventricle (with choroid plexus)

Parietal lobe

Falx cerebri

Occipital lobe

Superior sagittal sinus

Superior sagittal sinus

Frontal bone

Genu of corpus callosum

Coronal suture

Anterior limb of internal capsule

Frontal horn of lateral ventricle

Fornix

Posterior limb of internal capsule

Thalamus

Splenium of corpus callosum

Straight sinus

Parietal bone

Lambdoid suture

Occipital bone

Interhemispheric fissure

Falx cerebri

Frontal lobe

Caudate nucleus (head)

Septum pellucidum

Putamen

Insular cortex

Massa intermedia

Internal cerebral v.

Posterior horn of lateral ventricle (with choroid plexus)

Parietal lobe

Falx cerebri

Occipital lobe

Superior sagittal sinus

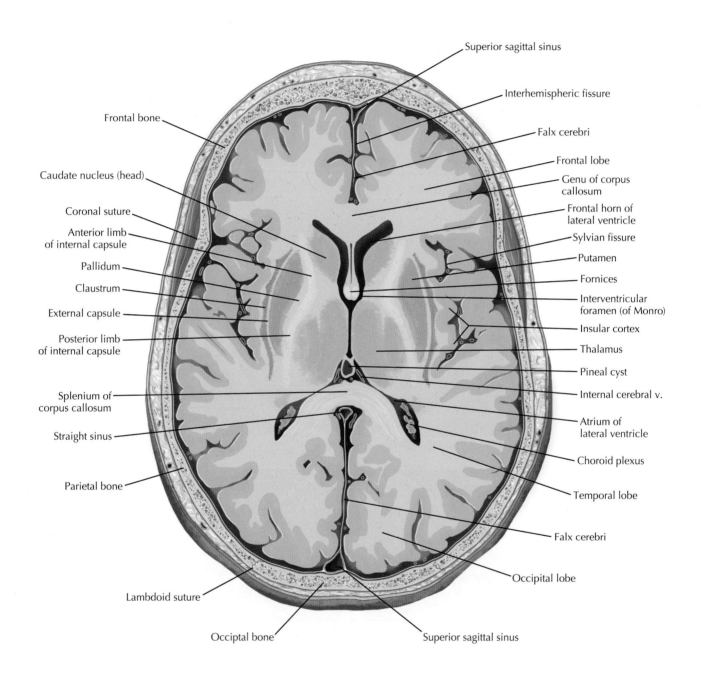

Superior sagittal sinus

Interhemispheric fissure

Frontal bone

Falx cerebri

Frontal lobe

Caudate nucleus (head)

Genu of corpus callosum

Coronal suture

Frontal horn of lateral ventricle

Anterior limb of internal capsule

Sylvian fissure

Putamen

Pallidum

Fornices

Claustrum

Interventricular foramen (of Monro)

External capsule

Insular cortex

Posterior limb of internal capsule

Thalamus

Pineal cyst

Splenium of corpus callosum

Internal cerebral v.

Straight sinus

Atrium of lateral ventricle

Choroid plexus

Parietal bone

Temporal lobe

Falx cerebri

Occipital lobe

Lambdoid suture

Occipital bone

Superior sagittal sinus

PATHOLOGIC PROCESS

The foramen of Monro (interventricular foramen) can be an important point of obstruction of cerebrospinal fluid (CSF) flow. A small colloid cyst can occasionally be found at this location and could cause obstruction in a relatively short time, rapidly becoming fatal if untreated. CSF is produced at a rate of about 500 mL/day and the subarachnoid space around the brain and spinal cord can contain only 150 mL. CSF intracranially and within the spinal canal turns over about four times a day.

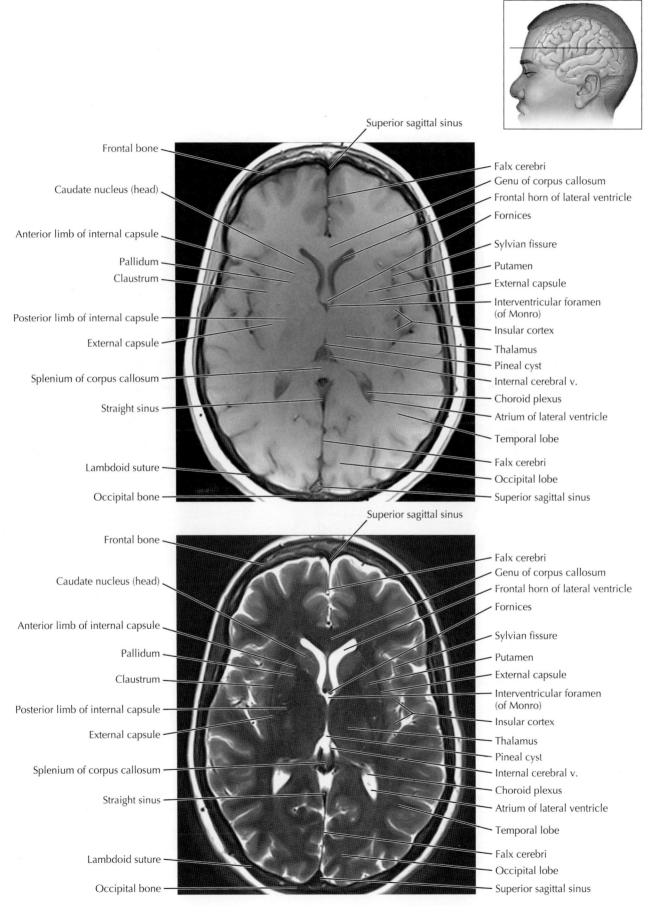

Superior sagittal sinus

Frontal bone

Caudate nucleus (head)

Anterior limb of internal capsule

Pallidum

Claustrum

Posterior limb of internal capsule

External capsule

Splenium of corpus callosum

Straight sinus

Lambdoid suture

Occipital bone

Falx cerebri
Genu of corpus callosum
Frontal horn of lateral ventricle
Fornices

Sylvian fissure

Putamen

External capsule

Interventricular foramen
(of Monro)

Insular cortex

Thalamus

Pineal cyst

Internal cerebral v.

Choroid plexus

Atrium of lateral ventricle

Temporal lobe

Falx cerebri

Occipital lobe

Superior sagittal sinus

Superior sagittal sinus

Frontal bone

Caudate nucleus (head)

Anterior limb of internal capsule

Pallidum

Claustrum

Posterior limb of internal capsule

External capsule

Splenium of corpus callosum

Straight sinus

Lambdoid suture

Occipital bone

Falx cerebri
Genu of corpus callosum
Frontal horn of lateral ventricle

Fornices

Sylvian fissure

Putamen

External capsule

Interventricular foramen
(of Monro)

Insular cortex

Thalamus

Pineal cyst

Internal cerebral v.

Choroid plexus

Atrium of lateral ventricle

Temporal lobe

Falx cerebri

Occipital lobe

Superior sagittal sinus

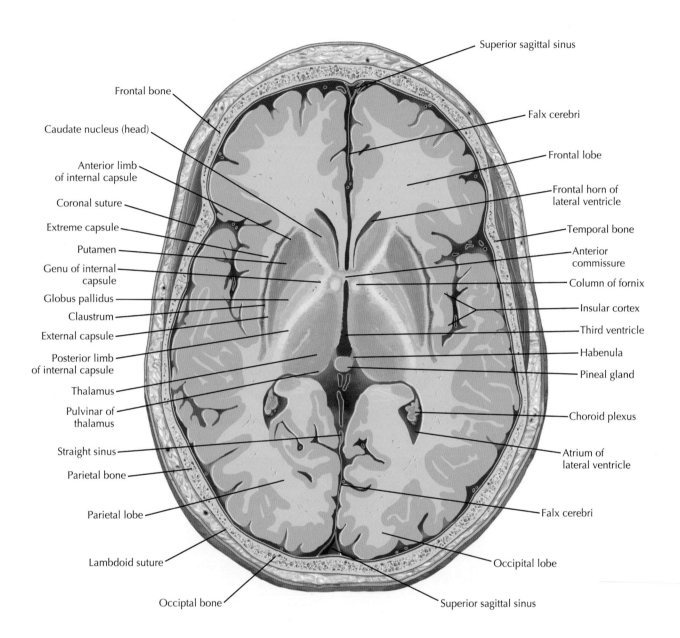

Superior sagittal sinus

Frontal bone

Caudate nucleus (head)

Anterior limb of internal capsule

Coronal suture

Extreme capsule

Putamen

Genu of internal capsule

Globus pallidus

Claustrum

External capsule

Posterior limb of internal capsule

Thalamus

Pulvinar of thalamus

Straight sinus

Parietal bone

Parietal lobe

Lambdoid suture

Occiptal bone

Falx cerebri

Frontal lobe

Frontal horn of lateral ventricle

Temporal bone

Anterior commissure

Column of fornix

Insular cortex

Third ventricle

Habenula

Pineal gland

Choroid plexus

Atrium of lateral ventricle

Falx cerebri

Occipital lobe

Superior sagittal sinus

NORMAL ANATOMY

The habenula (Latin *habena*, "rein") originally referred to the pineal gland stalk but is now commonly used to indicate a nearby group of neurons in the dorsal and caudal thalamus. The insular cortex is often the first location where an infarct in the area of the middle cerebral artery will become evident on unenhanced computed tomography (CT) of the head. Loss of differentiation of the insular gray matter from the subinsular white matter should always be evaluated.

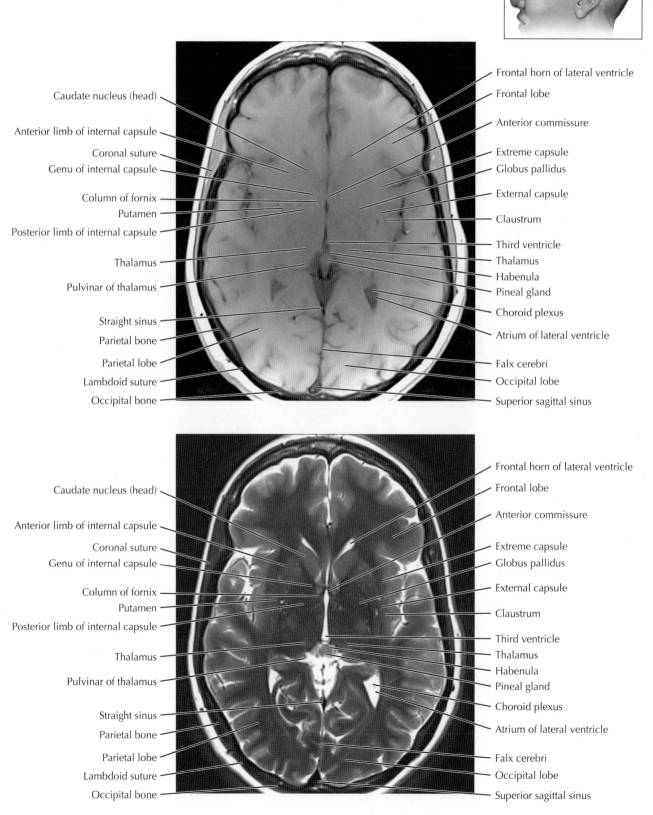

Caudate nucleus (head)

Anterior limb of internal capsule

Coronal suture

Genu of internal capsule

Column of fornix

Putamen

Posterior limb of internal capsule

Thalamus

Pulvinar of thalamus

Straight sinus

Parietal bone

Parietal lobe

Lambdoid suture

Occipital bone

Frontal horn of lateral ventricle

Frontal lobe

Anterior commissure

Extreme capsule

Globus pallidus

External capsule

Claustrum

Third ventricle

Thalamus

Habenula

Pineal gland

Choroid plexus

Atrium of lateral ventricle

Falx cerebri

Occipital lobe

Superior sagittal sinus

Caudate nucleus (head)

Anterior limb of internal capsule

Coronal suture

Genu of internal capsule

Column of fornix

Putamen

Posterior limb of internal capsule

Thalamus

Pulvinar of thalamus

Straight sinus

Parietal bone

Parietal lobe

Lambdoid suture

Occipital bone

Frontal horn of lateral ventricle

Frontal lobe

Anterior commissure

Extreme capsule

Globus pallidus

External capsule

Claustrum

Third ventricle

Thalamus

Habenula

Pineal gland

Choroid plexus

Atrium of lateral ventricle

Falx cerebri

Occipital lobe

Superior sagittal sinus

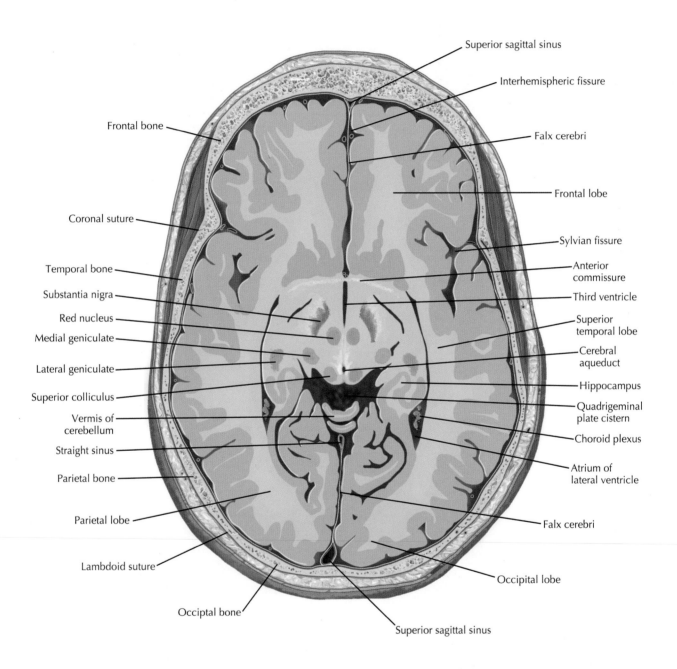

Superior sagittal sinus

Interhemispheric fissure

Frontal bone

Falx cerebri

Frontal lobe

Coronal suture

Sylvian fissure

Temporal bone

Anterior commissure

Substantia nigra

Third ventricle

Red nucleus

Superior temporal lobe

Medial geniculate

Cerebral aqueduct

Lateral geniculate

Hippocampus

Superior colliculus

Quadrigeminal plate cistern

Vermis of cerebellum

Choroid plexus

Straight sinus

Atrium of lateral ventricle

Parietal bone

Parietal lobe

Falx cerebri

Lambdoid suture

Occipital lobe

Occipital bone

Superior sagittal sinus

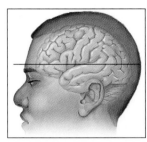

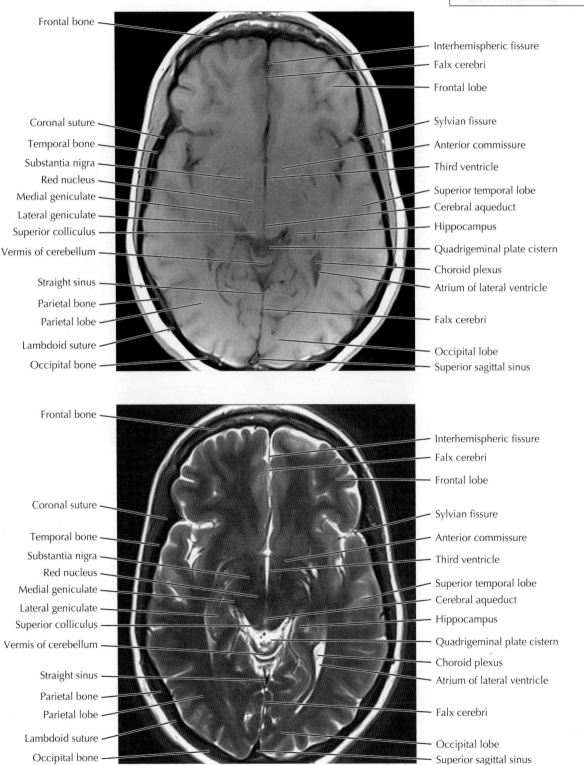

Frontal bone

Coronal suture
Temporal bone
Substantia nigra
Red nucleus
Medial geniculate
Lateral geniculate
Superior colliculus
Vermis of cerebellum

Straight sinus
Parietal bone
Parietal lobe
Lambdoid suture
Occipital bone

Interhemispheric fissure
Falx cerebri
Frontal lobe

Sylvian fissure
Anterior commissure
Third ventricle
Superior temporal lobe
Cerebral aqueduct
Hippocampus
Quadrigeminal plate cistern
Choroid plexus
Atrium of lateral ventricle

Falx cerebri

Occipital lobe
Superior sagittal sinus

Frontal bone

Coronal suture
Temporal bone
Substantia nigra
Red nucleus
Medial geniculate
Lateral geniculate
Superior colliculus
Vermis of cerebellum

Straight sinus
Parietal bone
Parietal lobe
Lambdoid suture
Occipital bone

Interhemispheric fissure
Falx cerebri
Frontal lobe

Sylvian fissure
Anterior commissure
Third ventricle
Superior temporal lobe
Cerebral aqueduct
Hippocampus
Quadrigeminal plate cistern
Choroid plexus
Atrium of lateral ventricle

Falx cerebri

Occipital lobe
Superior sagittal sinus

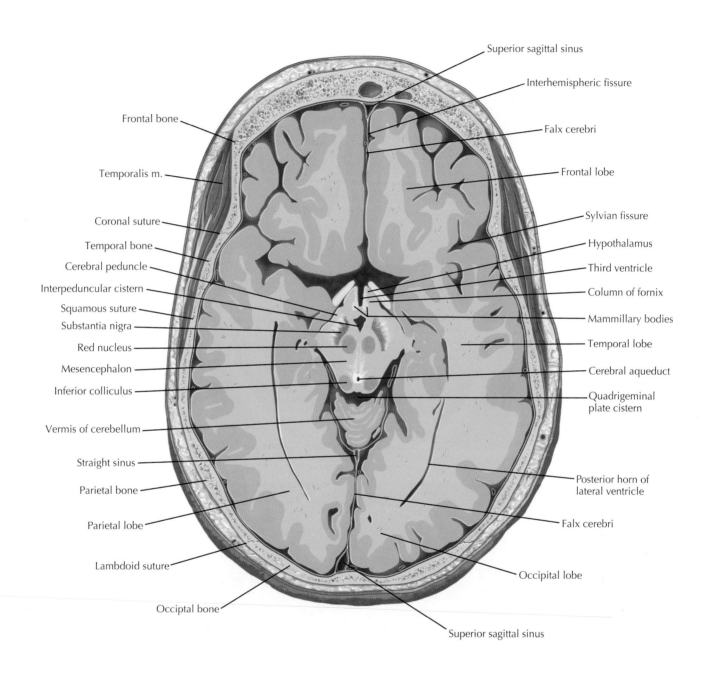

Superior sagittal sinus

Interhemispheric fissure

Frontal bone

Falx cerebri

Temporalis m.

Frontal lobe

Coronal suture

Sylvian fissure

Temporal bone

Hypothalamus

Cerebral peduncle

Third ventricle

Interpeduncular cistern

Column of fornix

Squamous suture

Mammillary bodies

Substantia nigra

Temporal lobe

Red nucleus

Cerebral aqueduct

Mesencephalon

Inferior colliculus

Quadrigeminal plate cistern

Vermis of cerebellum

Straight sinus

Parietal bone

Posterior horn of lateral ventricle

Parietal lobe

Falx cerebri

Lambdoid suture

Occiptal bone

Occipital lobe

Superior sagittal sinus

NORMAL ANATOMY

Note the small but conspicuous paired mammillary bodies anterior to the interpeduncular cistern, at the anterior end of the fornices. The mammillary bodies are part of the limbic system and are believed to add the element of smell to memories. The bodies can be enlarged and T2-weighted bright in Wernicke's encephalopathy. Do not confuse the mammillary bodies with the paired inferior and superior colliculi, which are located on the posterior surface of the brainstem.

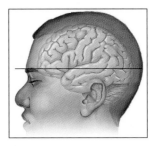

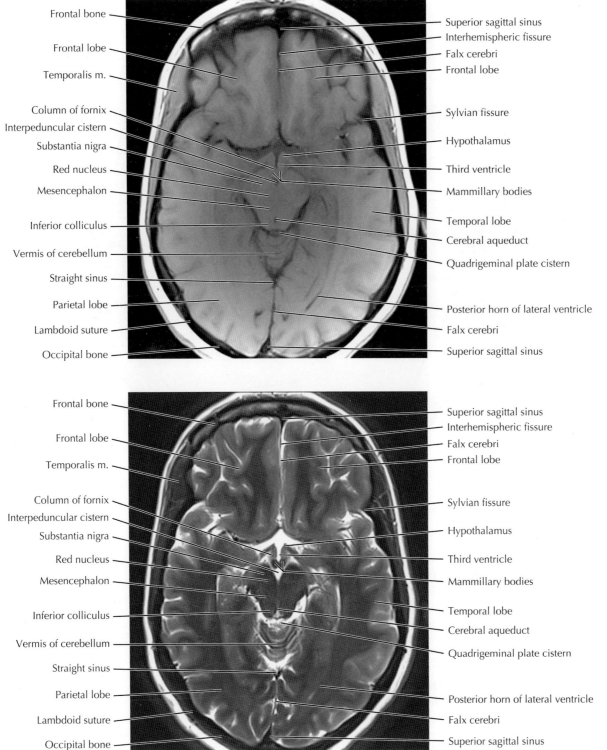

Frontal bone

Frontal lobe

Temporalis m.

Column of fornix

Interpeduncular cistern

Substantia nigra

Red nucleus

Mesencephalon

Inferior colliculus

Vermis of cerebellum

Straight sinus

Parietal lobe

Lambdoid suture

Occipital bone

Superior sagittal sinus

Interhemispheric fissure

Falx cerebri

Frontal lobe

Sylvian fissure

Hypothalamus

Third ventricle

Mammillary bodies

Temporal lobe

Cerebral aqueduct

Quadrigeminal plate cistern

Posterior horn of lateral ventricle

Falx cerebri

Superior sagittal sinus

Frontal bone

Frontal lobe

Temporalis m.

Column of fornix

Interpeduncular cistern

Substantia nigra

Red nucleus

Mesencephalon

Inferior colliculus

Vermis of cerebellum

Straight sinus

Parietal lobe

Lambdoid suture

Occipital bone

Superior sagittal sinus

Interhemispheric fissure

Falx cerebri

Frontal lobe

Sylvian fissure

Hypothalamus

Third ventricle

Mammillary bodies

Temporal lobe

Cerebral aqueduct

Quadrigeminal plate cistern

Posterior horn of lateral ventricle

Falx cerebri

Superior sagittal sinus

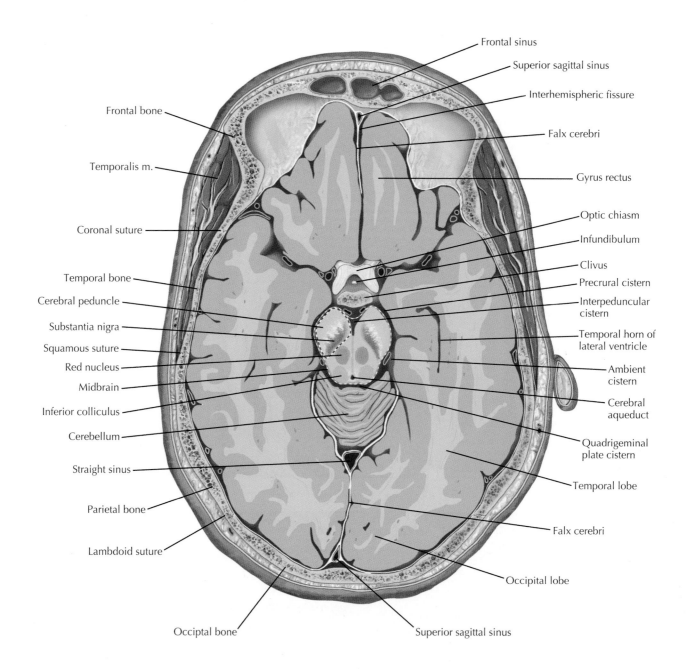

Frontal sinus

Superior sagittal sinus

Interhemispheric fissure

Frontal bone

Falx cerebri

Temporalis m.

Gyrus rectus

Optic chiasm

Coronal suture

Infundibulum

Clivus

Temporal bone

Precrural cistern

Cerebral peduncle

Interpeduncular cistern

Substantia nigra

Temporal horn of lateral ventricle

Squamous suture

Red nucleus

Ambient cistern

Midbrain

Cerebral aqueduct

Inferior colliculus

Cerebellum

Quadrigeminal plate cistern

Straight sinus

Temporal lobe

Parietal bone

Lambdoid suture

Falx cerebri

Occipital lobe

Occipital bone

Superior sagittal sinus

NORMAL ANATOMY

Note that the basal cisterns are composed of the suprasellar cistern, which resembles a six-pointed star, and the smile-shaped quadrgeminal plate cistern (see also Axial 14). The six points of the suprasellar cistern include the interhemispheric fissure, two Sylvian cisterns, two ambient cisterns, and the interpeduncular cistern.

PATHOLOGIC PROCESS

The interpeduncular cistern is a good anatomic feature to scrutinize; this location often first reveals subarachnoid hemorrhage when a brain aneurysm ruptures. This usually occurs from the area of the circle of Willis, which is prone to many anatomic vascular variations.

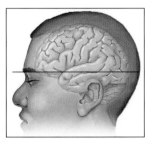

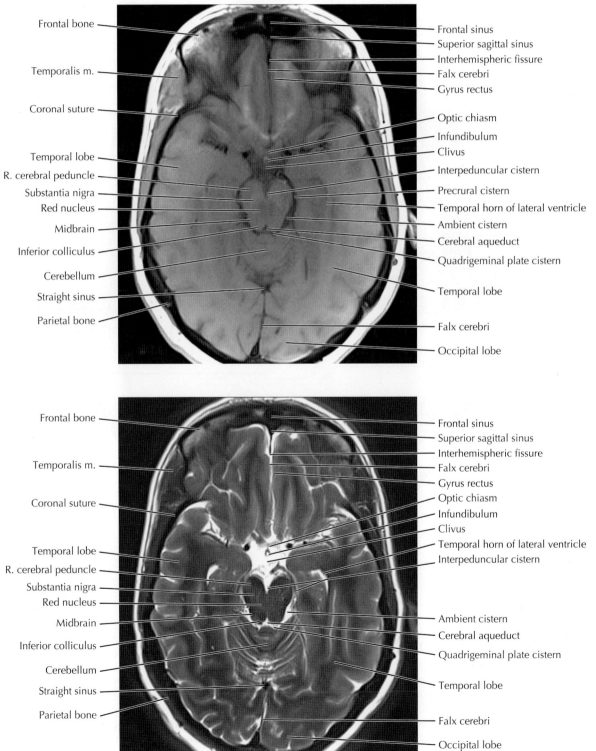

Frontal bone — Frontal sinus
Superior sagittal sinus
Interhemispheric fissure
Temporalis m. — Falx cerebri
Gyrus rectus
Coronal suture —
Optic chiasm
Infundibulum
Temporal lobe — Clivus
R. cerebral peduncle — Interpeduncular cistern
Substantia nigra — Precrural cistern
Red nucleus — Temporal horn of lateral ventricle
Midbrain — Ambient cistern
Inferior colliculus — Cerebral aqueduct
Quadrigeminal plate cistern
Cerebellum —
Straight sinus — Temporal lobe
Parietal bone —
Falx cerebri
Occipital lobe

Frontal bone — Frontal sinus
Superior sagittal sinus
Interhemispheric fissure
Temporalis m. — Falx cerebri
Gyrus rectus
Coronal suture — Optic chiasm
Infundibulum
Clivus
Temporal lobe — Temporal horn of lateral ventricle
R. cerebral peduncle — Interpeduncular cistern
Substantia nigra —
Red nucleus —
Midbrain — Ambient cistern
Inferior colliculus — Cerebral aqueduct
Quadrigeminal plate cistern
Cerebellum —
Straight sinus — Temporal lobe
Parietal bone —
Falx cerebri
Occipital lobe

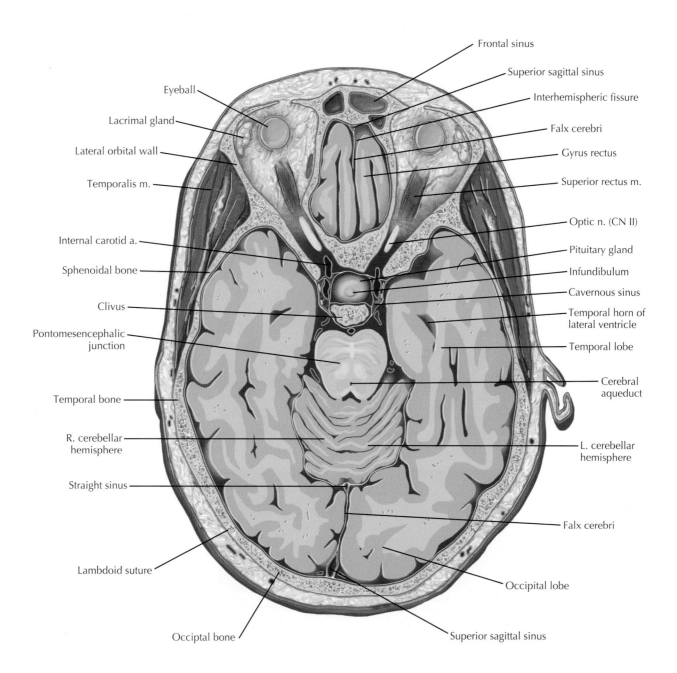

Frontal sinus

Superior sagittal sinus

Interhemispheric fissure

Eyeball

Lacrimal gland

Falx cerebri

Lateral orbital wall

Gyrus rectus

Temporalis m.

Superior rectus m.

Optic n. (CN II)

Internal carotid a.

Pituitary gland

Sphenoidal bone

Infundibulum

Clivus

Cavernous sinus

Pontomesencephalic junction

Temporal horn of lateral ventricle

Temporal lobe

Temporal bone

Cerebral aqueduct

R. cerebellar hemisphere

L. cerebellar hemisphere

Straight sinus

Falx cerebri

Occipital lobe

Lambdoid suture

Occiptal bone

Superior sagittal sinus

DIAGNOSTIC CONSIDERATION

The temporal horns can be useful to help differentiate true hydrocephalus from ex vacuo dilation of the ventricles from central white matter volume loss. In the former case, the temporal horns are dilated and in the latter case they are not. The body of the lateral ventricles can sometimes look prominent but with normal-sized temporal horns where there is central white matter volume loss from chronic microangiopathic disease. Since the body and temporal horns are continuous structures, both should be dilated in true hydrocephalus.

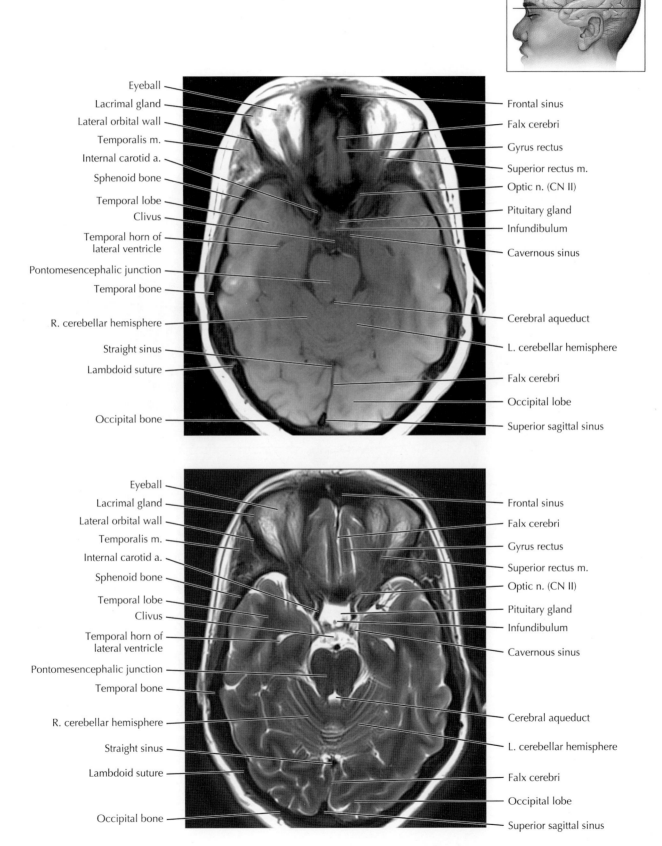

Eyeball
Lacrimal gland
Lateral orbital wall
Temporalis m.
Internal carotid a.
Sphenoid bone
Temporal lobe
Clivus
Temporal horn of lateral ventricle
Pontomesencephalic junction
Temporal bone
R. cerebellar hemisphere
Straight sinus
Lambdoid suture
Occipital bone

Frontal sinus
Falx cerebri
Gyrus rectus
Superior rectus m.
Optic n. (CN II)
Pituitary gland
Infundibulum
Cavernous sinus
Cerebral aqueduct
L. cerebellar hemisphere
Falx cerebri
Occipital lobe
Superior sagittal sinus

Eyeball
Lacrimal gland
Lateral orbital wall
Temporalis m.
Internal carotid a.
Sphenoid bone
Temporal lobe
Clivus
Temporal horn of lateral ventricle
Pontomesencephalic junction
Temporal bone
R. cerebellar hemisphere
Straight sinus
Lambdoid suture
Occipital bone

Frontal sinus
Falx cerebri
Gyrus rectus
Superior rectus m.
Optic n. (CN II)
Pituitary gland
Infundibulum
Cavernous sinus
Cerebral aqueduct
L. cerebellar hemisphere
Falx cerebri
Occipital lobe
Superior sagittal sinus

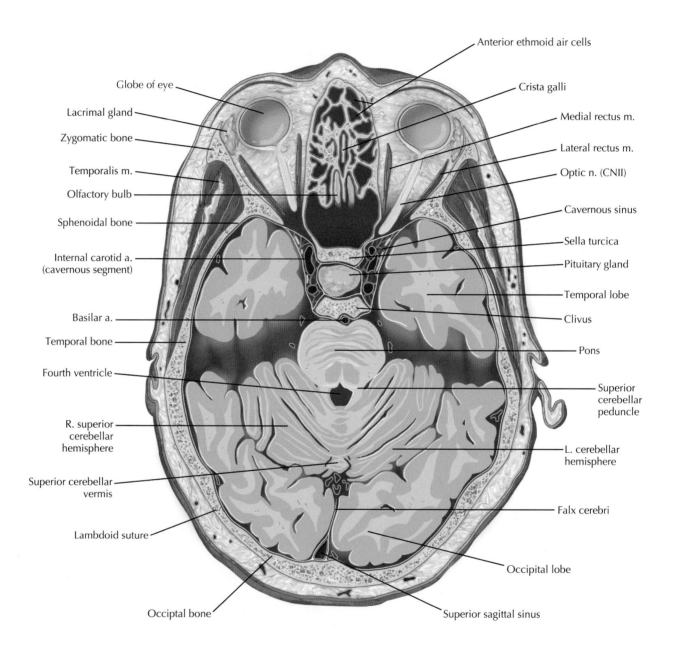

Globe of eye

Lacrimal gland

Zygomatic bone

Temporalis m.

Olfactory bulb

Sphenoidal bone

Internal carotid a.
(cavernous segment)

Basilar a.

Temporal bone

Fourth ventricle

R. superior
cerebellar
hemisphere

Superior cerebellar
vermis

Lambdoid suture

Occiptal bone

Anterior ethmoid air cells

Crista galli

Medial rectus m.

Lateral rectus m.

Optic n. (CNII)

Cavernous sinus

Sella turcica

Pituitary gland

Temporal lobe

Clivus

Pons

Superior
cerebellar
peduncle

L. cerebellar
hemisphere

Falx cerebri

Occipital lobe

Superior sagittal sinus

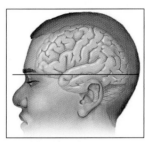

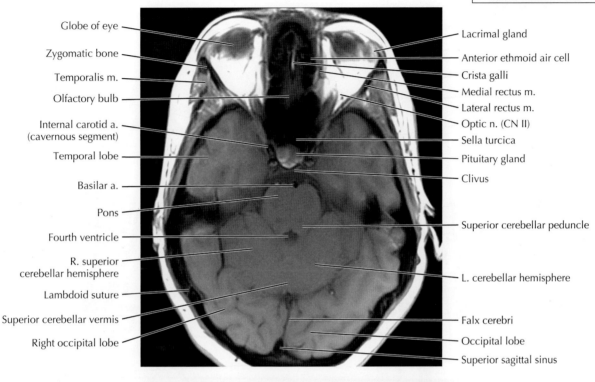

Globe of eye — Lacrimal gland
Zygomatic bone — Anterior ethmoid air cell
Temporalis m. — Crista galli
Olfactory bulb — Medial rectus m.
— Lateral rectus m.
Internal carotid a. (cavernous segment) — Optic n. (CN II)
— Sella turcica
Temporal lobe — Pituitary gland
— Clivus
Basilar a. —
Pons —
Fourth ventricle — Superior cerebellar peduncle
R. superior cerebellar hemisphere —
Lambdoid suture — L. cerebellar hemisphere
Superior cerebellar vermis — Falx cerebri
Right occipital lobe — Occipital lobe
— Superior sagittal sinus

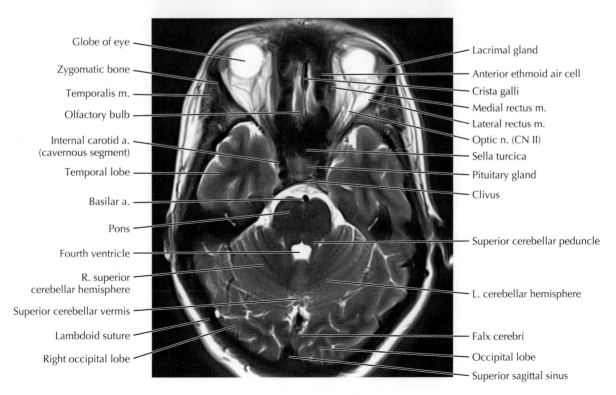

Globe of eye — Lacrimal gland
Zygomatic bone — Anterior ethmoid air cell
Temporalis m. — Crista galli
Olfactory bulb — Medial rectus m.
— Lateral rectus m.
Internal carotid a. (cavernous segment) — Optic n. (CN II)
— Sella turcica
Temporal lobe — Pituitary gland
— Clivus
Basilar a. —
Pons —
Fourth ventricle — Superior cerebellar peduncle
R. superior cerebellar hemisphere —
Superior cerebellar vermis — L. cerebellar hemisphere
Lambdoid suture —
Right occipital lobe — Falx cerebri
— Occipital lobe
— Superior sagittal sinus

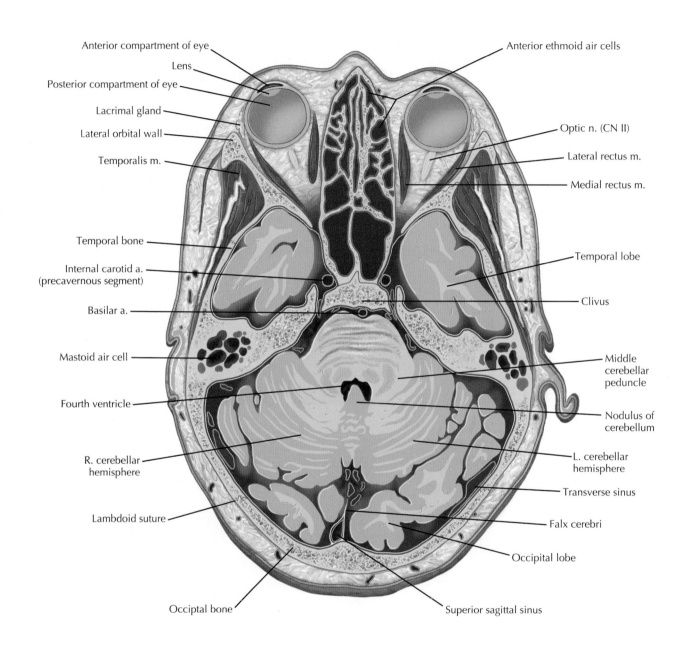

Anterior compartment of eye

Lens

Posterior compartment of eye

Lacrimal gland

Lateral orbital wall

Temporalis m.

Temporal bone

Internal carotid a.
(precavernous segment)

Basilar a.

Mastoid air cell

Fourth ventricle

R. cerebellar
hemisphere

Lambdoid suture

Occiptal bone

Anterior ethmoid air cells

Optic n. (CN II)

Lateral rectus m.

Medial rectus m.

Temporal lobe

Clivus

Middle
cerebellar
peduncle

Nodulus of
cerebellum

L. cerebellar
hemisphere

Transverse sinus

Falx cerebri

Occipital lobe

Superior sagittal sinus

DIAGNOSTIC CONSIDERATION

A subtle but important finding is loss of the normal dark flow void in the basilar artery, which may indicate a clot.

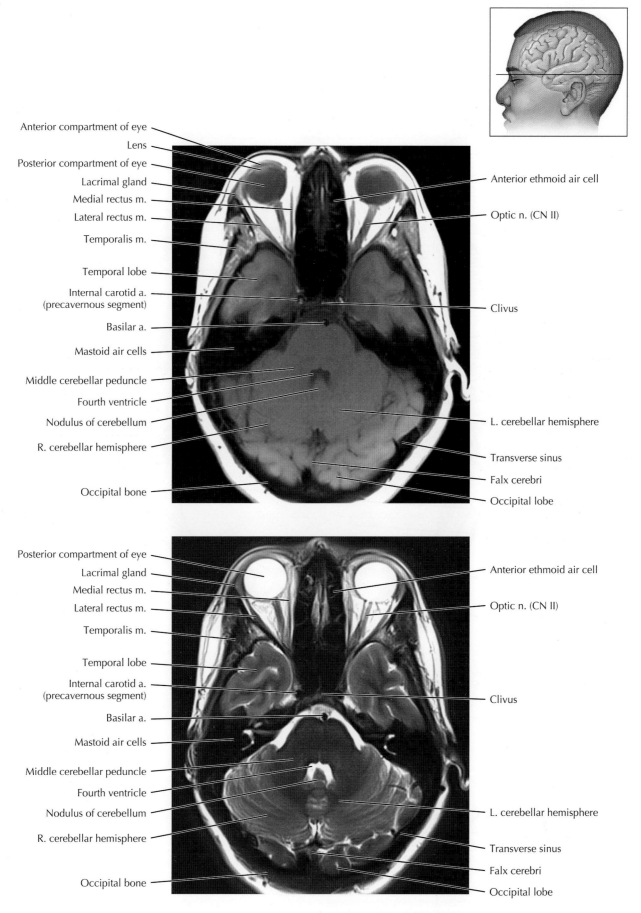

Anterior compartment of eye
Lens
Posterior compartment of eye
Lacrimal gland
Medial rectus m.
Lateral rectus m.
Temporalis m.
Temporal lobe
Internal carotid a. (precavernous segment)
Basilar a.
Mastoid air cells
Middle cerebellar peduncle
Fourth ventricle
Nodulus of cerebellum
R. cerebellar hemisphere
Occipital bone

Anterior ethmoid air cell
Optic n. (CN II)
Clivus
L. cerebellar hemisphere
Transverse sinus
Falx cerebri
Occipital lobe

Posterior compartment of eye
Lacrimal gland
Medial rectus m.
Lateral rectus m.
Temporalis m.
Temporal lobe
Internal carotid a. (precavernous segment)
Basilar a.
Mastoid air cells
Middle cerebellar peduncle
Fourth ventricle
Nodulus of cerebellum
R. cerebellar hemisphere
Occipital bone

Anterior ethmoid air cell
Optic n. (CN II)
Clivus
L. cerebellar hemisphere
Transverse sinus
Falx cerebri
Occipital lobe

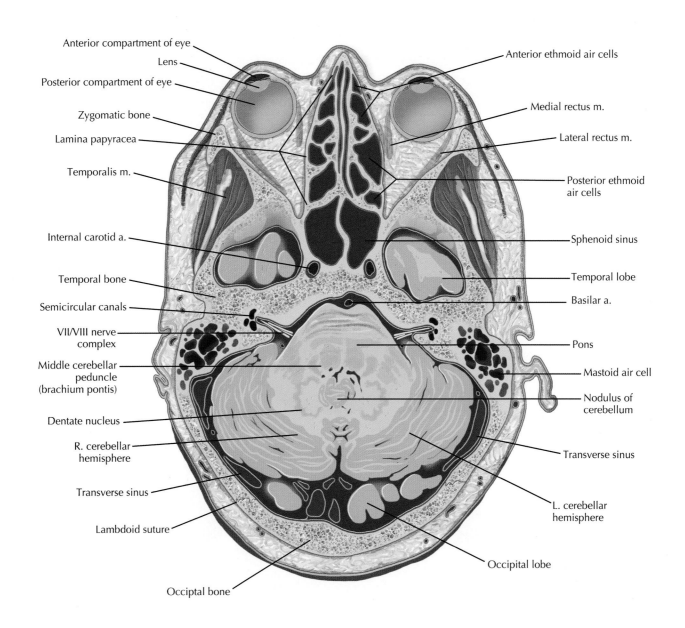

Anterior compartment of eye

Lens

Posterior compartment of eye

Zygomatic bone

Lamina papyracea

Temporalis m.

Internal carotid a.

Temporal bone

Semicircular canals

VII/VIII nerve complex

Middle cerebellar peduncle (brachium pontis)

Dentate nucleus

R. cerebellar hemisphere

Transverse sinus

Lambdoid suture

Occiptal bone

Anterior ethmoid air cells

Medial rectus m.

Lateral rectus m.

Posterior ethmoid air cells

Sphenoid sinus

Temporal lobe

Basilar a.

Pons

Mastoid air cell

Nodulus of cerebellum

Transverse sinus

L. cerebellar hemisphere

Occipital lobe

NORMAL ANATOMY

Note the regions with bright T2 fluid signal, including the vitreous humor, CSF in Meckel's cave, prepontine cistern, and endolymph fluid in the cochlea, semicircular canals, and internal auditory canals. Recall that fat is also bright on fast spin-echo T2-weighted MRI.

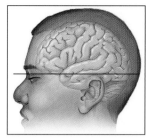

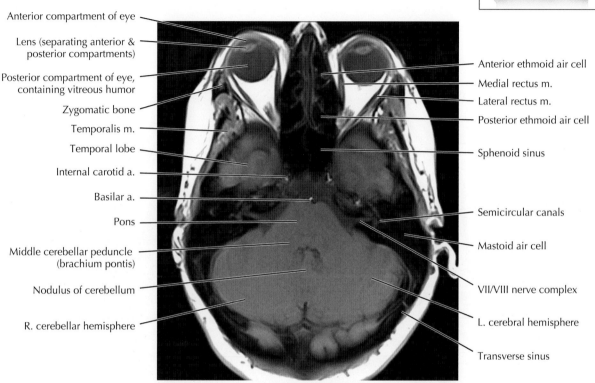

Anterior compartment of eye

Lens (separating anterior & posterior compartments)

Posterior compartment of eye, containing vitreous humor

Zygomatic bone

Temporalis m.

Temporal lobe

Internal carotid a.

Basilar a.

Pons

Middle cerebellar peduncle (brachium pontis)

Nodulus of cerebellum

R. cerebellar hemisphere

Anterior ethmoid air cell

Medial rectus m.

Lateral rectus m.

Posterior ethmoid air cell

Sphenoid sinus

Semicircular canals

Mastoid air cell

VII/VIII nerve complex

L. cerebral hemisphere

Transverse sinus

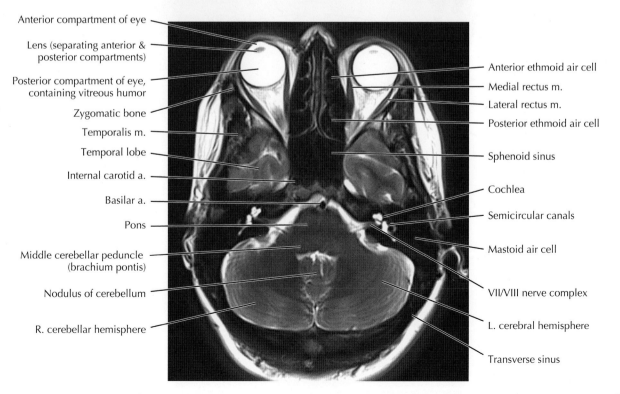

Anterior compartment of eye

Lens (separating anterior & posterior compartments)

Posterior compartment of eye, containing vitreous humor

Zygomatic bone

Temporalis m.

Temporal lobe

Internal carotid a.

Basilar a.

Pons

Middle cerebellar peduncle (brachium pontis)

Nodulus of cerebellum

R. cerebellar hemisphere

Anterior ethmoid air cell

Medial rectus m.

Lateral rectus m.

Posterior ethmoid air cell

Sphenoid sinus

Cochlea

Semicircular canals

Mastoid air cell

VII/VIII nerve complex

L. cerebral hemisphere

Transverse sinus

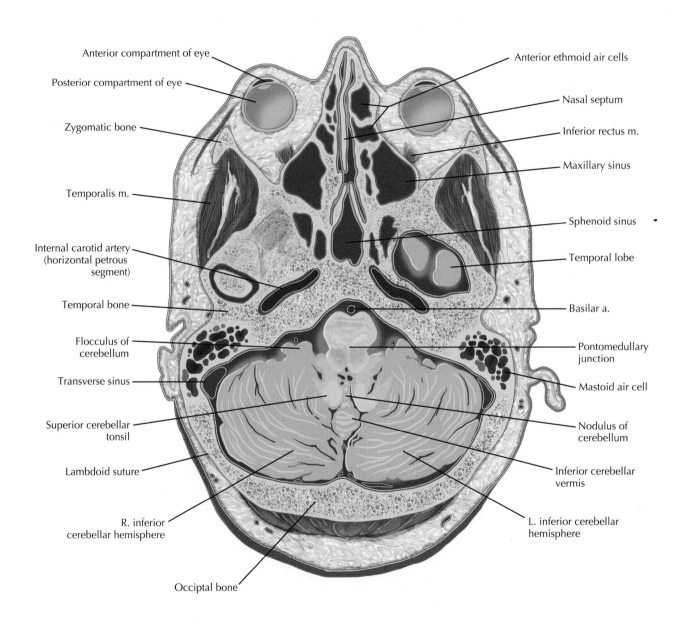

Anterior compartment of eye

Posterior compartment of eye

Zygomatic bone

Temporalis m.

Internal carotid artery
(horizontal petrous
segment)

Temporal bone

Flocculus of
cerebellum

Transverse sinus

Superior cerebellar
tonsil

Lambdoid suture

R. inferior
cerebellar hemisphere

Occiptal bone

Anterior ethmoid air cells

Nasal septum

Inferior rectus m.

Maxillary sinus

Sphenoid sinus

Temporal lobe

Basilar a.

Pontomedullary
junction

Mastoid air cell

Nodulus of
cerebellum

Inferior cerebellar
vermis

L. inferior cerebellar
hemisphere

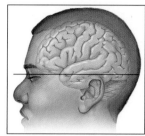

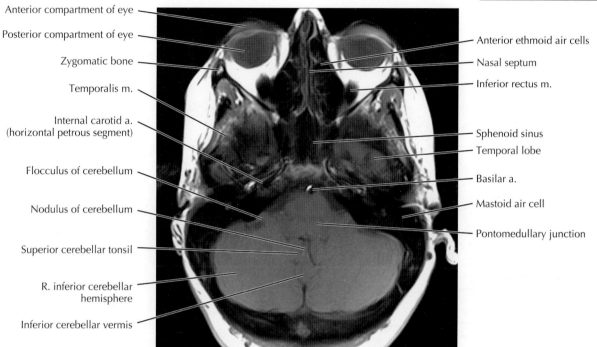

Anterior compartment of eye
Posterior compartment of eye
Zygomatic bone
Temporalis m.
Internal carotid a. (horizontal petrous segment)
Flocculus of cerebellum
Nodulus of cerebellum
Superior cerebellar tonsil
R. inferior cerebellar hemisphere
Inferior cerebellar vermis

Anterior ethmoid air cells
Nasal septum
Inferior rectus m.
Sphenoid sinus
Temporal lobe
Basilar a.
Mastoid air cell
Pontomedullary junction

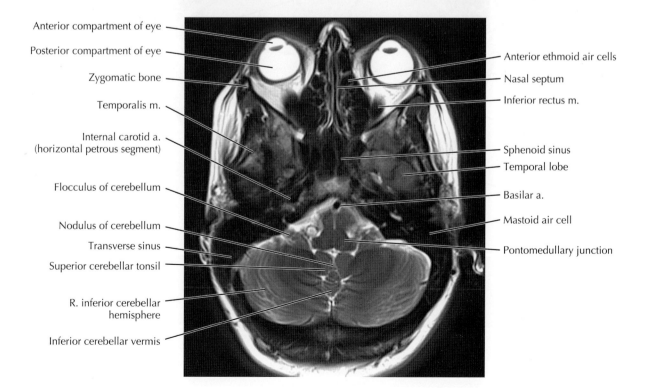

Anterior compartment of eye
Posterior compartment of eye
Zygomatic bone
Temporalis m.
Internal carotid a. (horizontal petrous segment)
Flocculus of cerebellum
Nodulus of cerebellum
Transverse sinus
Superior cerebellar tonsil
R. inferior cerebellar hemisphere
Inferior cerebellar vermis

Anterior ethmoid air cells
Nasal septum
Inferior rectus m.
Sphenoid sinus
Temporal lobe
Basilar a.
Mastoid air cell
Pontomedullary junction

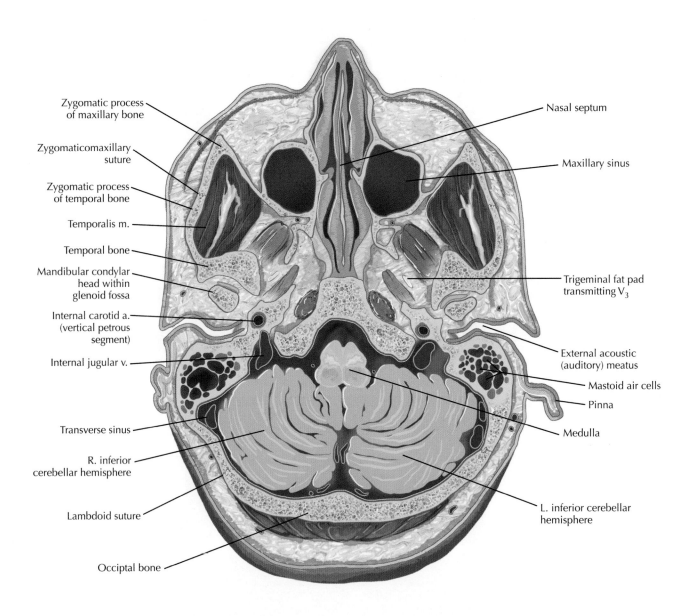

Zygomatic process of maxillary bone

Zygomaticomaxillary suture

Zygomatic process of temporal bone

Temporalis m.

Temporal bone

Mandibular condylar head within glenoid fossa

Internal carotid a. (vertical petrous segment)

Internal jugular v.

Transverse sinus

R. inferior cerebellar hemisphere

Lambdoid suture

Occiptal bone

Nasal septum

Maxillary sinus

Trigeminal fat pad transmitting V_3

External acoustic (auditory) meatus

Mastoid air cells

Pinna

Medulla

L. inferior cerebellar hemisphere

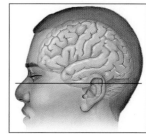

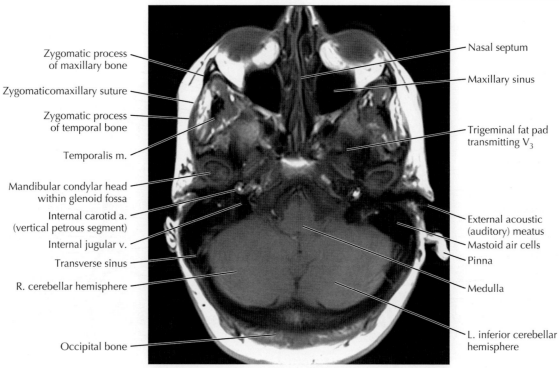

Zygomatic process
of maxillary bone

Zygomaticomaxillary suture

Zygomatic process
of temporal bone

Temporalis m.

Mandibular condylar head
within glenoid fossa

Internal carotid a.
(vertical petrous segment)

Internal jugular v.

Transverse sinus

R. cerebellar hemisphere

Occipital bone

Nasal septum

Maxillary sinus

Trigeminal fat pad
transmitting V₃

External acoustic
(auditory) meatus

Mastoid air cells

Pinna

Medulla

L. inferior cerebellar
hemisphere

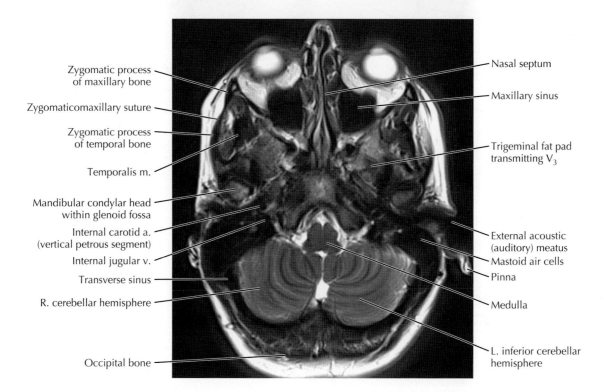

Zygomatic process
of maxillary bone

Zygomaticomaxillary suture

Zygomatic process
of temporal bone

Temporalis m.

Mandibular condylar head
within glenoid fossa

Internal carotid a.
(vertical petrous segment)

Internal jugular v.

Transverse sinus

R. cerebellar hemisphere

Occipital bone

Nasal septum

Maxillary sinus

Trigeminal fat pad
transmitting V₃

External acoustic
(auditory) meatus

Mastoid air cells

Pinna

Medulla

L. inferior cerebellar
hemisphere

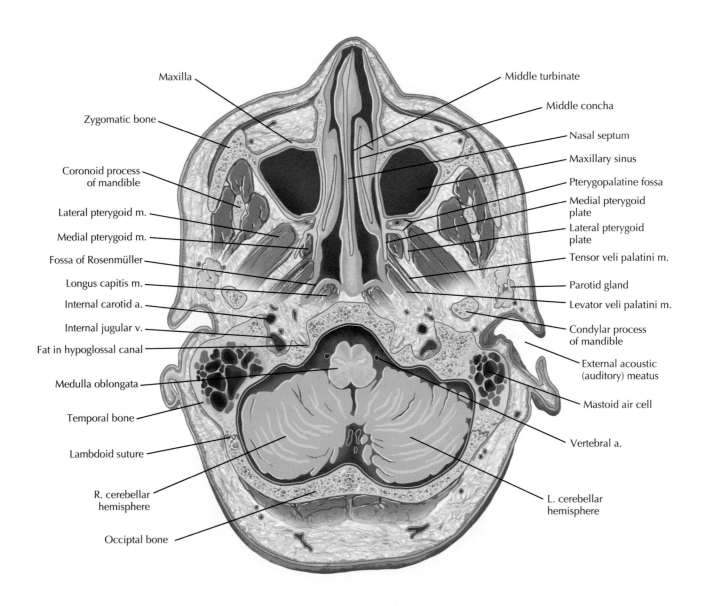

Maxilla

Zygomatic bone

Coronoid process of mandible

Lateral pterygoid m.

Medial pterygoid m.

Fossa of Rosenmüller

Longus capitis m.

Internal carotid a.

Internal jugular v.

Fat in hypoglossal canal

Medulla oblongata

Temporal bone

Lambdoid suture

R. cerebellar hemisphere

Occiptal bone

Middle turbinate

Middle concha

Nasal septum

Maxillary sinus

Pterygopalatine fossa

Medial pterygoid plate

Lateral pterygoid plate

Tensor veli palatini m.

Parotid gland

Levator veli palatini m.

Condylar process of mandible

External acoustic (auditory) meatus

Mastoid air cell

Vertebral a.

L. cerebellar hemisphere

PATHOLOGIC PROCESS

Note the vessels and nerves in the pterygopalatine fossa surrounded by bright fat. Loss of this normal fat signal can be a sign of perineural spread of disease along the maxillary branch of the trigeminal nerve (V_2). Meckel's ganglion (pterygopalatine ganglion) sits in this fossa, as opposed to the Gasserian ganglion, which sits more posteriorly, in Meckel's cave.

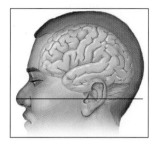

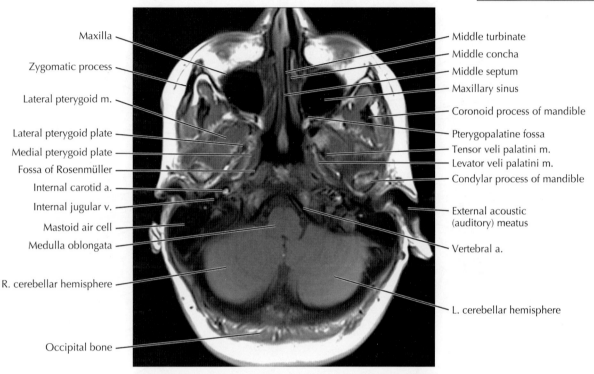

Maxilla

Zygomatic process

Lateral pterygoid m.

Lateral pterygoid plate

Medial pterygoid plate

Fossa of Rosenmüller

Internal carotid a.

Internal jugular v.

Mastoid air cell

Medulla oblongata

R. cerebellar hemisphere

Occipital bone

Middle turbinate

Middle concha

Middle septum

Maxillary sinus

Coronoid process of mandible

Pterygopalatine fossa

Tensor veli palatini m.

Levator veli palatini m.

Condylar process of mandible

External acoustic (auditory) meatus

Vertebral a.

L. cerebellar hemisphere

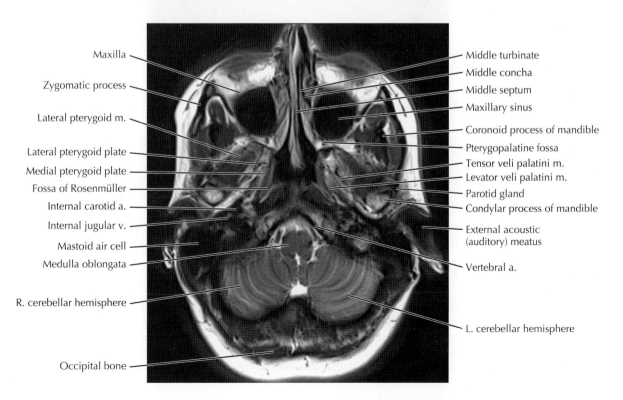

Maxilla

Zygomatic process

Lateral pterygoid m.

Lateral pterygoid plate

Medial pterygoid plate

Fossa of Rosenmüller

Internal carotid a.

Internal jugular v.

Mastoid air cell

Medulla oblongata

R. cerebellar hemisphere

Occipital bone

Middle turbinate

Middle concha

Middle septum

Maxillary sinus

Coronoid process of mandible

Pterygopalatine fossa

Tensor veli palatini m.

Levator veli palatini m.

Parotid gland

Condylar process of mandible

External acoustic (auditory) meatus

Vertebral a.

L. cerebellar hemisphere

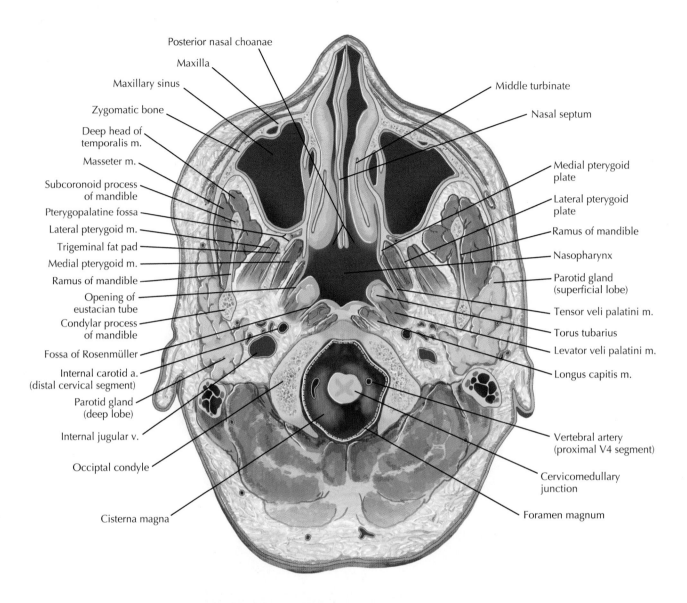

Posterior nasal choanae

Maxilla

Maxillary sinus

Zygomatic bone

Deep head of temporalis m.

Masseter m.

Subcoronoid process of mandible

Pterygopalatine fossa

Lateral pterygoid m.

Trigeminal fat pad

Medial pterygoid m.

Ramus of mandible

Opening of eustacian tube

Condylar process of mandible

Fossa of Rosenmüller

Internal carotid a. (distal cervical segment)

Parotid gland (deep lobe)

Internal jugular v.

Occiptal condyle

Cisterna magna

Middle turbinate

Nasal septum

Medial pterygoid plate

Lateral pterygoid plate

Ramus of mandible

Nasopharynx

Parotid gland (superficial lobe)

Tensor veli palatini m.

Torus tubarius

Levator veli palatini m.

Longus capitis m.

Vertebral artery (proximal V4 segment)

Cervicomedullary junction

Foramen magnum

DIAGNOSTIC CONSIDERATIONS

On most head studies, the most inferior axial image will show the upper aspect of neck structures such as the parotid glands and nasopharynx. These are often "blind spots" for the unwary neuroradiologist. Loss of the normal "divot" caused by the blind-ending fossa of Rosenmüller between the longus capitis muscle and the torus tubarius in an adult patient may be a sign of nasopharyngeal carcinoma. This can also lead to obstruction of the Eustachian tube opening with fluid in the mastoid air cells. Parotid lesions, even benign tumors such as pleomorphic adenoma, are often resected, unlike thyroid lesions, most of which do not cause symptoms.

IMAGING TECHNIQUE CONSIDERATION

On fast spin-echo T2-weighted imaging, fat is bright, as on T1-weighted imaging. The best way to differentiate is to look at fluid, such as the CSF around the brainstem, which will be bright on T2-weighted imaging and gray on T1-weighted imaging. Please note that there is entry-slice phenomenon causing the lumina of the vertebral arteries to appear bright on T1-weighted imaging due to unsaturated blood entering the imaging slice; no contrast was given.

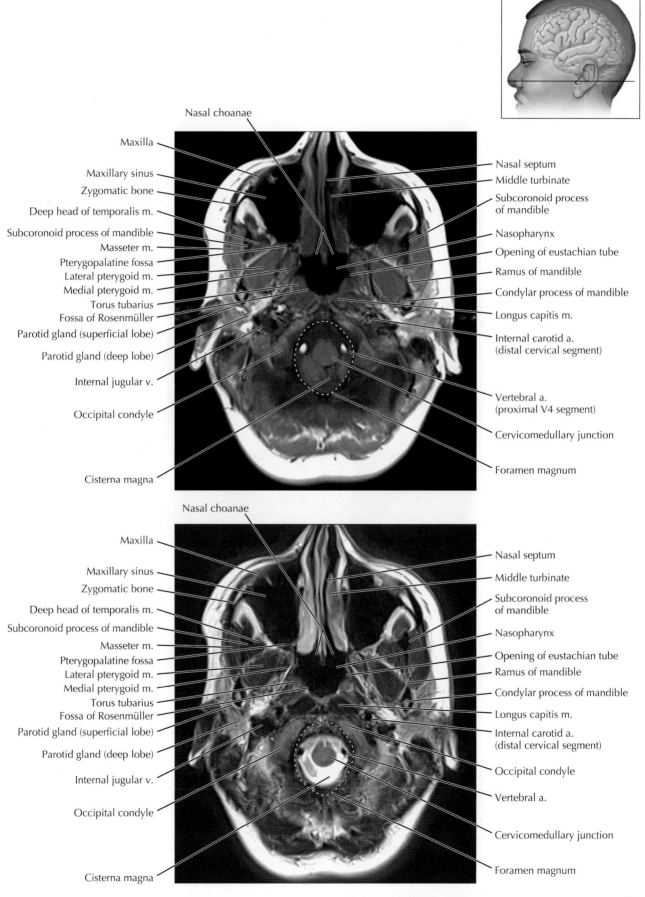

Nasal choanae

Maxilla

Maxillary sinus

Zygomatic bone

Deep head of temporalis m.

Subcoronoid process of mandible

Masseter m.

Pterygopalatine fossa

Lateral pterygoid m.

Medial pterygoid m.

Torus tubarius

Fossa of Rosenmüller

Parotid gland (superficial lobe)

Parotid gland (deep lobe)

Internal jugular v.

Occipital condyle

Cisterna magna

Nasal septum

Middle turbinate

Subcoronoid process of mandible

Nasopharynx

Opening of eustachian tube

Ramus of mandible

Condylar process of mandible

Longus capitis m.

Internal carotid a. (distal cervical segment)

Vertebral a. (proximal V4 segment)

Cervicomedullary junction

Foramen magnum

Nasal choanae

Maxilla

Maxillary sinus

Zygomatic bone

Deep head of temporalis m.

Subcoronoid process of mandible

Masseter m.

Pterygopalatine fossa

Lateral pterygoid m.

Medial pterygoid m.

Torus tubarius

Fossa of Rosenmüller

Parotid gland (superficial lobe)

Parotid gland (deep lobe)

Internal jugular v.

Occipital condyle

Cisterna magna

Nasal septum

Middle turbinate

Subcoronoid process of mandible

Nasopharynx

Opening of eustachian tube

Ramus of mandible

Condylar process of mandible

Longus capitis m.

Internal carotid a. (distal cervical segment)

Occipital condyle

Vertebral a.

Cervicomedullary junction

Foramen magnum

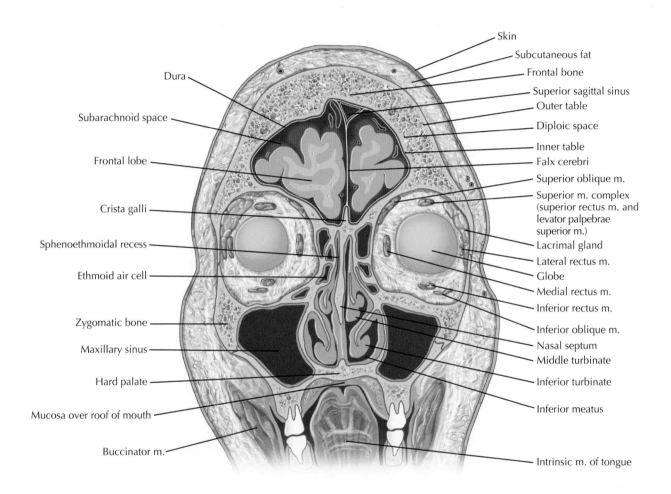

Skin
Subcutaneous fat
Frontal bone
Superior sagittal sinus
Outer table
Diploic space
Inner table
Falx cerebri
Superior oblique m.
Superior m. complex (superior rectus m. and levator palpebrae superior m.)
Lacrimal gland
Lateral rectus m.
Globe
Medial rectus m.
Inferior rectus m.
Inferior oblique m.
Nasal septum
Middle turbinate
Inferior turbinate
Inferior meatus
Intrinsic m. of tongue

Dura
Subarachnoid space
Frontal lobe
Crista galli
Sphenoethmoidal recess
Ethmoid air cell
Zygomatic bone
Maxillary sinus
Hard palate
Mucosa over roof of mouth
Buccinator m.

NORMAL ANATOMY

The *crista galli* (Latin, "crest of the cock") is a ridge of bone arising in the midline from the cribriform plate. The crista galli is the anterior attachment point of the falx to the skull. The olfactory nerves lie to either side of the crista galli within the olfactory grooves.

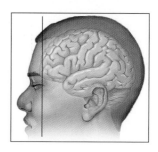

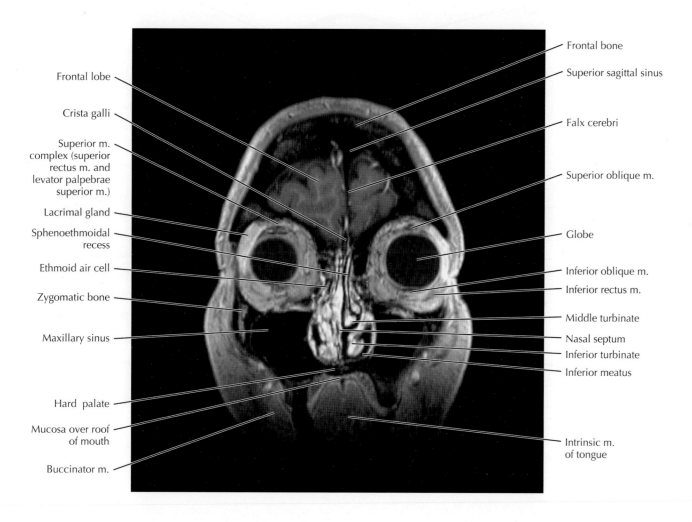

Frontal lobe

Crista galli

Superior m. complex (superior rectus m. and levator palpebrae superior m.)

Lacrimal gland

Sphenoethmoidal recess

Ethmoid air cell

Zygomatic bone

Maxillary sinus

Hard palate

Mucosa over roof of mouth

Buccinator m.

Frontal bone

Superior sagittal sinus

Falx cerebri

Superior oblique m.

Globe

Inferior oblique m.

Inferior rectus m.

Middle turbinate

Nasal septum

Inferior turbinate

Inferior meatus

Intrinsic m. of tongue

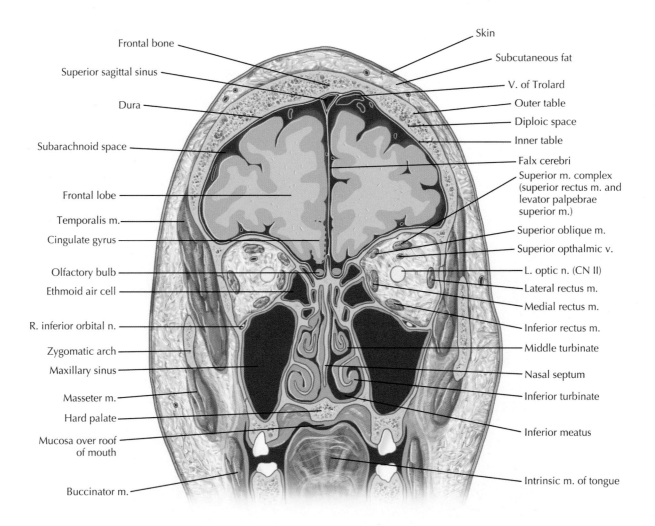

Frontal bone

Superior sagittal sinus

Dura

Subarachnoid space

Frontal lobe

Temporalis m.

Cingulate gyrus

Olfactory bulb

Ethmoid air cell

R. inferior orbital n.

Zygomatic arch

Maxillary sinus

Masseter m.

Hard palate

Mucosa over roof
of mouth

Buccinator m.

Skin

Subcutaneous fat

V. of Trolard

Outer table

Diploic space

Inner table

Falx cerebri

Superior m. complex
(superior rectus m. and
levator palpebrae
superior m.)

Superior oblique m.

Superior opthalmic v.

L. optic n. (CN II)

Lateral rectus m.

Medial rectus m.

Inferior rectus m.

Middle turbinate

Nasal septum

Inferior turbinate

Inferior meatus

Intrinsic m. of tongue

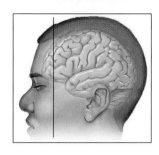

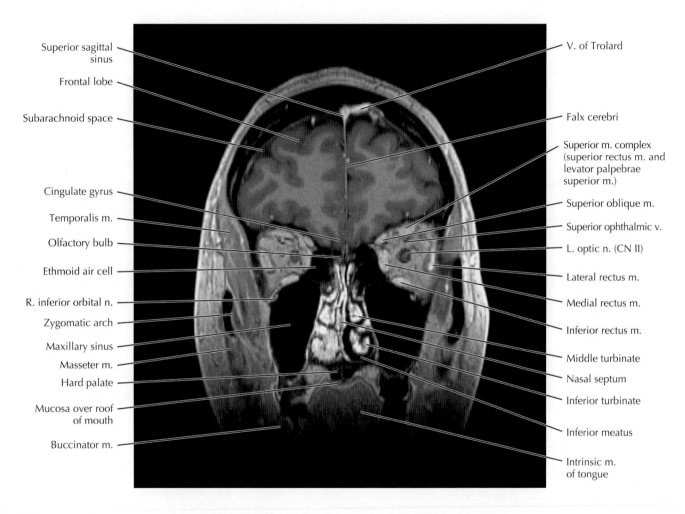

Superior sagittal sinus

Frontal lobe

Subarachnoid space

Cingulate gyrus

Temporalis m.

Olfactory bulb

Ethmoid air cell

R. inferior orbital n.

Zygomatic arch

Maxillary sinus

Masseter m.

Hard palate

Mucosa over roof of mouth

Buccinator m.

V. of Trolard

Falx cerebri

Superior m. complex (superior rectus m. and levator palpebrae superior m.)

Superior oblique m.

Superior ophthalmic v.

L. optic n. (CN II)

Lateral rectus m.

Medial rectus m.

Inferior rectus m.

Middle turbinate

Nasal septum

Inferior turbinate

Inferior meatus

Intrinsic m. of tongue

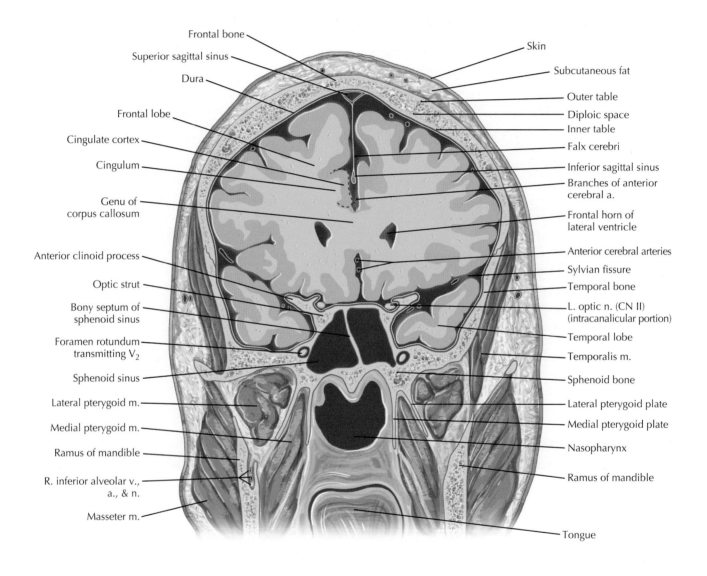

Frontal bone

Superior sagittal sinus

Dura

Frontal lobe

Cingulate cortex

Cingulum

Genu of
corpus callosum

Anterior clinoid process

Optic strut

Bony septum of
sphenoid sinus

Foramen rotundum
transmitting V_2

Sphenoid sinus

Lateral pterygoid m.

Medial pterygoid m.

Ramus of mandible

R. inferior alveolar v.,
a., & n.

Masseter m.

Skin

Subcutaneous fat

Outer table

Diploic space

Inner table

Falx cerebri

Inferior sagittal sinus

Branches of anterior
cerebral a.

Frontal horn of
lateral ventricle

Anterior cerebral arteries

Sylvian fissure

Temporal bone

L. optic n. (CN II)
(intracanalicular portion)

Temporal lobe

Temporalis m.

Sphenoid bone

Lateral pterygoid plate

Medial pterygoid plate

Nasopharynx

Ramus of mandible

Tongue

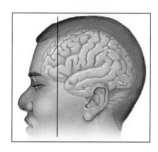

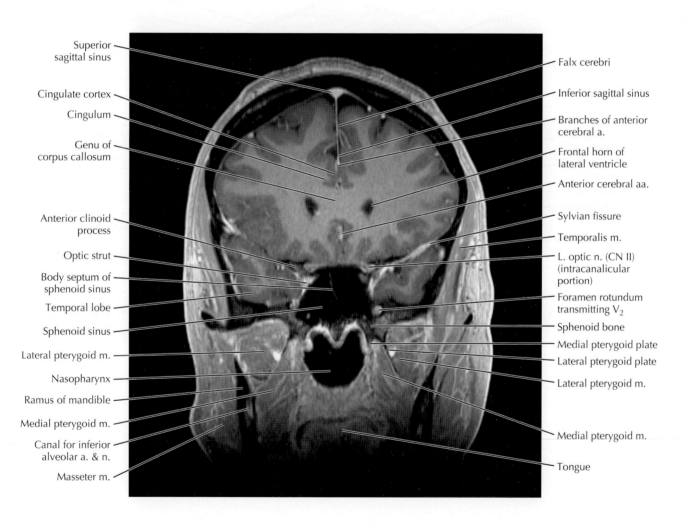

Superior sagittal sinus

Cingulate cortex

Cingulum

Genu of corpus callosum

Anterior clinoid process

Optic strut

Body septum of sphenoid sinus

Temporal lobe

Sphenoid sinus

Lateral pterygoid m.

Nasopharynx

Ramus of mandible

Medial pterygoid m.

Canal for inferior alveolar a. & n.

Masseter m.

Falx cerebri

Inferior sagittal sinus

Branches of anterior cerebral a.

Frontal horn of lateral ventricle

Anterior cerebral aa.

Sylvian fissure

Temporalis m.

L. optic n. (CN II) (intracanalicular portion)

Foramen rotundum transmitting V$_2$

Sphenoid bone

Medial pterygoid plate

Lateral pterygoid plate

Lateral pterygoid m.

Medial pterygoid m.

Tongue

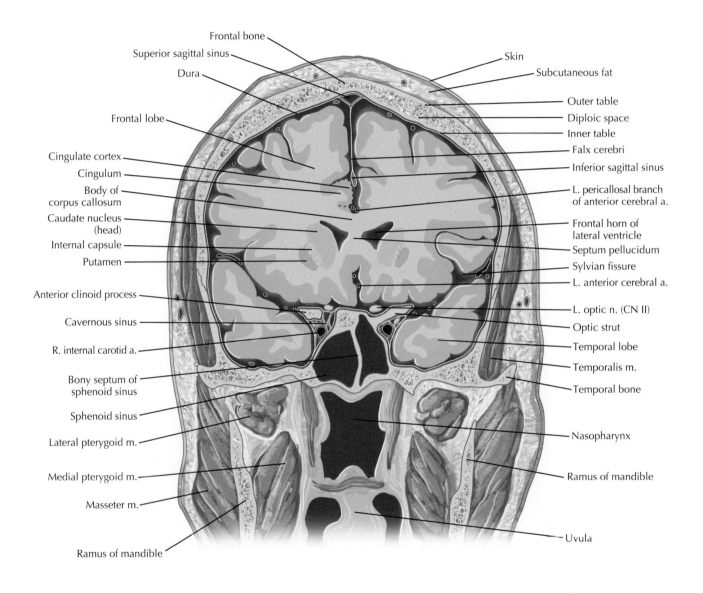

Frontal bone

Superior sagittal sinus

Dura

Frontal lobe

Cingulate cortex

Cingulum

Body of corpus callosum

Caudate nucleus (head)

Internal capsule

Putamen

Anterior clinoid process

Cavernous sinus

R. internal carotid a.

Bony septum of sphenoid sinus

Sphenoid sinus

Lateral pterygoid m.

Medial pterygoid m.

Masseter m.

Ramus of mandible

Skin

Subcutaneous fat

Outer table

Diploic space

Inner table

Falx cerebri

Inferior sagittal sinus

L. pericallosal branch of anterior cerebral a.

Frontal horn of lateral ventricle

Septum pellucidum

Sylvian fissure

L. anterior cerebral a.

L. optic n. (CN II)

Optic strut

Temporal lobe

Temporalis m.

Temporal bone

Nasopharynx

Ramus of mandible

Uvula

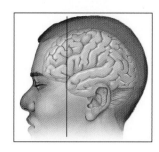

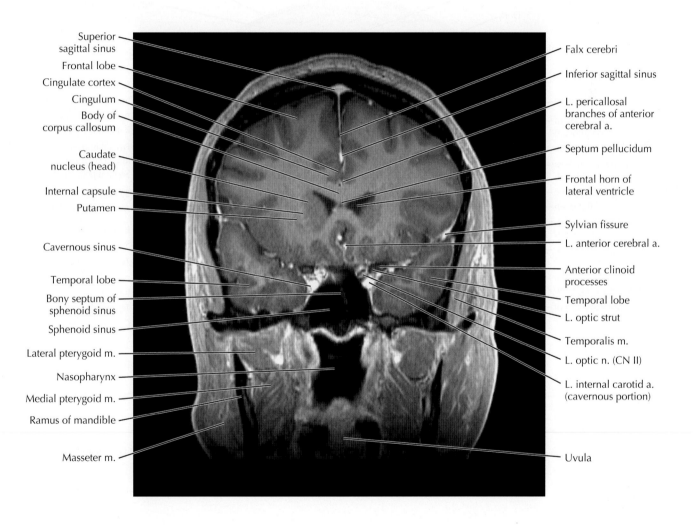

Superior sagittal sinus

Frontal lobe

Cingulate cortex

Cingulum

Body of corpus callosum

Caudate nucleus (head)

Internal capsule

Putamen

Cavernous sinus

Temporal lobe

Bony septum of sphenoid sinus

Sphenoid sinus

Lateral pterygoid m.

Nasopharynx

Medial pterygoid m.

Ramus of mandible

Masseter m.

Falx cerebri

Inferior sagittal sinus

L. pericallosal branches of anterior cerebral a.

Septum pellucidum

Frontal horn of lateral ventricle

Sylvian fissure

L. anterior cerebral a.

Anterior clinoid processes

Temporal lobe

L. optic strut

Temporalis m.

L. optic n. (CN II)

L. internal carotid a. (cavernous portion)

Uvula

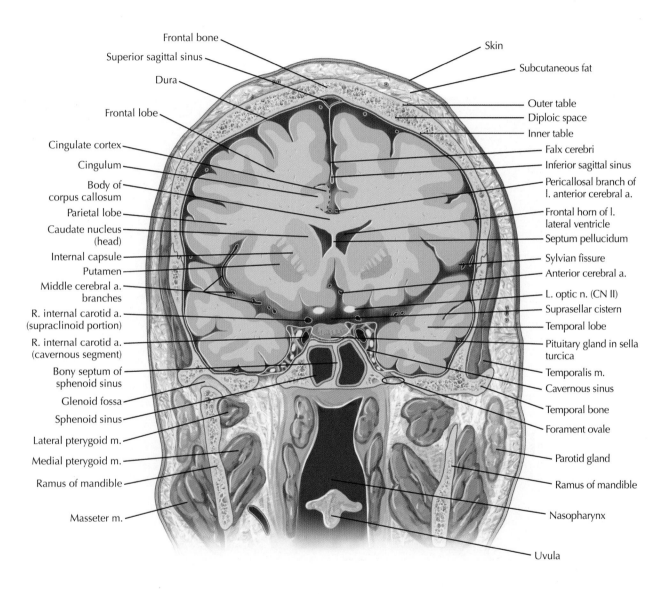

Frontal bone

Superior sagittal sinus

Dura

Frontal lobe

Cingulate cortex

Cingulum

Body of corpus callosum

Parietal lobe

Caudate nucleus (head)

Internal capsule

Putamen

Middle cerebral a. branches

R. internal carotid a. (supraclinoid portion)

R. internal carotid a. (cavernous segment)

Bony septum of sphenoid sinus

Glenoid fossa

Sphenoid sinus

Lateral pterygoid m.

Medial pterygoid m.

Ramus of mandible

Masseter m.

Skin

Subcutaneous fat

Outer table

Diploic space

Inner table

Falx cerebri

Inferior sagittal sinus

Pericallosal branch of l. anterior cerebral a.

Frontal horn of l. lateral ventricle

Septum pellucidum

Sylvian fissure

Anterior cerebral a.

L. optic n. (CN II)

Suprasellar cistern

Temporal lobe

Pituitary gland in sella turcica

Temporalis m.

Cavernous sinus

Temporal bone

Forament ovale

Parotid gland

Ramus of mandible

Nasopharynx

Uvula

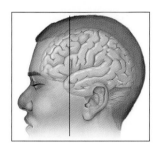

Superior sagittal sinus

Cingulate cortex

Cingulum

Body of corpus callosum

Caudate nucleus (head)

Internal capsule

Putamen

Middle cerebral a.

R. internal carotid a. (supraclinoid portion)

R. internal carotid a. (cavernous segment)

Temporal lobe

Body septum of sphenoid sinus

Sphenoid sinus

Lateral pterygoid m.

Nasopharynx

Medial pterygoid m.

Ramus of mandible

Masseter m.

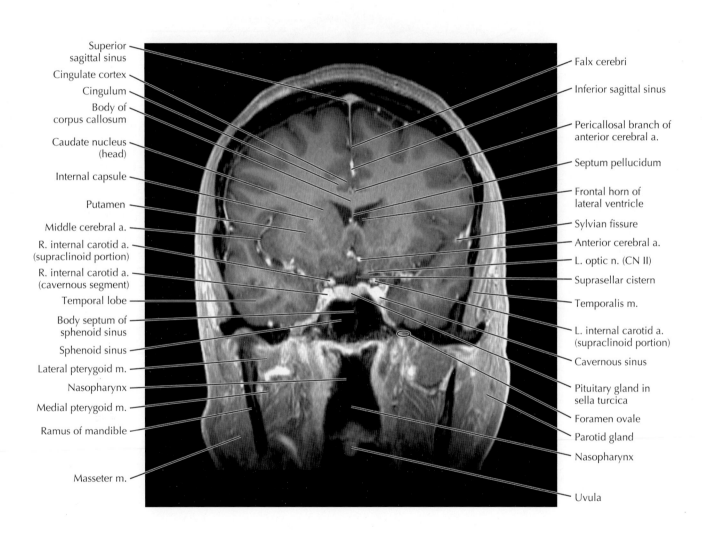

Falx cerebri

Inferior sagittal sinus

Pericallosal branch of anterior cerebral a.

Septum pellucidum

Frontal horn of lateral ventricle

Sylvian fissure

Anterior cerebral a.

L. optic n. (CN II)

Suprasellar cistern

Temporalis m.

L. internal carotid a. (supraclinoid portion)

Cavernous sinus

Pituitary gland in sella turcica

Foramen ovale

Parotid gland

Nasopharynx

Uvula

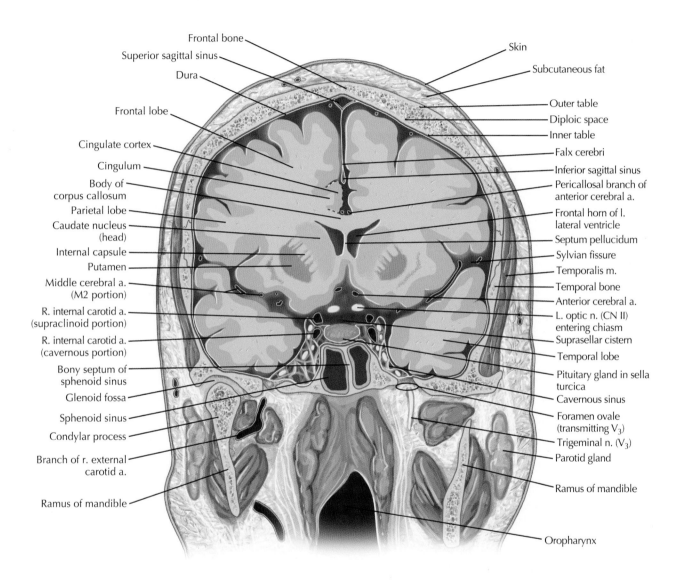

Frontal bone

Superior sagittal sinus

Dura

Frontal lobe

Cingulate cortex

Cingulum

Body of corpus callosum

Parietal lobe

Caudate nucleus (head)

Internal capsule

Putamen

Middle cerebral a. (M2 portion)

R. internal carotid a. (supraclinoid portion)

R. internal carotid a. (cavernous portion)

Bony septum of sphenoid sinus

Glenoid fossa

Sphenoid sinus

Condylar process

Branch of r. external carotid a.

Ramus of mandible

Skin

Subcutaneous fat

Outer table

Diploic space

Inner table

Falx cerebri

Inferior sagittal sinus

Pericallosal branch of anterior cerebral a.

Frontal horn of l. lateral ventricle

Septum pellucidum

Sylvian fissure

Temporalis m.

Temporal bone

Anterior cerebral a.

L. optic n. (CN II) entering chiasm

Suprasellar cistern

Temporal lobe

Pituitary gland in sella turcica

Cavernous sinus

Foramen ovale (transmitting V₃)

Trigeminal n. (V₃)

Parotid gland

Ramus of mandible

Oropharynx

NORMAL ANATOMY

Note the mandibular branch of the trigeminal nerve (V₃) descending from Meckel's cave into the foramen ovale.

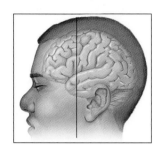

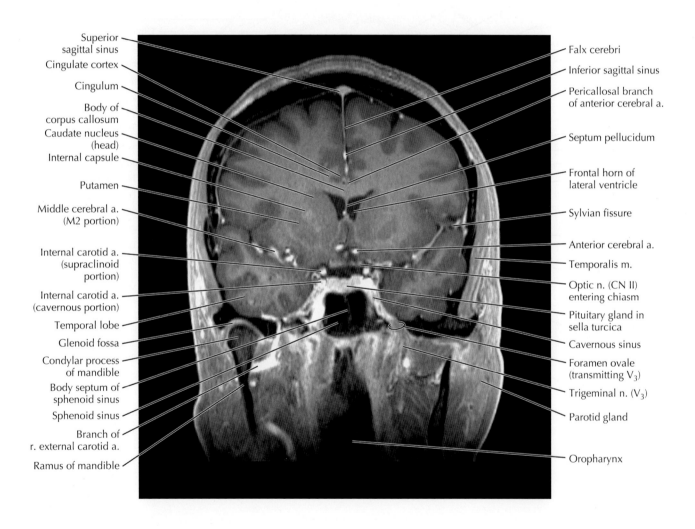

Superior sagittal sinus

Cingulate cortex

Cingulum

Body of corpus callosum

Caudate nucleus (head)

Internal capsule

Putamen

Middle cerebral a. (M2 portion)

Internal carotid a. (supraclinoid portion)

Internal carotid a. (cavernous portion)

Temporal lobe

Glenoid fossa

Condylar process of mandible

Body septum of sphenoid sinus

Sphenoid sinus

Branch of r. external carotid a.

Ramus of mandible

Falx cerebri

Inferior sagittal sinus

Pericallosal branch of anterior cerebral a.

Septum pellucidum

Frontal horn of lateral ventricle

Sylvian fissure

Anterior cerebral a.

Temporalis m.

Optic n. (CN II) entering chiasm

Pituitary gland in sella turcica

Cavernous sinus

Foramen ovale (transmitting V_3)

Trigeminal n. (V_3)

Parotid gland

Oropharynx

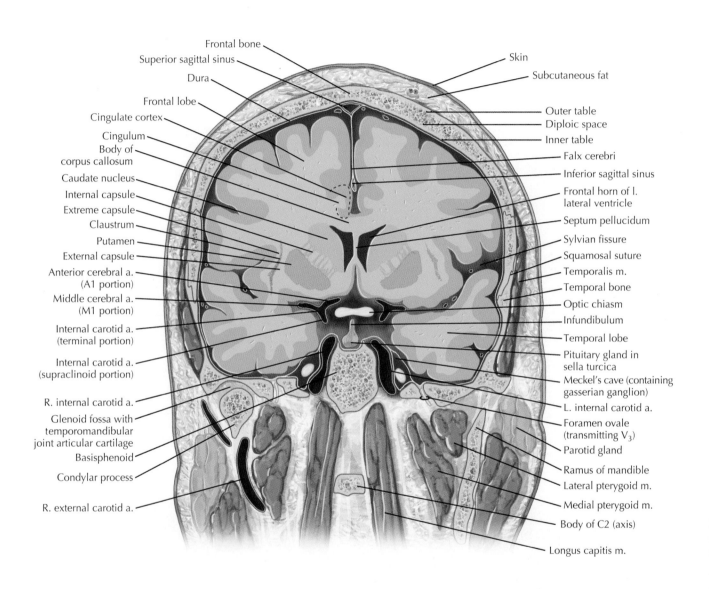

Frontal bone

Superior sagittal sinus

Dura

Frontal lobe

Cingulate cortex

Cingulum

Body of corpus callosum

Caudate nucleus

Internal capsule

Extreme capsule

Claustrum

Putamen

External capsule

Anterior cerebral a. (A1 portion)

Middle cerebral a. (M1 portion)

Internal carotid a. (terminal portion)

Internal carotid a. (supraclinoid portion)

R. internal carotid a.

Glenoid fossa with temporomandibular joint articular cartilage

Basisphenoid

Condylar process

R. external carotid a.

Skin

Subcutaneous fat

Outer table

Diploic space

Inner table

Falx cerebri

Inferior sagittal sinus

Frontal horn of l. lateral ventricle

Septum pellucidum

Sylvian fissure

Squamosal suture

Temporalis m.

Temporal bone

Optic chiasm

Infundibulum

Temporal lobe

Pituitary gland in sella turcica

Meckel's cave (containing gasserian ganglion)

L. internal carotid a.

Foramen ovale (transmitting V₃)

Parotid gland

Ramus of mandible

Lateral pterygoid m.

Medial pterygoid m.

Body of C2 (axis)

Longus capitis m.

NORMAL ANATOMY

The coronal view is often the best view for assessing the pituitary gland, infundibulum, and optic chiasm. The infundibulum may be asymmetric in some cases, as in this image, where it is slightly deviated to the right as a normal variant, but in some cases it can be deviated from a pituitary mass. A large mass can extend into the suprasellar region and compress the optic chiasm, leading to bitemporal hemianopsia.

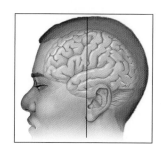

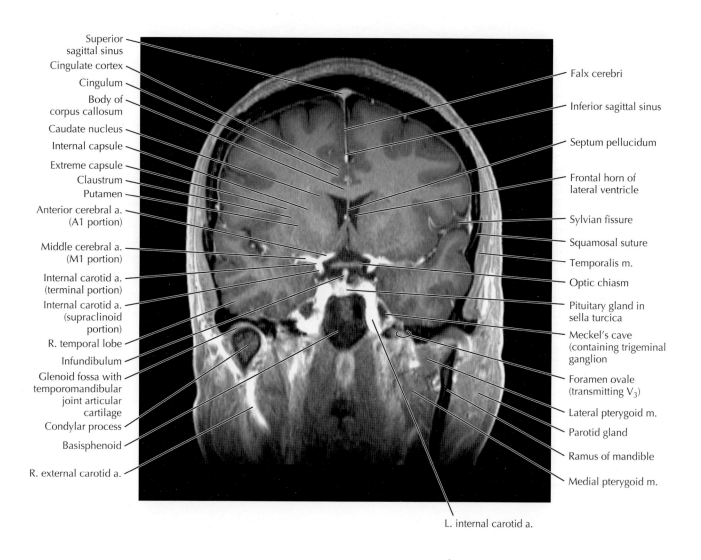

Superior sagittal sinus

Cingulate cortex

Cingulum

Body of corpus callosum

Caudate nucleus

Internal capsule

Extreme capsule

Claustrum

Putamen

Anterior cerebral a. (A1 portion)

Middle cerebral a. (M1 portion)

Internal carotid a. (terminal portion)

Internal carotid a. (supraclinoid portion)

R. temporal lobe

Infundibulum

Glenoid fossa with temporomandibular joint articular cartilage

Condylar process

Basisphenoid

R. external carotid a.

Falx cerebri

Inferior sagittal sinus

Septum pellucidum

Frontal horn of lateral ventricle

Sylvian fissure

Squamosal suture

Temporalis m.

Optic chiasm

Pituitary gland in sella turcica

Meckel's cave (containing trigeminal ganglion

Foramen ovale (transmitting V_3)

Lateral pterygoid m.

Parotid gland

Ramus of mandible

Medial pterygoid m.

L. internal carotid a.

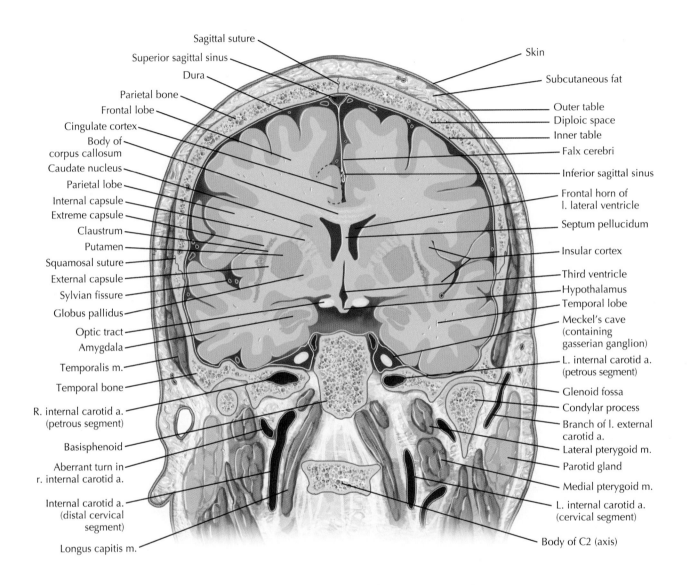

Sagittal suture
Superior sagittal sinus
Dura
Parietal bone
Frontal lobe
Cingulate cortex
Body of corpus callosum
Caudate nucleus
Parietal lobe
Internal capsule
Extreme capsule
Claustrum
Putamen
Squamosal suture
External capsule
Sylvian fissure
Globus pallidus
Optic tract
Amygdala
Temporalis m.
Temporal bone
R. internal carotid a. (petrous segment)
Basisphenoid
Aberrant turn in r. internal carotid a.
Internal carotid a. (distal cervical segment)
Longus capitis m.

Skin
Subcutaneous fat
Outer table
Diploic space
Inner table
Falx cerebri
Inferior sagittal sinus
Frontal horn of l. lateral ventricle
Septum pellucidum
Insular cortex
Third ventricle
Hypothalamus
Temporal lobe
Meckel's cave (containing gasserian ganglion)
L. internal carotid a. (petrous segment)
Glenoid fossa
Condylar process
Branch of l. external carotid a.
Lateral pterygoid m.
Parotid gland
Medial pterygoid m.
L. internal carotid a. (cervical segment)
Body of C2 (axis)

NORMAL ANATOMY

From the Greek meaning "under inner chamber," the hypothalamus forms the floor of the third ventricle and contains small nuclei with a variety of functions. One of the most important functions is to provide signals from the nervous system to the endocrine system through the pituitary gland.

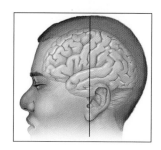

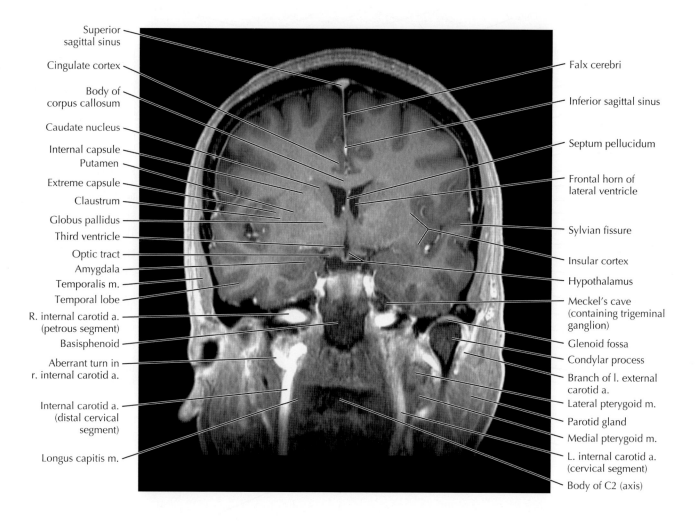

Superior sagittal sinus

Cingulate cortex

Body of corpus callosum

Caudate nucleus

Internal capsule

Putamen

Extreme capsule

Claustrum

Globus pallidus

Third ventricle

Optic tract

Amygdala

Temporalis m.

Temporal lobe

R. internal carotid a. (petrous segment)

Basisphenoid

Aberrant turn in r. internal carotid a.

Internal carotid a. (distal cervical segment)

Longus capitis m.

Falx cerebri

Inferior sagittal sinus

Septum pellucidum

Frontal horn of lateral ventricle

Sylvian fissure

Insular cortex

Hypothalamus

Meckel's cave (containing trigeminal ganglion)

Glenoid fossa

Condylar process

Branch of l. external carotid a.

Lateral pterygoid m.

Parotid gland

Medial pterygoid m.

L. internal carotid a. (cervical segment)

Body of C2 (axis)

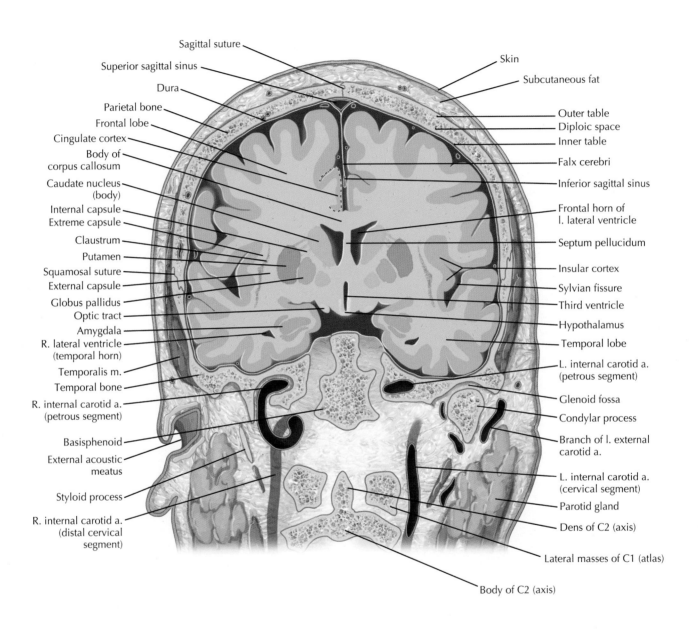

Sagittal suture

Superior sagittal sinus

Dura

Parietal bone

Frontal lobe

Cingulate cortex

Body of corpus callosum

Caudate nucleus (body)

Internal capsule

Extreme capsule

Claustrum

Putamen

Squamosal suture

External capsule

Globus pallidus

Optic tract

Amygdala

R. lateral ventricle (temporal horn)

Temporalis m.

Temporal bone

R. internal carotid a. (petrous segment)

Basisphenoid

External acoustic meatus

Styloid process

R. internal carotid a. (distal cervical segment)

Skin

Subcutaneous fat

Outer table

Diploic space

Inner table

Falx cerebri

Inferior sagittal sinus

Frontal horn of l. lateral ventricle

Septum pellucidum

Insular cortex

Sylvian fissure

Third ventricle

Hypothalamus

Temporal lobe

L. internal carotid a. (petrous segment)

Glenoid fossa

Condylar process

Branch of l. external carotid a.

L. internal carotid a. (cervical segment)

Parotid gland

Dens of C2 (axis)

Lateral masses of C1 (atlas)

Body of C2 (axis)

NORMAL ANATOMY

The cingulate cortex is located on the medial surface of the cerebral hemisphere adjacent to the corpus callosum. The cingulate cortex is usually considered part of the limbic system, which is involved with emotion, learning, and memory. The combination of these three functions makes the cingulate cortex extremely influential in associating behavioral outcomes to motivation.

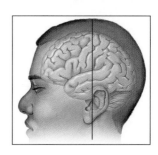

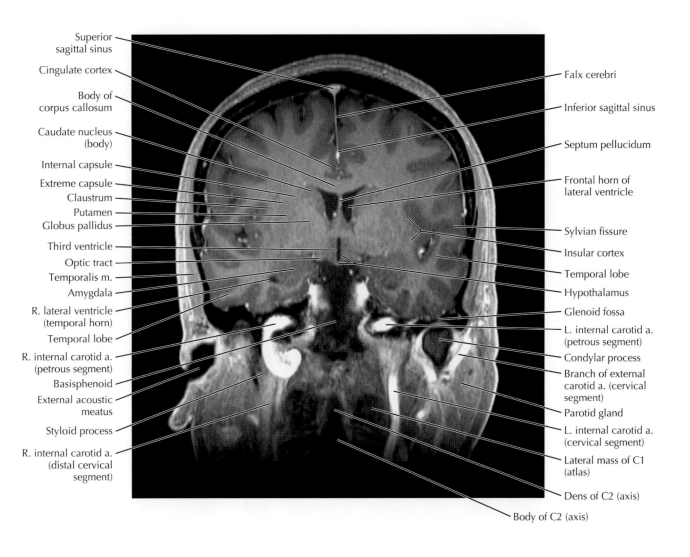

Superior sagittal sinus

Cingulate cortex

Body of corpus callosum

Caudate nucleus (body)

Internal capsule

Extreme capsule

Claustrum

Putamen

Globus pallidus

Third ventricle

Optic tract

Temporalis m.

Amygdala

R. lateral ventricle (temporal horn)

Temporal lobe

R. internal carotid a. (petrous segment)

Basisphenoid

External acoustic meatus

Styloid process

R. internal carotid a. (distal cervical segment)

Falx cerebri

Inferior sagittal sinus

Septum pellucidum

Frontal horn of lateral ventricle

Sylvian fissure

Insular cortex

Temporal lobe

Hypothalamus

Glenoid fossa

L. internal carotid a. (petrous segment)

Condylar process

Branch of external carotid a. (cervical segment)

Parotid gland

L. internal carotid a. (cervical segment)

Lateral mass of C1 (atlas)

Dens of C2 (axis)

Body of C2 (axis)

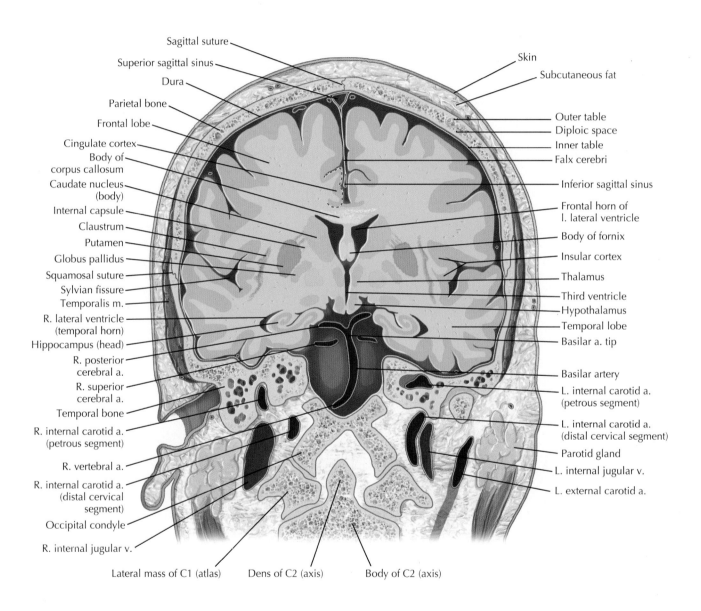

Sagittal suture

Superior sagittal sinus

Dura

Parietal bone

Frontal lobe

Cingulate cortex

Body of corpus callosum

Caudate nucleus (body)

Internal capsule

Claustrum

Putamen

Globus pallidus

Squamosal suture

Sylvian fissure

Temporalis m.

R. lateral ventricle (temporal horn)

Hippocampus (head)

R. posterior cerebral a.

R. superior cerebral a.

Temporal bone

R. internal carotid a. (petrous segment)

R. vertebral a.

R. internal carotid a. (distal cervical segment)

Occipital condyle

R. internal jugular v.

Skin

Subcutaneous fat

Outer table

Diploic space

Inner table

Falx cerebri

Inferior sagittal sinus

Frontal horn of l. lateral ventricle

Body of fornix

Insular cortex

Thalamus

Third ventricle

Hypothalamus

Temporal lobe

Basilar a. tip

Basilar artery

L. internal carotid a. (petrous segment)

L. internal carotid a. (distal cervical segment)

Parotid gland

L. internal jugular v.

L. external carotid a.

Lateral mass of C1 (atlas)   Dens of C2 (axis)   Body of C2 (axis)

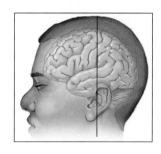

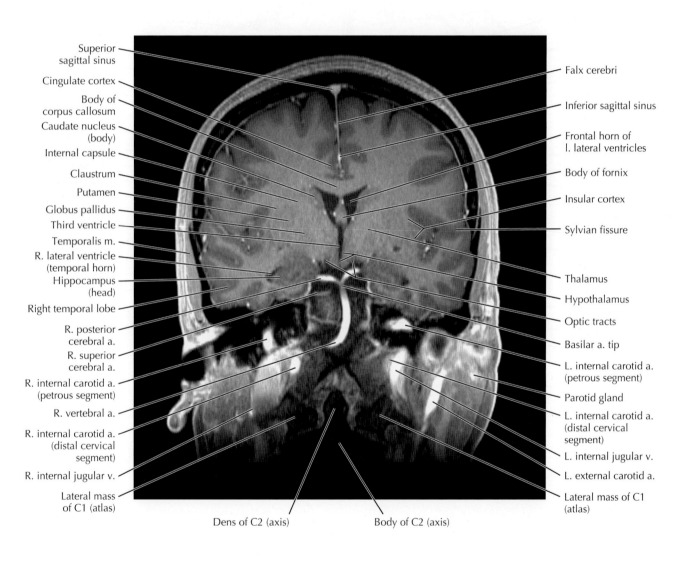

Superior sagittal sinus

Cingulate cortex

Body of corpus callosum

Caudate nucleus (body)

Internal capsule

Claustrum

Putamen

Globus pallidus

Third ventricle

Temporalis m.

R. lateral ventricle (temporal horn)

Hippocampus (head)

Right temporal lobe

R. posterior cerebral a.

R. superior cerebral a.

R. internal carotid a. (petrous segment)

R. vertebral a.

R. internal carotid a. (distal cervical segment)

R. internal jugular v.

Lateral mass of C1 (atlas)

Falx cerebri

Inferior sagittal sinus

Frontal horn of l. lateral ventricles

Body of fornix

Insular cortex

Sylvian fissure

Thalamus

Hypothalamus

Optic tracts

Basilar a. tip

L. internal carotid a. (petrous segment)

Parotid gland

L. internal carotid a. (distal cervical segment)

L. internal jugular v.

L. external carotid a.

Lateral mass of C1 (atlas)

Dens of C2 (axis)

Body of C2 (axis)

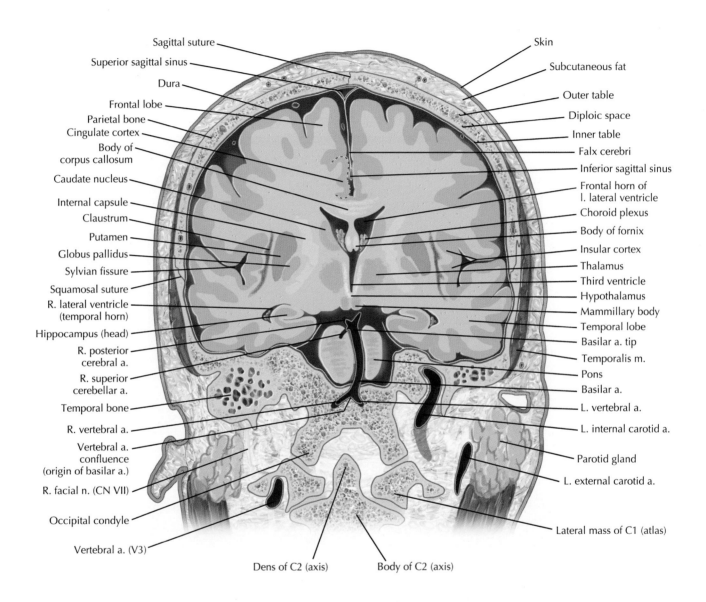

Sagittal suture
Superior sagittal sinus
Dura
Frontal lobe
Parietal bone
Cingulate cortex
Body of corpus callosum
Caudate nucleus
Internal capsule
Claustrum
Putamen
Globus pallidus
Sylvian fissure
Squamosal suture
R. lateral ventricle (temporal horn)
Hippocampus (head)
R. posterior cerebral a.
R. superior cerebellar a.
Temporal bone
R. vertebral a.
Vertebral a. confluence (origin of basilar a.)
R. facial n. (CN VII)
Occipital condyle
Vertebral a. (V3)

Dens of C2 (axis)
Body of C2 (axis)

Skin
Subcutaneous fat
Outer table
Diploic space
Inner table
Falx cerebri
Inferior sagittal sinus
Frontal horn of l. lateral ventricle
Choroid plexus
Body of fornix
Insular cortex
Thalamus
Third ventricle
Hypothalamus
Mammillary body
Temporal lobe
Basilar a. tip
Temporalis m.
Pons
Basilar a.
L. vertebral a.
L. internal carotid a.
Parotid gland
L. external carotid a.
Lateral mass of C1 (atlas)

NORMAL ANATOMY

The coronal plane is an excellent view for obtaining an overview of the vertebrobasilar system in assessing for stenoses or aneurysms. In just a few coronal images, the neuroradiologist can often seen both vertebral arteries with the posterior inferior cerebellar artery origins, the anterior inferior cerebellar artery and superior cerebellar artery origins from the basilar artery, and the proximal posterior cerebral arteries originating from the basilar artery tip.

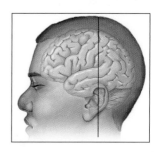

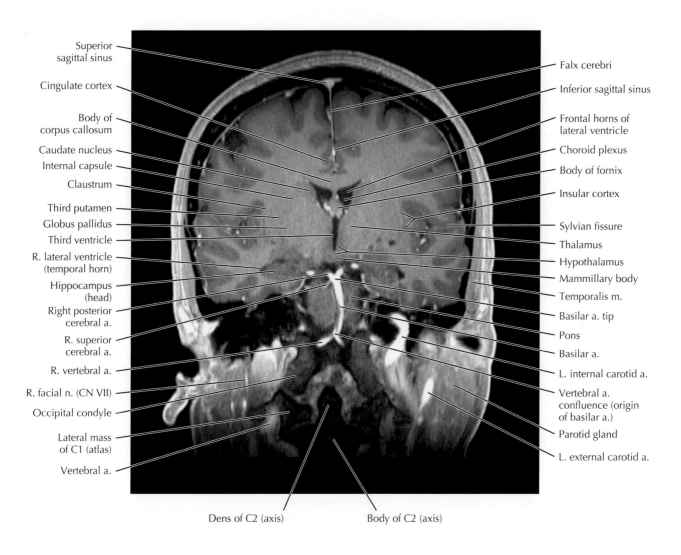

Superior sagittal sinus

Cingulate cortex

Body of corpus callosum

Caudate nucleus

Internal capsule

Claustrum

Third putamen

Globus pallidus

Third ventricle

R. lateral ventricle (temporal horn)

Hippocampus (head)

Right posterior cerebral a.

R. superior cerebral a.

R. vertebral a.

R. facial n. (CN VII)

Occipital condyle

Lateral mass of C1 (atlas)

Vertebral a.

Falx cerebri

Inferior sagittal sinus

Frontal horns of lateral ventricle

Choroid plexus

Body of fornix

Insular cortex

Sylvian fissure

Thalamus

Hypothalamus

Mammillary body

Temporalis m.

Basilar a. tip

Pons

Basilar a.

L. internal carotid a.

Vertebral a. confluence (origin of basilar a.)

Parotid gland

L. external carotid a.

Dens of C2 (axis)

Body of C2 (axis)

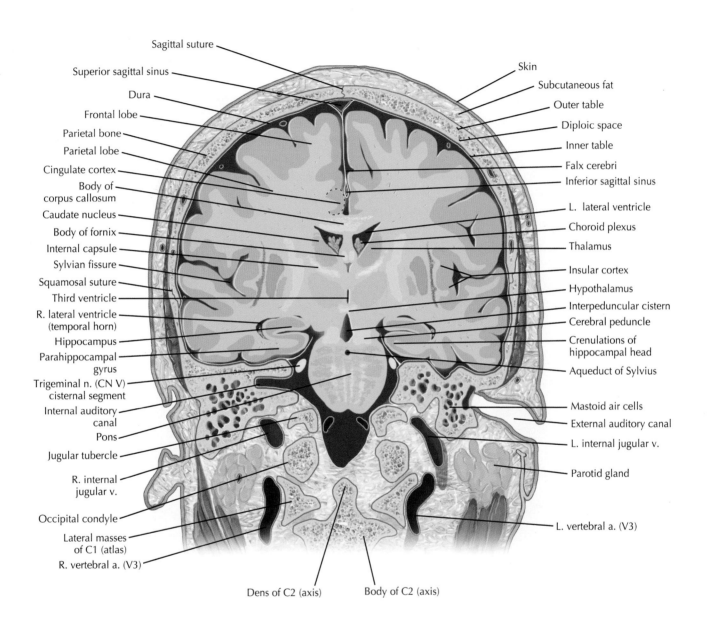

Sagittal suture
Superior sagittal sinus
Dura
Frontal lobe
Parietal bone
Parietal lobe
Cingulate cortex
Body of corpus callosum
Caudate nucleus
Body of fornix
Internal capsule
Sylvian fissure
Squamosal suture
Third ventricle
R. lateral ventricle (temporal horn)
Hippocampus
Parahippocampal gyrus
Trigeminal n. (CN V) cisternal segment
Internal auditory canal
Pons
Jugular tubercle
R. internal jugular v.
Occipital condyle
Lateral masses of C1 (atlas)
R. vertebral a. (V3)

Skin
Subcutaneous fat
Outer table
Diploic space
Inner table
Falx cerebri
Inferior sagittal sinus
L. lateral ventricle
Choroid plexus
Thalamus
Insular cortex
Hypothalamus
Interpeduncular cistern
Cerebral peduncle
Crenulations of hippocampal head
Aqueduct of Sylvius
Mastoid air cells
External auditory canal
L. internal jugular v.
Parotid gland
L. vertebral a. (V3)

Dens of C2 (axis)
Body of C2 (axis)

DIAGNOSTIC CONSIDERATION

Injury to the cruciate ligaments with laxity of the odontoid ("toothlike") process of the second cervical vertebra (C2; dens axis) is more definitively assessed with voluntary flexion and extension radiographs. However, such injury may be suspected from asymmetric positioning of the odontoid process relative to the lateral masses on coronal MR view.

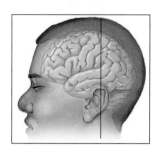

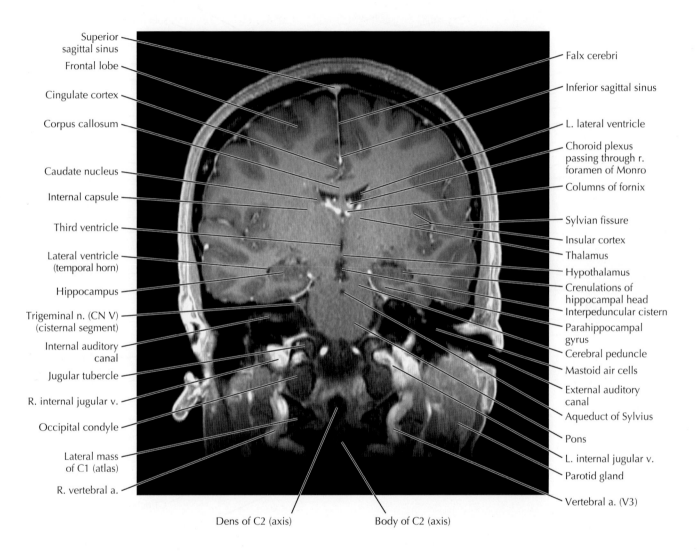

Superior sagittal sinus

Frontal lobe

Cingulate cortex

Corpus callosum

Caudate nucleus

Internal capsule

Third ventricle

Lateral ventricle (temporal horn)

Hippocampus

Trigeminal n. (CN V) (cisternal segment)

Internal auditory canal

Jugular tubercle

R. internal jugular v.

Occipital condyle

Lateral mass of C1 (atlas)

R. vertebral a.

Falx cerebri

Inferior sagittal sinus

L. lateral ventricle

Choroid plexus passing through r. foramen of Monro

Columns of fornix

Sylvian fissure

Insular cortex

Thalamus

Hypothalamus

Crenulations of hippocampal head

Interpeduncular cistern

Parahippocampal gyrus

Cerebral peduncle

Mastoid air cells

External auditory canal

Aqueduct of Sylvius

Pons

L. internal jugular v.

Parotid gland

Vertebral a. (V3)

Dens of C2 (axis)

Body of C2 (axis)

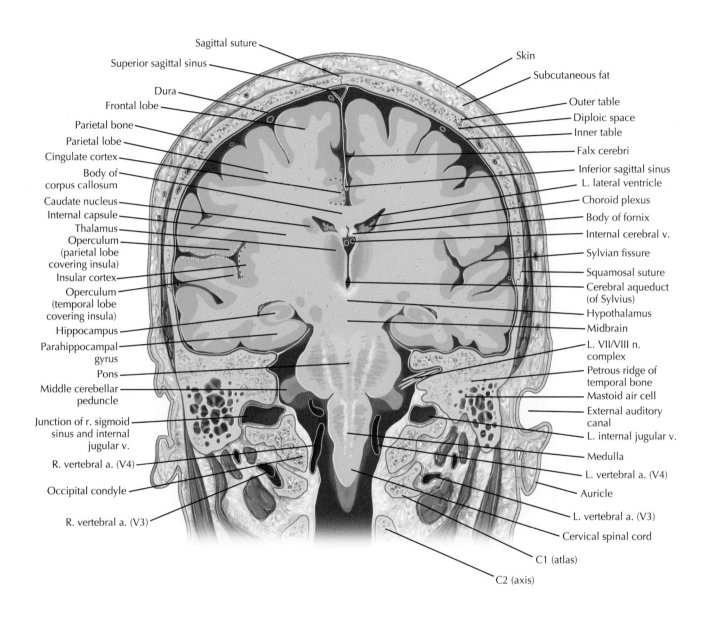

Sagittal suture
Superior sagittal sinus
Dura
Frontal lobe
Parietal bone
Parietal lobe
Cingulate cortex
Body of corpus callosum
Caudate nucleus
Internal capsule
Thalamus
Operculum (parietal lobe covering insula)
Insular cortex
Operculum (temporal lobe covering insula)
Hippocampus
Parahippocampal gyrus
Pons
Middle cerebellar peduncle
Junction of r. sigmoid sinus and internal jugular v.
R. vertebral a. (V4)
Occipital condyle
R. vertebral a. (V3)

Skin
Subcutaneous fat
Outer table
Diploic space
Inner table
Falx cerebri
Inferior sagittal sinus
L. lateral ventricle
Choroid plexus
Body of fornix
Internal cerebral v.
Sylvian fissure
Squamosal suture
Cerebral aqueduct (of Sylvius)
Hypothalamus
Midbrain
L. VII/VIII n. complex
Petrous ridge of temporal bone
Mastoid air cell
External auditory canal
L. internal jugular v.
Medulla
L. vertebral a. (V4)
Auricle
L. vertebral a. (V3)
Cervical spinal cord
C1 (atlas)
C2 (axis)

DIAGNOSTIC CONSIDERATION

Coronal imaging is the best way to assess the hippocampi, although size and abnormal signal are best assessed with T2-weighted fluid-attenuated inversion recovery (FLAIR) sequence (see Chapter 4).

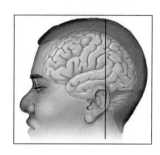

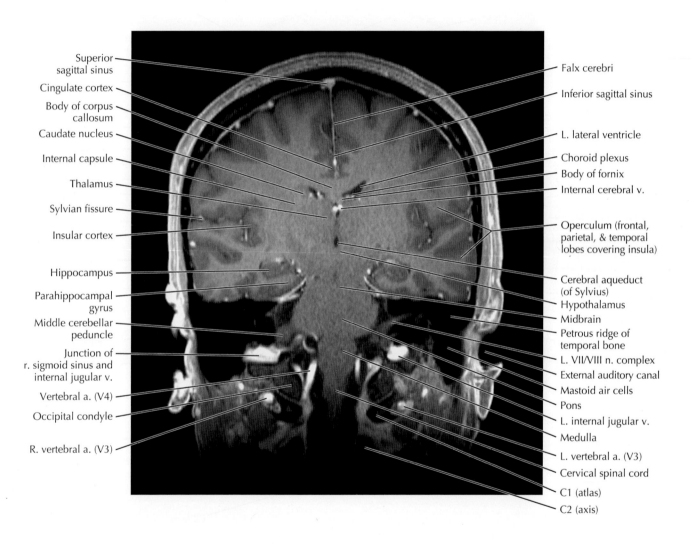

Superior sagittal sinus

Cingulate cortex

Body of corpus callosum

Caudate nucleus

Internal capsule

Thalamus

Sylvian fissure

Insular cortex

Hippocampus

Parahippocampal gyrus

Middle cerebellar peduncle

Junction of r. sigmoid sinus and internal jugular v.

Vertebral a. (V4)

Occipital condyle

R. vertebral a. (V3)

Falx cerebri

Inferior sagittal sinus

L. lateral ventricle

Choroid plexus

Body of fornix

Internal cerebral v.

Operculum (frontal, parietal, & temporal lobes covering insula)

Cerebral aqueduct (of Sylvius)

Hypothalamus

Midbrain

Petrous ridge of temporal bone

L. VII/VIII n. complex

External auditory canal

Mastoid air cells

Pons

L. internal jugular v.

Medulla

L. vertebral a. (V3)

Cervical spinal cord

C1 (atlas)

C2 (axis)

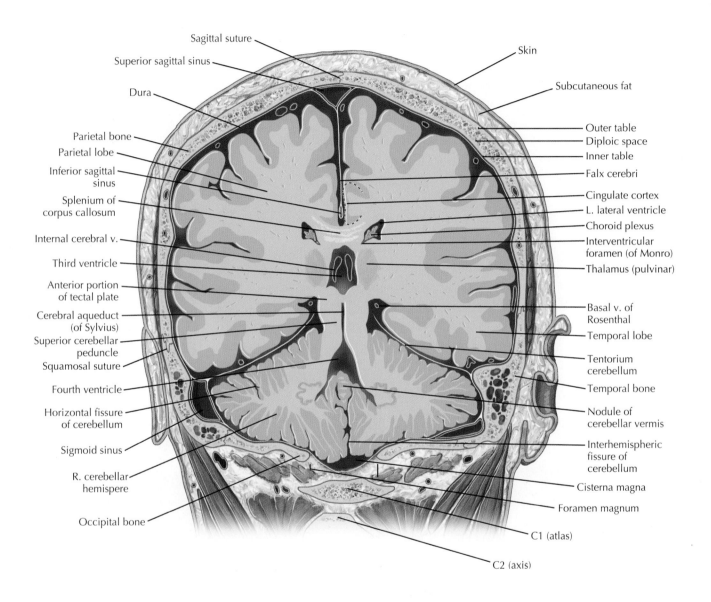

Sagittal suture

Superior sagittal sinus

Dura

Parietal bone

Parietal lobe

Inferior sagittal sinus

Splenium of corpus callosum

Internal cerebral v.

Third ventricle

Anterior portion of tectal plate

Cerebral aqueduct (of Sylvius)

Superior cerebellar peduncle

Squamosal suture

Fourth ventricle

Horizontal fissure of cerebellum

Sigmoid sinus

R. cerebellar hemisphere

Occipital bone

Skin

Subcutaneous fat

Outer table

Diploic space

Inner table

Falx cerebri

Cingulate cortex

L. lateral ventricle

Choroid plexus

Interventricular foramen (of Monro)

Thalamus (pulvinar)

Basal v. of Rosenthal

Temporal lobe

Tentorium cerebellum

Temporal bone

Nodule of cerebellar vermis

Interhemispheric fissure of cerebellum

Cisterna magna

Foramen magnum

C1 (atlas)

C2 (axis)

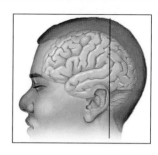

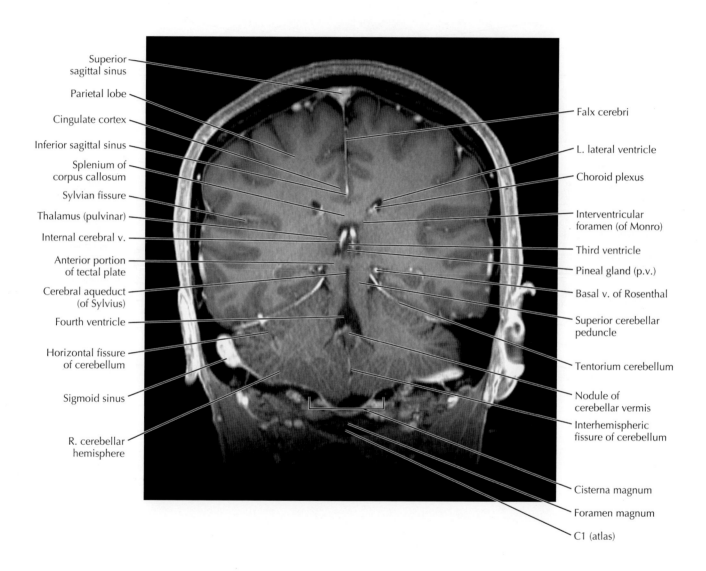

Superior sagittal sinus

Parietal lobe

Cingulate cortex

Inferior sagittal sinus

Splenium of corpus callosum

Sylvian fissure

Thalamus (pulvinar)

Internal cerebral v.

Anterior portion of tectal plate

Cerebral aqueduct (of Sylvius)

Fourth ventricle

Horizontal fissure of cerebellum

Sigmoid sinus

R. cerebellar hemisphere

Falx cerebri

L. lateral ventricle

Choroid plexus

Interventricular foramen (of Monro)

Third ventricle

Pineal gland (p.v.)

Basal v. of Rosenthal

Superior cerebellar peduncle

Tentorium cerebellum

Nodule of cerebellar vermis

Interhemispheric fissure of cerebellum

Cisterna magnum

Foramen magnum

C1 (atlas)

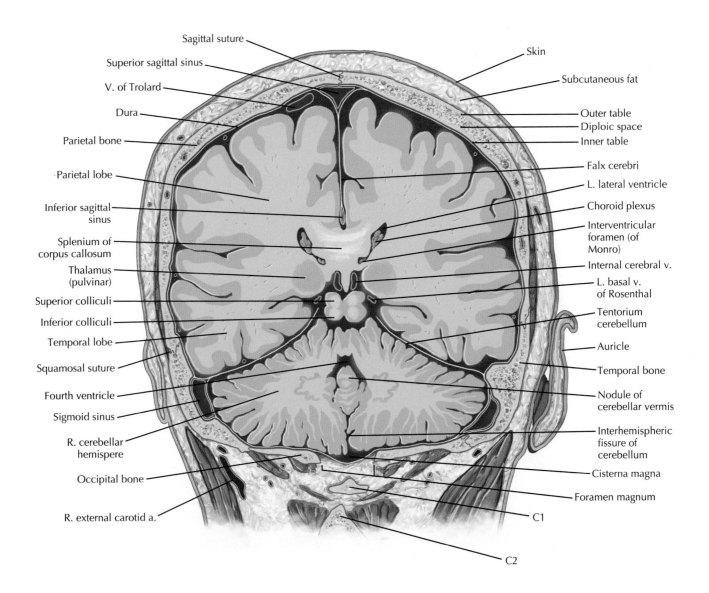

Sagittal suture

Superior sagittal sinus

V. of Trolard

Dura

Parietal bone

Parietal lobe

Inferior sagittal sinus

Splenium of corpus callosum

Thalamus (pulvinar)

Superior colliculi

Inferior colliculi

Temporal lobe

Squamosal suture

Fourth ventricle

Sigmoid sinus

R. cerebellar hemispere

Occipital bone

R. external carotid a.

Skin

Subcutaneous fat

Outer table

Diploic space

Inner table

Falx cerebri

L. lateral ventricle

Choroid plexus

Interventricular foramen (of Monro)

Internal cerebral v.

L. basal v. of Rosenthal

Tentorium cerebellum

Auricle

Temporal bone

Nodule of cerebellar vermis

Interhemispheric fissure of cerebellum

Cisterna magna

Foramen magnum

C1

C2

NORMAL ANATOMY

The internal cerebral veins, or deep cerebral veins, drain the deep portions of the hemisphere and are paired structures. Each internal cerebral vein is formed near the interventricular foramen, or foramen of Monro, by the union of the terminal and choroid veins. The veins course beneath the splenium of the corpus callosum and unite to form a short trunk, the great cerebral vein (of Galen). Just before this union, each cerebral vein receives the corresponding basal vein of Rosenthal. The basal vein is formed by the union of a small anterior cerebral vein, the deep middle cerebral vein (deep Sylvian vein), and the inferior striate veins.

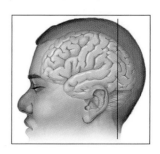

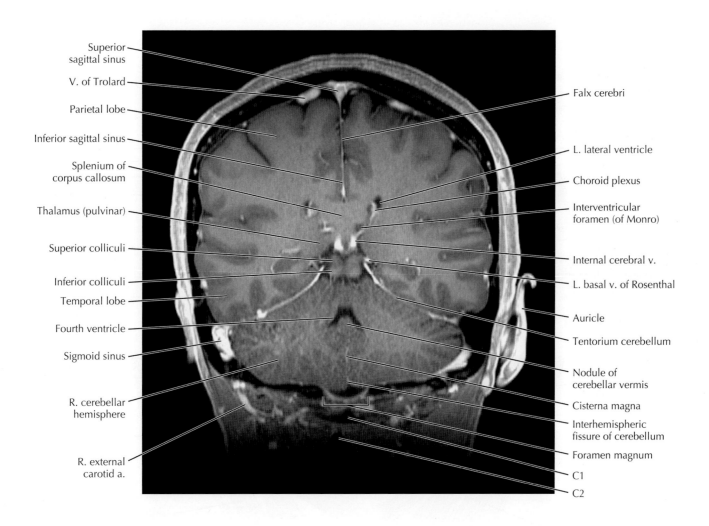

Superior sagittal sinus

V. of Trolard

Parietal lobe

Inferior sagittal sinus

Splenium of corpus callosum

Thalamus (pulvinar)

Superior colliculi

Inferior colliculi

Temporal lobe

Fourth ventricle

Sigmoid sinus

R. cerebellar hemisphere

R. external carotid a.

Falx cerebri

L. lateral ventricle

Choroid plexus

Interventricular foramen (of Monro)

Internal cerebral v.

L. basal v. of Rosenthal

Auricle

Tentorium cerebellum

Nodule of cerebellar vermis

Cisterna magna

Interhemispheric fissure of cerebellum

Foramen magnum

C1

C2

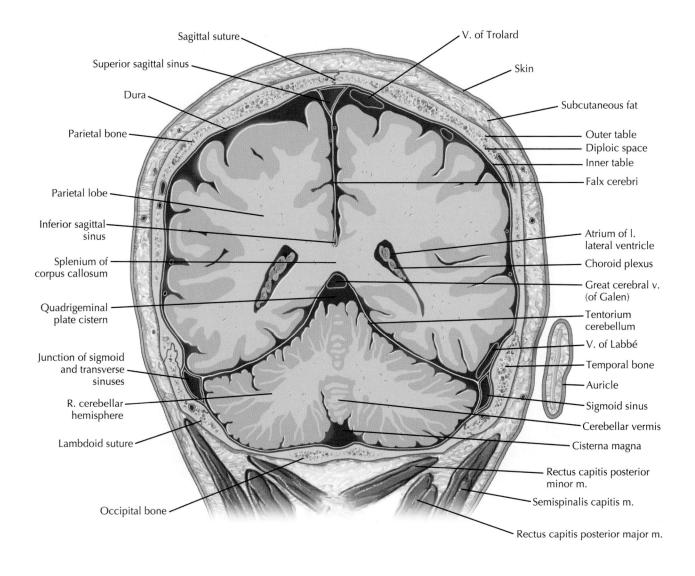

Sagittal suture

Superior sagittal sinus

Dura

Parietal bone

Parietal lobe

Inferior sagittal sinus

Splenium of corpus callosum

Quadrigeminal plate cistern

Junction of sigmoid and transverse sinuses

R. cerebellar hemisphere

Lambdoid suture

Occipital bone

V. of Trolard

Skin

Subcutaneous fat

Outer table
Diploic space
Inner table

Falx cerebri

Atrium of l. lateral ventricle

Choroid plexus

Great cerebral v. (of Galen)

Tentorium cerebellum

V. of Labbé

Temporal bone

Auricle

Sigmoid sinus

Cerebellar vermis

Cisterna magna

Rectus capitis posterior minor m.

Semispinalis capitis m.

Rectus capitis posterior major m.

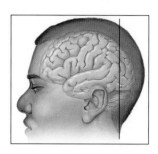

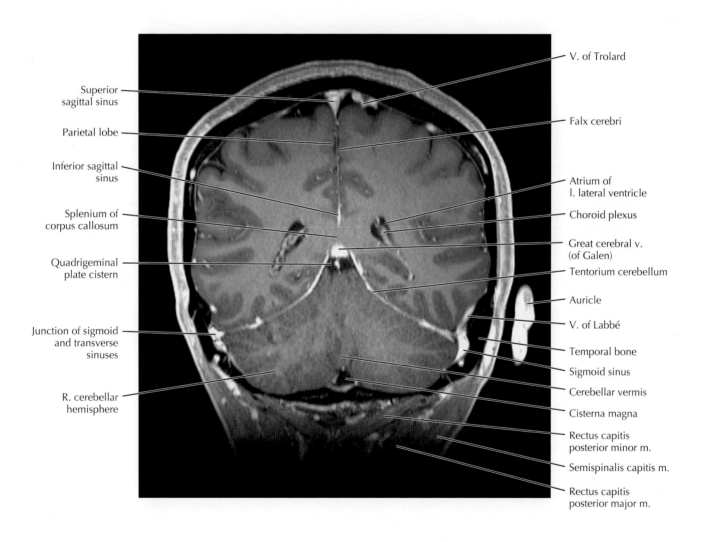

Superior sagittal sinus

Parietal lobe

Inferior sagittal sinus

Splenium of corpus callosum

Quadrigeminal plate cistern

Junction of sigmoid and transverse sinuses

R. cerebellar hemisphere

V. of Trolard

Falx cerebri

Atrium of l. lateral ventricle

Choroid plexus

Great cerebral v. (of Galen)

Tentorium cerebellum

Auricle

V. of Labbé

Temporal bone

Sigmoid sinus

Cerebellar vermis

Cisterna magna

Rectus capitis posterior minor m.

Semispinalis capitis m.

Rectus capitis posterior major m.

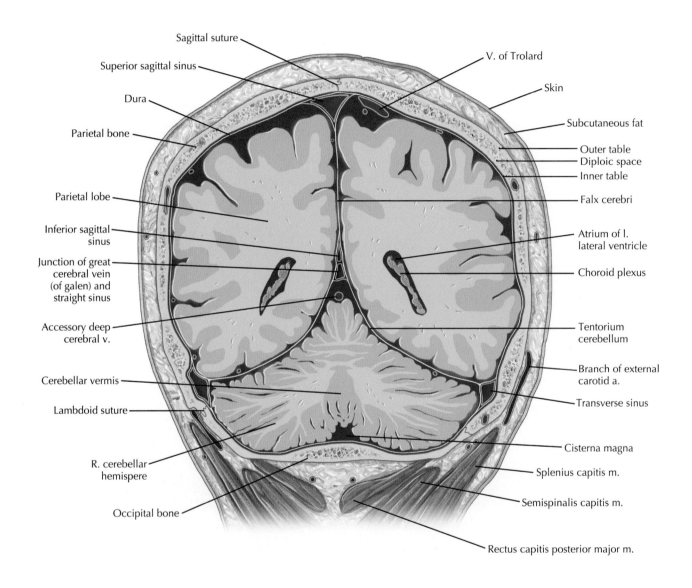

Sagittal suture

Superior sagittal sinus

Dura

Parietal bone

Parietal lobe

Inferior sagittal sinus

Junction of great cerebral vein (of galen) and straight sinus

Accessory deep cerebral v.

Cerebellar vermis

Lambdoid suture

R. cerebellar hemispere

Occipital bone

V. of Trolard

Skin

Subcutaneous fat

Outer table
Diploic space
Inner table

Falx cerebri

Atrium of l. lateral ventricle

Choroid plexus

Tentorium cerebellum

Branch of external carotid a.

Transverse sinus

Cisterna magna

Splenius capitis m.

Semispinalis capitis m.

Rectus capitis posterior major m.

NORMAL ANATOMY

The cisterna magna in this view is within normal limits of size. An enlarged cisterna magna can be seen with arachnoid cysts and mega–cisterna magna.

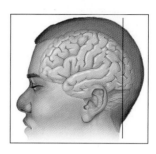

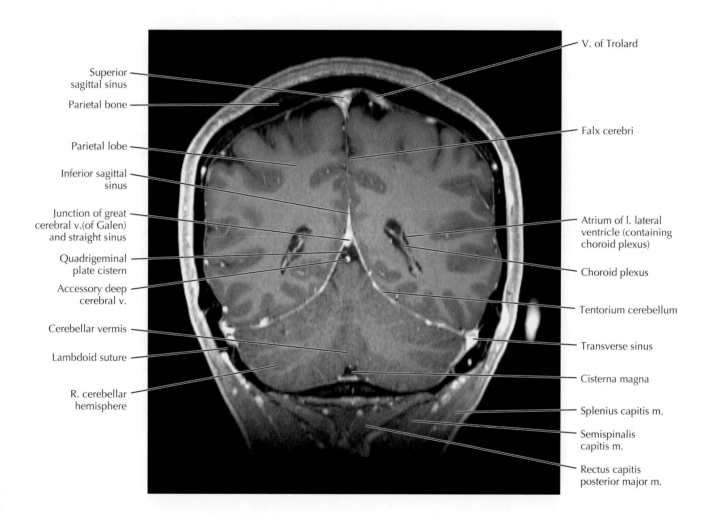

Superior sagittal sinus

Parietal bone

Parietal lobe

Inferior sagittal sinus

Junction of great cerebral v.(of Galen) and straight sinus

Quadrigeminal plate cistern

Accessory deep cerebral v.

Cerebellar vermis

Lambdoid suture

R. cerebellar hemisphere

V. of Trolard

Falx cerebri

Atrium of l. lateral ventricle (containing choroid plexus)

Choroid plexus

Tentorium cerebellum

Transverse sinus

Cisterna magna

Splenius capitis m.

Semispinalis capitis m.

Rectus capitis posterior major m.

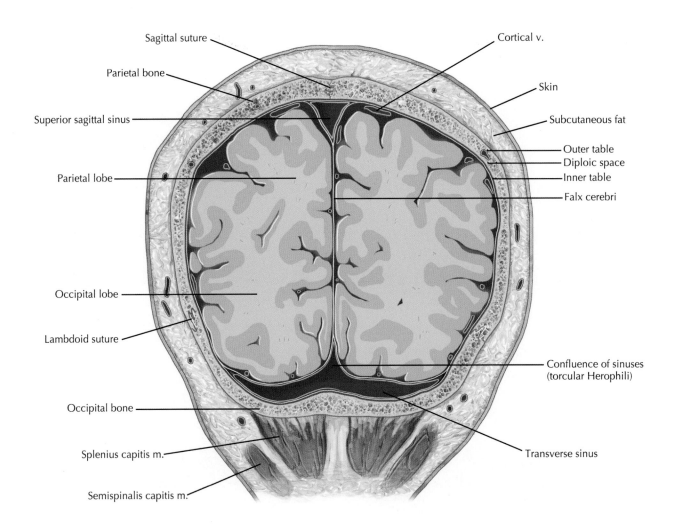

Sagittal suture

Parietal bone

Superior sagittal sinus

Parietal lobe

Occipital lobe

Lambdoid suture

Occipital bone

Splenius capitis m.

Semispinalis capitis m.

Cortical v.

Skin

Subcutaneous fat

Outer table

Diploic space

Inner table

Falx cerebri

Confluence of sinuses
(torcular Herophili)

Transverse sinus

DIAGNOSTIC CONSIDERATION

The coronal view is perpendicular to most of the superior sagittal sinus and is often the best view for assessment of venous thrombosis in the sinus. In this view there is a small, rounded filling defect in the right transverse sinus close to midline consistent with an arachnoid granulation.

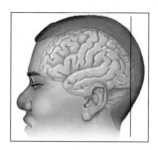

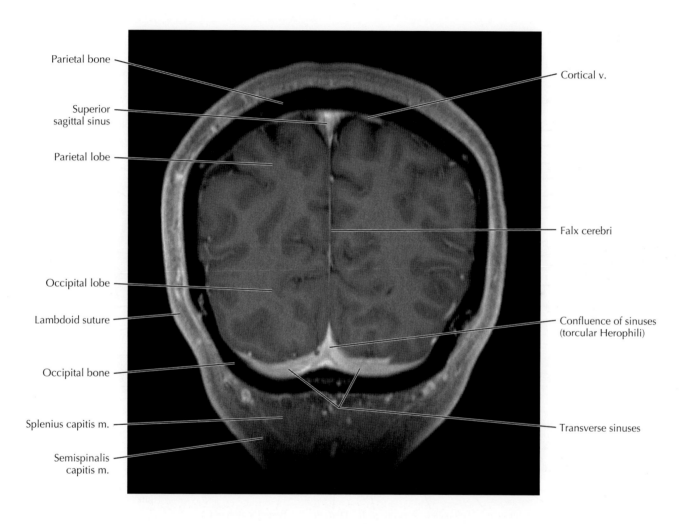

Parietal bone

Superior
sagittal sinus

Parietal lobe

Occipital lobe

Lambdoid suture

Occipital bone

Splenius capitis m.

Semispinalis
capitis m.

Cortical v.

Falx cerebri

Confluence of sinuses
(torcular Herophili)

Transverse sinuses

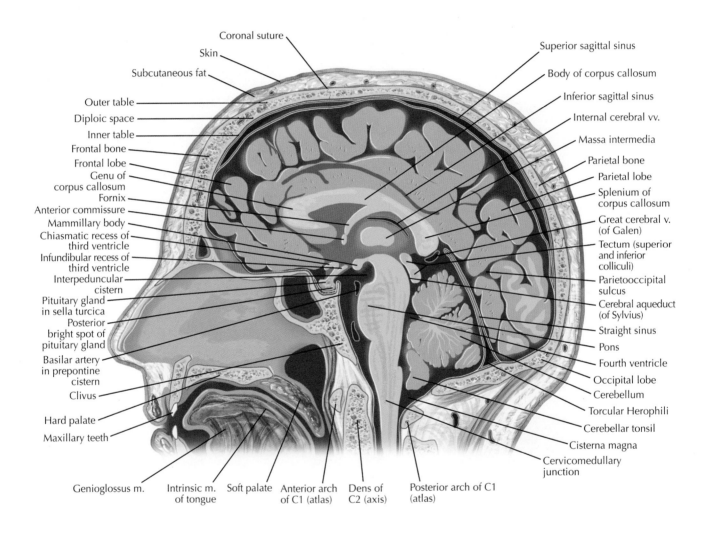

Coronal suture

Skin

Subcutaneous fat

Outer table

Diploic space

Inner table

Frontal bone

Frontal lobe

Genu of corpus callosum

Fornix

Anterior commissure

Mammillary body

Chiasmatic recess of third ventricle

Infundibular recess of third ventricle

Interpeduncular cistern

Pituitary gland in sella turcica

Posterior bright spot of pituitary gland

Basilar artery in prepontine cistern

Clivus

Hard palate

Maxillary teeth

Genioglossus m.

Intrinsic m. of tongue

Soft palate

Anterior arch of C1 (atlas)

Dens of C2 (axis)

Posterior arch of C1 (atlas)

Superior sagittal sinus

Body of corpus callosum

Inferior sagittal sinus

Internal cerebral vv.

Massa intermedia

Parietal bone

Parietal lobe

Splenium of corpus callosum

Great cerebral v. (of Galen)

Tectum (superior and inferior colliculi)

Parietooccipital sulcus

Cerebral aqueduct (of Sylvius)

Straight sinus

Pons

Fourth ventricle

Occipital lobe

Cerebellum

Torcular Herophili

Cerebellar tonsil

Cisterna magna

Cervicomedullary junction

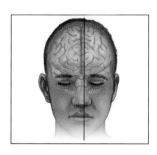

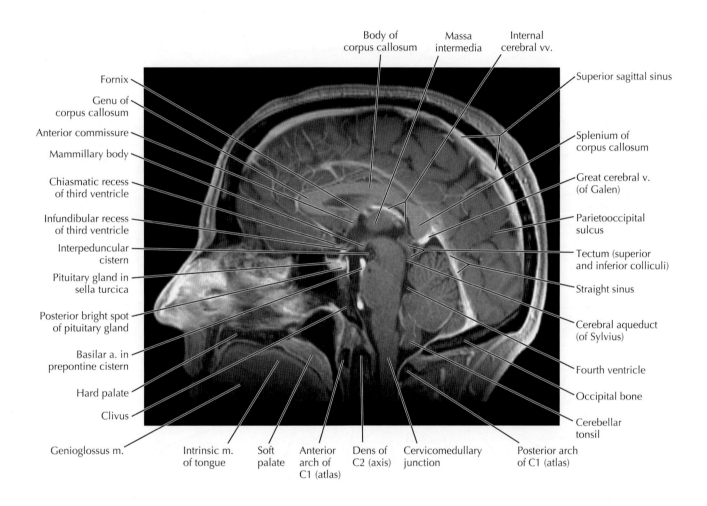

Body of corpus callosum

Massa intermedia

Internal cerebral vv.

Fornix

Genu of corpus callosum

Anterior commissure

Mammillary body

Chiasmatic recess of third ventricle

Infundibular recess of third ventricle

Interpeduncular cistern

Pituitary gland in sella turcica

Posterior bright spot of pituitary gland

Basilar a. in prepontine cistern

Hard palate

Clivus

Genioglossus m.

Superior sagittal sinus

Splenium of corpus callosum

Great cerebral v. (of Galen)

Parietooccipital sulcus

Tectum (superior and inferior colliculi)

Straight sinus

Cerebral aqueduct (of Sylvius)

Fourth ventricle

Occipital bone

Cerebellar tonsil

Intrinsic m. of tongue

Soft palate

Anterior arch of C1 (atlas)

Dens of C2 (axis)

Cervicomedullary junction

Posterior arch of C1 (atlas)

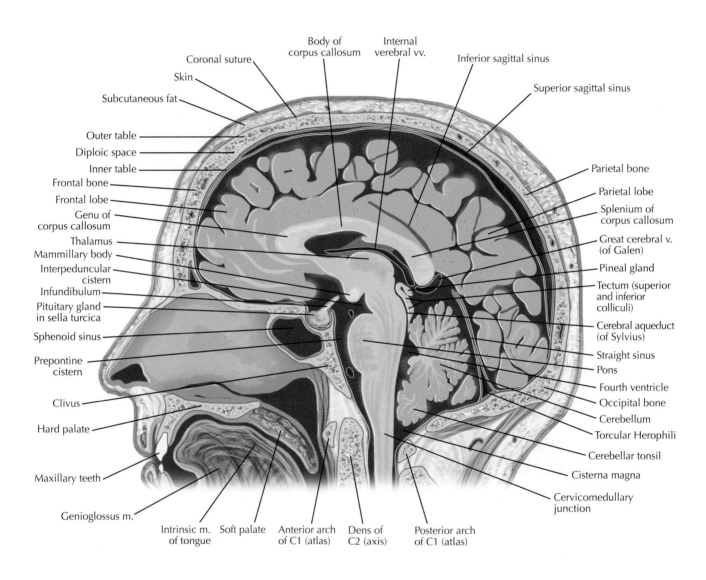

Body of corpus callosum

Internal verebral vv.

Inferior sagittal sinus

Coronal suture

Superior sagittal sinus

Skin

Subcutaneous fat

Outer table

Diploic space

Inner table

Parietal bone

Frontal bone

Parietal lobe

Frontal lobe

Splenium of corpus callosum

Genu of corpus callosum

Great cerebral v. (of Galen)

Thalamus

Pineal gland

Mammillary body

Tectum (superior and inferior colliculi)

Interpeduncular cistern

Infundibulum

Cerebral aqueduct (of Sylvius)

Pituitary gland in sella turcica

Sphenoid sinus

Straight sinus

Prepontine cistern

Pons

Fourth ventricle

Occipital bone

Clivus

Cerebellum

Hard palate

Torcular Herophili

Cerebellar tonsil

Maxillary teeth

Cisterna magna

Cervicomedullary junction

Genioglossus m.

Intrinsic m. of tongue

Soft palate

Anterior arch of C1 (atlas)

Dens of C2 (axis)

Posterior arch of C1 (atlas)

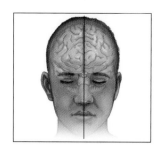

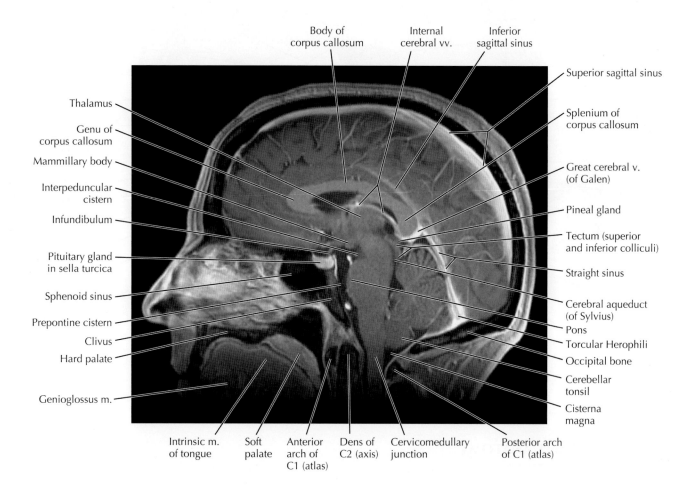

Body of corpus callosum

Internal cerebral vv.

Inferior sagittal sinus

Superior sagittal sinus

Thalamus

Genu of corpus callosum

Mammillary body

Interpeduncular cistern

Infundibulum

Pituitary gland in sella turcica

Sphenoid sinus

Prepontine cistern

Clivus

Hard palate

Genioglossus m.

Splenium of corpus callosum

Great cerebral v. (of Galen)

Pineal gland

Tectum (superior and inferior colliculi)

Straight sinus

Cerebral aqueduct (of Sylvius)

Pons

Torcular Herophili

Occipital bone

Cerebellar tonsil

Cisterna magna

Intrinsic m. of tongue

Soft palate

Anterior arch of C1 (atlas)

Dens of C2 (axis)

Cervicomedullary junction

Posterior arch of C1 (atlas)

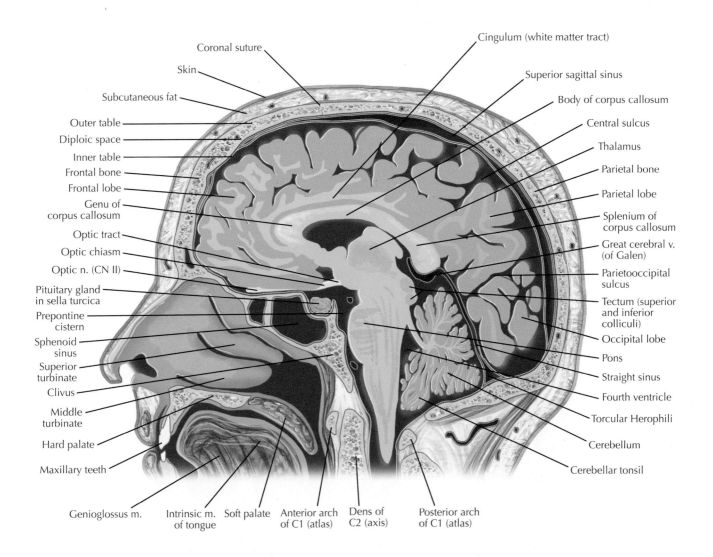

Coronal suture

Skin

Subcutaneous fat

Outer table

Diploic space

Inner table

Frontal bone

Frontal lobe

Genu of corpus callosum

Optic tract

Optic chiasm

Optic n. (CN II)

Pituitary gland in sella turcica

Prepontine cistern

Sphenoid sinus

Superior turbinate

Clivus

Middle turbinate

Hard palate

Maxillary teeth

Cingulum (white matter tract)

Superior sagittal sinus

Body of corpus callosum

Central sulcus

Thalamus

Parietal bone

Parietal lobe

Splenium of corpus callosum

Great cerebral v. (of Galen)

Parietooccipital sulcus

Tectum (superior and inferior colliculi)

Occipital lobe

Pons

Straight sinus

Fourth ventricle

Torcular Herophili

Cerebellum

Cerebellar tonsil

Genioglossus m.

Intrinsic m. of tongue

Soft palate

Anterior arch of C1 (atlas)

Dens of C2 (axis)

Posterior arch of C1 (atlas)

NORMAL ANATOMY

The lateral aspect of the cerebellar tonsils may lie lower than the midline vermis. In adults, up to 5 mm below the foramen magnum is within normal limits. The radiologist should also comment on whether the configuration is rounded or has an abnormal, pointed configuration.

DIAGNOSTIC CONSIDERATION

The superior sagittal sinus lies within the sagittal plane and thus may appear irregular because of volume-averaging effects. To assess for clots, a coronal or axial plane perpendicular to the superior sagittal sinus provides a more accurate view.

Note that the clivus lines up with the posterior aspect of the odontoid process, and the opisthion (posterior edge of foramen magnum) aligns with the anterior edge of the posterior arch of the first cervical vertebra (C1, atlas).

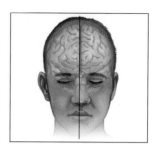

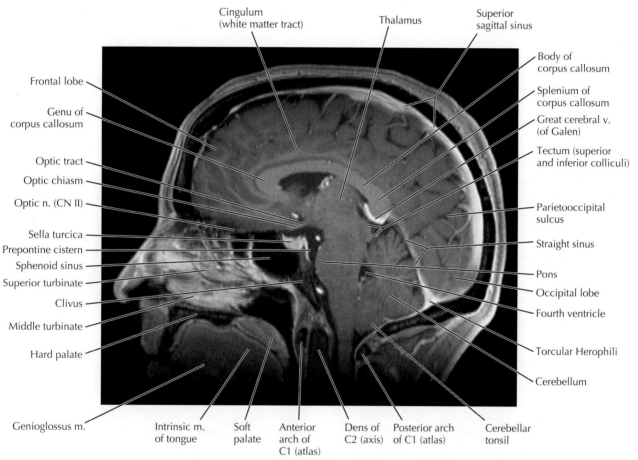

Cingulum
(white matter tract)

Thalamus

Superior
sagittal sinus

Frontal lobe

Genu of
corpus callosum

Optic tract

Optic chiasm

Optic n. (CN II)

Sella turcica

Prepontine cistern

Sphenoid sinus

Superior turbinate

Clivus

Middle turbinate

Hard palate

Genioglossus m.

Body of
corpus callosum

Splenium of
corpus callosum

Great cerebral v.
(of Galen)

Tectum (superior
and inferior colliculi)

Parietooccipital
sulcus

Straight sinus

Pons

Occipital lobe

Fourth ventricle

Torcular Herophili

Cerebellum

Intrinsic m.
of tongue

Soft
palate

Anterior
arch of
C1 (atlas)

Dens of
C2 (axis)

Posterior arch
of C1 (atlas)

Cerebellar
tonsil

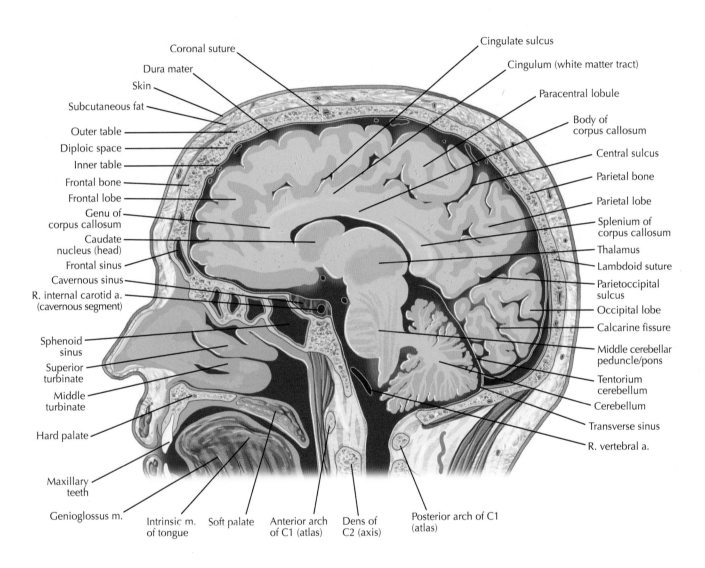

Coronal suture

Dura mater

Skin

Subcutaneous fat

Outer table

Diploic space

Inner table

Frontal bone

Frontal lobe

Genu of
corpus callosum

Caudate
nucleus (head)

Frontal sinus

Cavernous sinus

R. internal carotid a.
(cavernous segment)

Sphenoid
sinus

Superior
turbinate

Middle
turbinate

Hard palate

Maxillary
teeth

Genioglossus m.

Intrinsic m.
of tongue

Soft palate

Anterior arch
of C1 (atlas)

Dens of
C2 (axis)

Posterior arch of C1
(atlas)

Cingulate sulcus

Cingulum (white matter tract)

Paracentral lobule

Body of
corpus callosum

Central sulcus

Parietal bone

Parietal lobe

Splenium of
corpus callosum

Thalamus

Lambdoid suture

Parietoccipital
sulcus

Occipital lobe

Calcarine fissure

Middle cerebellar
peduncle/pons

Tentorium
cerebellum

Cerebellum

Transverse sinus

R. vertebral a.

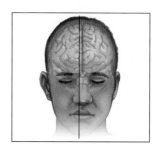

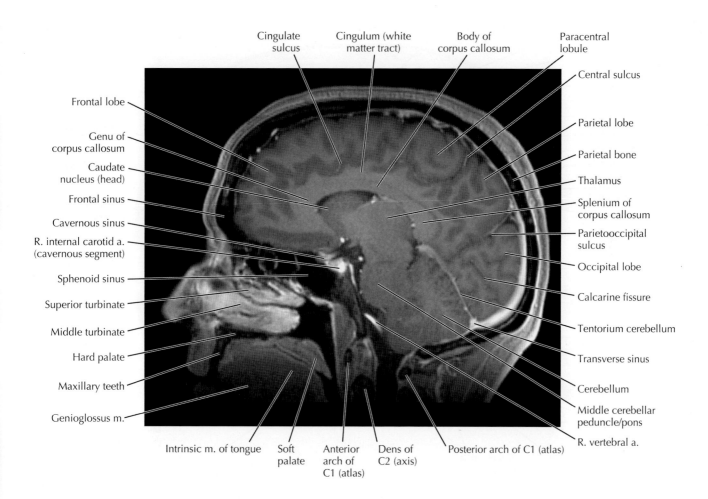

Cingulate sulcus

Cingulum (white matter tract)

Body of corpus callosum

Paracentral lobule

Central sulcus

Frontal lobe

Genu of corpus callosum

Caudate nucleus (head)

Frontal sinus

Cavernous sinus

R. internal carotid a. (cavernous segment)

Sphenoid sinus

Superior turbinate

Middle turbinate

Hard palate

Maxillary teeth

Genioglossus m.

Parietal lobe

Parietal bone

Thalamus

Splenium of corpus callosum

Parietooccipital sulcus

Occipital lobe

Calcarine fissure

Tentorium cerebellum

Transverse sinus

Cerebellum

Middle cerebellar peduncle/pons

R. vertebral a.

Intrinsic m. of tongue

Soft palate

Anterior arch of C1 (atlas)

Dens of C2 (axis)

Posterior arch of C1 (atlas)

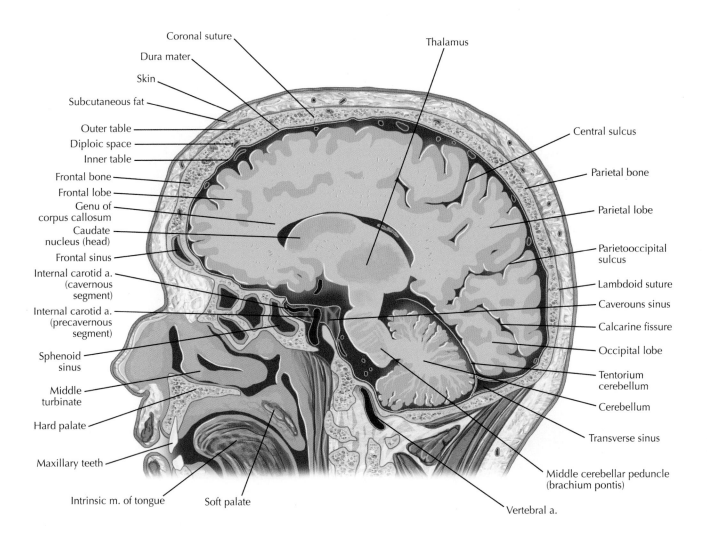

Coronal suture

Dura mater

Skin

Subcutaneous fat

Outer table

Diploic space

Inner table

Frontal bone

Frontal lobe

Genu of corpus callosum

Caudate nucleus (head)

Frontal sinus

Internal carotid a. (cavernous segment)

Internal carotid a. (precavernous segment)

Sphenoid sinus

Middle turbinate

Hard palate

Maxillary teeth

Intrinsic m. of tongue

Soft palate

Thalamus

Central sulcus

Parietal bone

Parietal lobe

Parietooccipital sulcus

Lambdoid suture

Caverouns sinus

Calcarine fissure

Occipital lobe

Tentorium cerebellum

Cerebellum

Transverse sinus

Middle cerebellar peduncle (brachium pontis)

Vertebral a.

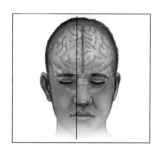

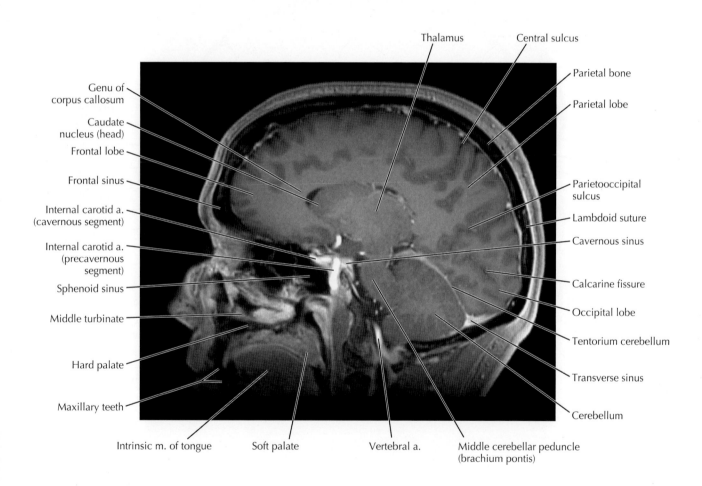

Thalamus

Central sulcus

Genu of corpus callosum

Caudate nucleus (head)

Frontal lobe

Frontal sinus

Internal carotid a. (cavernous segment)

Internal carotid a. (precavernous segment)

Sphenoid sinus

Middle turbinate

Hard palate

Maxillary teeth

Parietal bone

Parietal lobe

Parietooccipital sulcus

Lambdoid suture

Cavernous sinus

Calcarine fissure

Occipital lobe

Tentorium cerebellum

Transverse sinus

Cerebellum

Intrinsic m. of tongue   Soft palate   Vertebral a.   Middle cerebellar peduncle (brachium pontis)

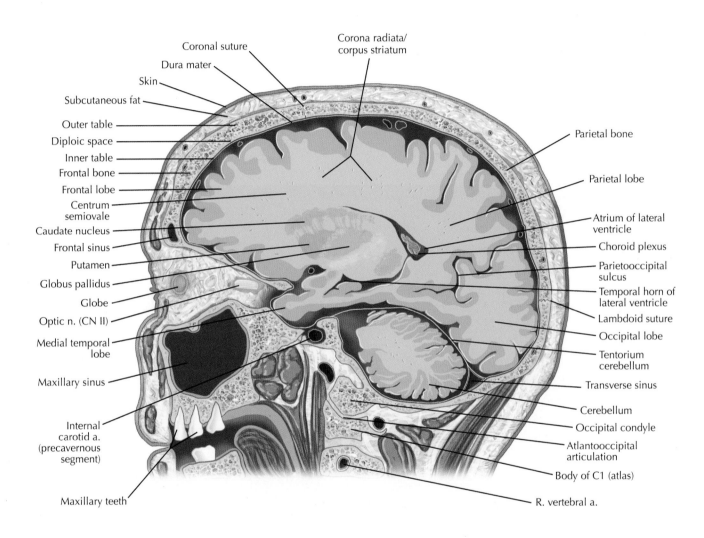

Coronal suture
Corona radiata/corpus striatum
Dura mater
Skin
Subcutaneous fat
Outer table
Diploic space
Inner table
Frontal bone
Frontal lobe
Centrum semiovale
Caudate nucleus
Frontal sinus
Putamen
Globus pallidus
Globe
Optic n. (CN II)
Medial temporal lobe
Maxillary sinus
Internal carotid a. (precavernous segment)
Maxillary teeth

Parietal bone
Parietal lobe
Atrium of lateral ventricle
Choroid plexus
Parietooccipital sulcus
Temporal horn of lateral ventricle
Lambdoid suture
Occipital lobe
Tentorium cerebellum
Transverse sinus
Cerebellum
Occipital condyle
Atlantooccipital articulation
Body of C1 (atlas)
R. vertebral a.

DIAGNOSTIC CONSIDERATIONS

As with the floor of the middle cranial fossa, which lies in the axial plane, the tentorium cerebellum can harbor a small meningioma or dural metastasis, which may be much more conspicuous on sagittal imaging.

Note also the clear view of the alveolar roots of the maxillary teeth. Inflammatory changes in the maxillary sinuses may result from periodontal disease, an area that can be overlooked in imaging of the head.

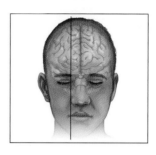

Corona radiata/
corpus striatum

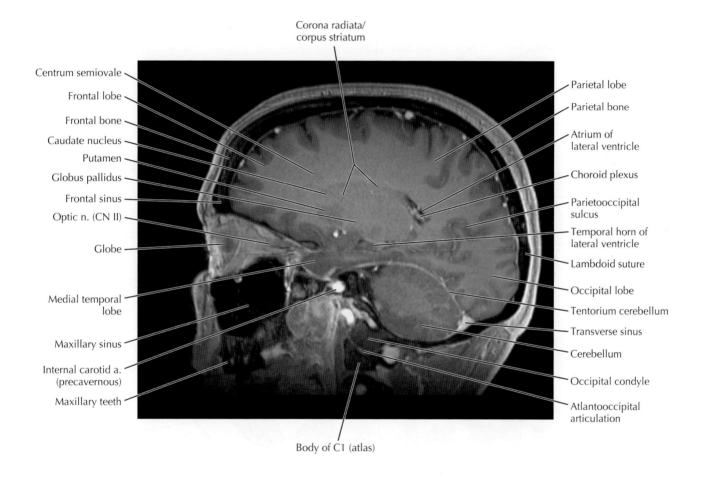

Centrum semiovale

Frontal lobe

Frontal bone

Caudate nucleus

Putamen

Globus pallidus

Frontal sinus

Optic n. (CN II)

Globe

Medial temporal
lobe

Maxillary sinus

Internal carotid a.
(precavernous)

Maxillary teeth

Parietal lobe

Parietal bone

Atrium of
lateral ventricle

Choroid plexus

Parietooccipital
sulcus

Temporal horn of
lateral ventricle

Lambdoid suture

Occipital lobe

Tentorium cerebellum

Transverse sinus

Cerebellum

Occipital condyle

Atlantooccipital
articulation

Body of C1 (atlas)

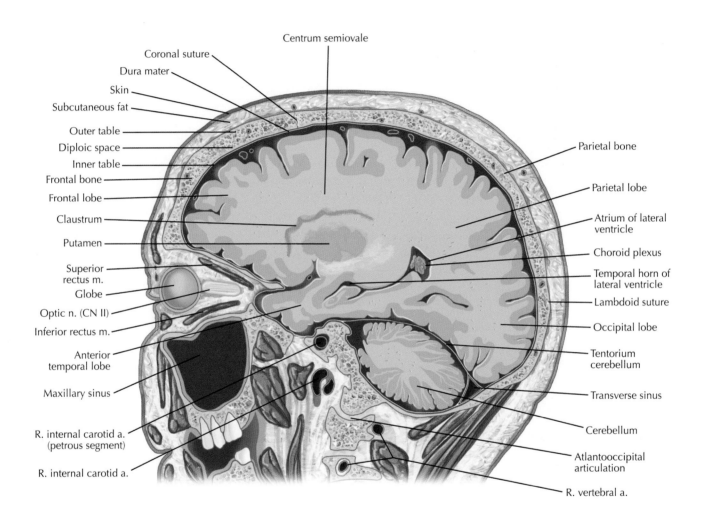

Centrum semiovale

Coronal suture

Dura mater

Skin

Subcutaneous fat

Outer table

Diploic space

Inner table

Frontal bone

Frontal lobe

Claustrum

Putamen

Superior rectus m.

Globe

Optic n. (CN II)

Inferior rectus m.

Anterior temporal lobe

Maxillary sinus

R. internal carotid a. (petrous segment)

R. internal carotid a.

Parietal bone

Parietal lobe

Atrium of lateral ventricle

Choroid plexus

Temporal horn of lateral ventricle

Lambdoid suture

Occipital lobe

Tentorium cerebellum

Transverse sinus

Cerebellum

Atlantooccipital articulation

R. vertebral a.

DIAGNOSTIC CONSIDERATION

It is important to assess the visualized portions of the upper cervical spine on any head study. In this view, the radiologist can see the atlantooccipital articulation. Dislocation or subluxation is often much more conspicuous on a sagittal than an axial view.

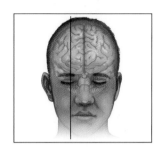

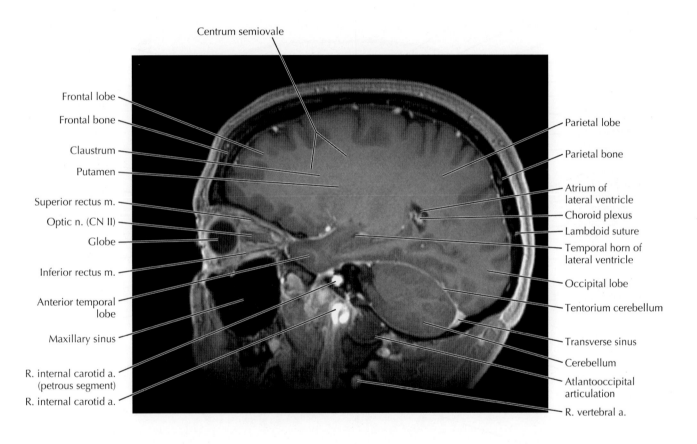

Centrum semiovale

Frontal lobe

Frontal bone

Claustrum

Putamen

Superior rectus m.

Optic n. (CN II)

Globe

Inferior rectus m.

Anterior temporal lobe

Maxillary sinus

R. internal carotid a. (petrous segment)

R. internal carotid a.

Parietal lobe

Parietal bone

Atrium of lateral ventricle

Choroid plexus

Lambdoid suture

Temporal horn of lateral ventricle

Occipital lobe

Tentorium cerebellum

Transverse sinus

Cerebellum

Atlantooccipital articulation

R. vertebral a.

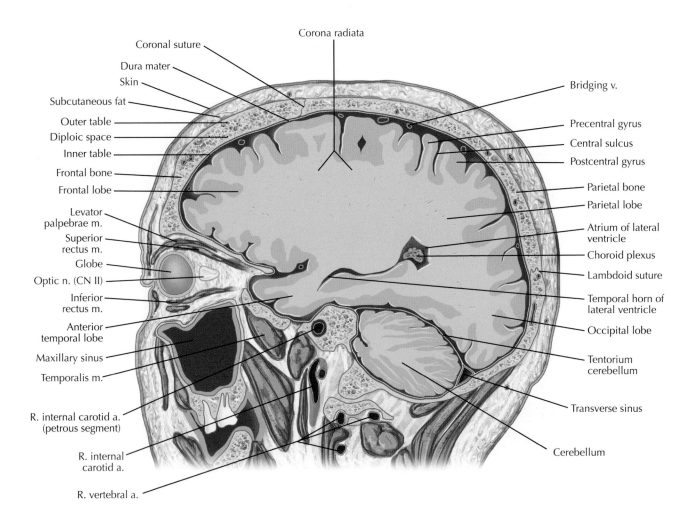

Corona radiata

Coronal suture

Dura mater

Skin

Subcutaneous fat

Outer table

Diploic space

Inner table

Frontal bone

Frontal lobe

Levator palpebrae m.

Superior rectus m.

Globe

Optic n. (CN II)

Inferior rectus m.

Anterior temporal lobe

Maxillary sinus

Temporalis m.

R. internal carotid a. (petrous segment)

R. internal carotid a.

R. vertebral a.

Bridging v.

Precentral gyrus

Central sulcus

Postcentral gyrus

Parietal bone

Parietal lobe

Atrium of lateral ventricle

Choroid plexus

Lambdoid suture

Temporal horn of lateral ventricle

Occipital lobe

Tentorium cerebellum

Transverse sinus

Cerebellum

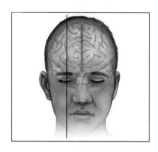

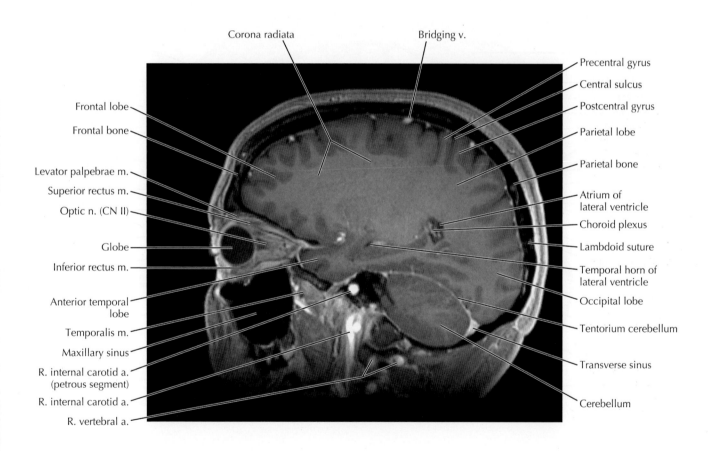

Corona radiata

Bridging v.

Precentral gyrus

Central sulcus

Frontal lobe

Postcentral gyrus

Frontal bone

Parietal lobe

Parietal bone

Levator palpebrae m.

Superior rectus m.

Atrium of
lateral ventricle

Optic n. (CN II)

Choroid plexus

Globe

Lambdoid suture

Inferior rectus m.

Temporal horn of
lateral ventricle

Anterior temporal
lobe

Occipital lobe

Temporalis m.

Tentorium cerebellum

Maxillary sinus

R. internal carotid a.
(petrous segment)

Transverse sinus

R. internal carotid a.

Cerebellum

R. vertebral a.

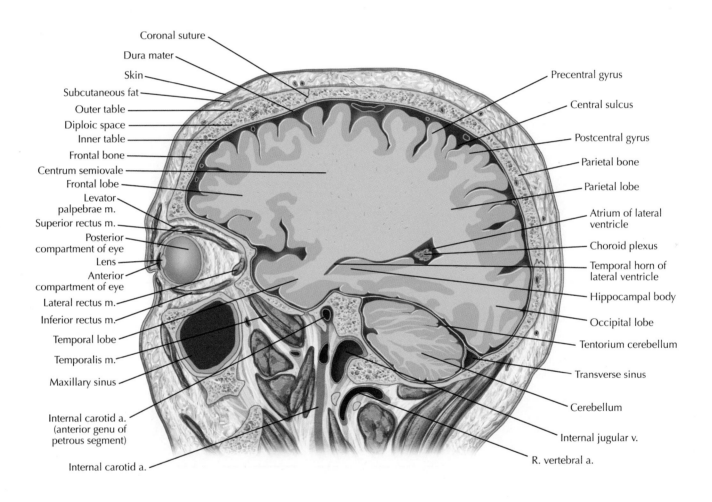

Coronal suture

Dura mater

Skin

Subcutaneous fat

Outer table

Diploic space

Inner table

Frontal bone

Centrum semiovale

Frontal lobe

Levator palpebrae m.

Superior rectus m.

Posterior compartment of eye

Lens

Anterior compartment of eye

Lateral rectus m.

Inferior rectus m.

Temporal lobe

Temporalis m.

Maxillary sinus

Internal carotid a. (anterior genu of petrous segment)

Internal carotid a.

Precentral gyrus

Central sulcus

Postcentral gyrus

Parietal bone

Parietal lobe

Atrium of lateral ventricle

Choroid plexus

Temporal horn of lateral ventricle

Hippocampal body

Occipital lobe

Tentorium cerebellum

Transverse sinus

Cerebellum

Internal jugular v.

R. vertebral a.

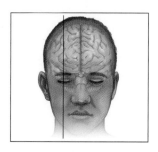

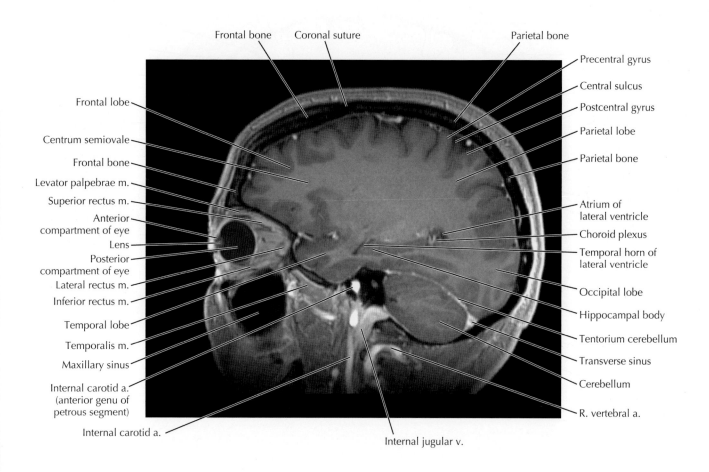

Frontal bone Coronal suture Parietal bone

Precentral gyrus

Central sulcus

Postcentral gyrus

Parietal lobe

Parietal bone

Frontal lobe

Centrum semiovale

Frontal bone

Levator palpebrae m.

Superior rectus m.

Anterior compartment of eye

Lens

Posterior compartment of eye

Lateral rectus m.

Inferior rectus m.

Temporal lobe

Temporalis m.

Maxillary sinus

Internal carotid a. (anterior genu of petrous segment)

Internal carotid a.

Atrium of lateral ventricle

Choroid plexus

Temporal horn of lateral ventricle

Occipital lobe

Hippocampal body

Tentorium cerebellum

Transverse sinus

Cerebellum

R. vertebral a.

Internal jugular v.

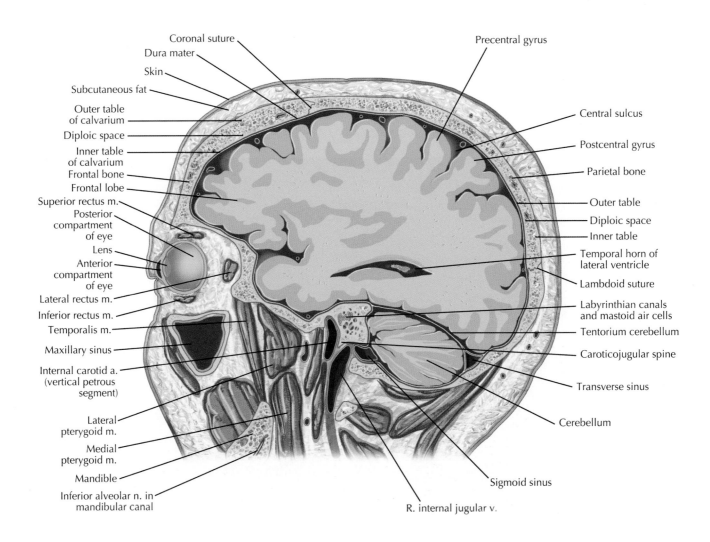

Coronal suture
Dura mater
Skin
Subcutaneous fat
Outer table of calvarium
Diploic space
Inner table of calvarium
Frontal bone
Frontal lobe
Superior rectus m.
Posterior compartment of eye
Lens
Anterior compartment of eye
Lateral rectus m.
Inferior rectus m.
Temporalis m.
Maxillary sinus
Internal carotid a. (vertical petrous segment)
Lateral pterygoid m.
Medial pterygoid m.
Mandible
Inferior alveolar n. in mandibular canal

Precentral gyrus
Central sulcus
Postcentral gyrus
Parietal bone
Outer table
Diploic space
Inner table
Temporal horn of lateral ventricle
Lambdoid suture
Labyrinthian canals and mastoid air cells
Tentorium cerebellum
Caroticojugular spine
Transverse sinus
Cerebellum
Sigmoid sinus
R. internal jugular v.

DIAGNOSTIC CONSIDERATION

For any patient presenting with headache, the neuroradiologist should carefully assess the dural venous sinuses (e.g., transverse and sigmoid sinuses) for evidence of a filling defect to indicate venous thrombosis. Often, a rounded filling defect with a focus of central enhancement is seen; this appearance is typical of arachnoid granulation, unlike the linear wormlike filling defect of venous clots.

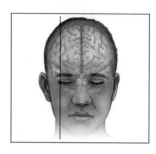

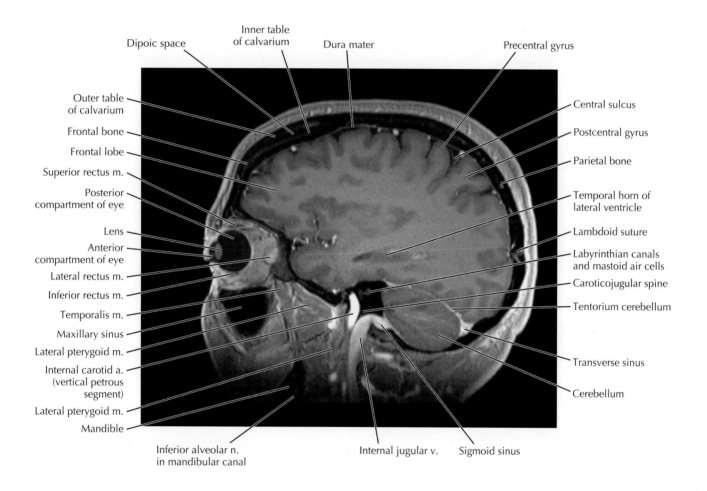

Dipoic space

Inner table of calvarium

Dura mater

Precentral gyrus

Outer table of calvarium

Frontal bone

Frontal lobe

Superior rectus m.

Posterior compartment of eye

Lens

Anterior compartment of eye

Lateral rectus m.

Inferior rectus m.

Temporalis m.

Maxillary sinus

Lateral pterygoid m.

Internal carotid a. (vertical petrous segment)

Lateral pterygoid m.

Mandible

Central sulcus

Postcentral gyrus

Parietal bone

Temporal horn of lateral ventricle

Lambdoid suture

Labyrinthian canals and mastoid air cells

Caroticojugular spine

Tentorium cerebellum

Transverse sinus

Cerebellum

Inferior alveolar n. in mandibular canal

Internal jugular v.

Sigmoid sinus

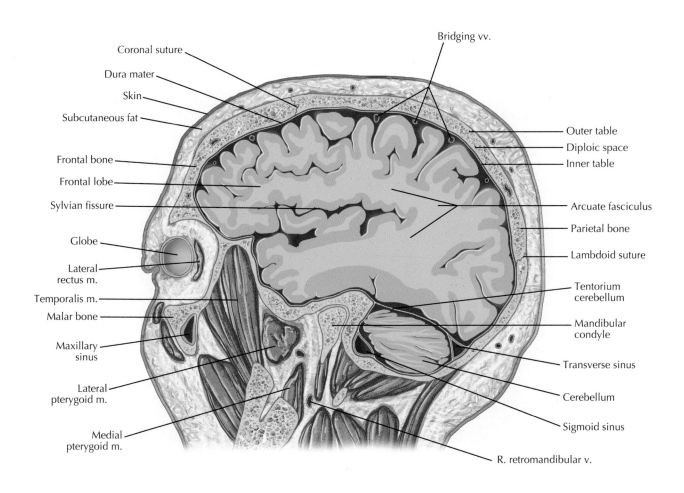

Coronal suture

Dura mater

Skin

Subcutaneous fat

Frontal bone

Frontal lobe

Sylvian fissure

Globe

Lateral rectus m.

Temporalis m.

Malar bone

Maxillary sinus

Lateral pterygoid m.

Medial pterygoid m.

Bridging vv.

Outer table

Diploic space

Inner table

Arcuate fasciculus

Parietal bone

Lambdoid suture

Tentorium cerebellum

Mandibular condyle

Transverse sinus

Cerebellum

Sigmoid sinus

R. retromandibular v.

DIAGNOSTIC CONSIDERATION

One of the most difficult diagnoses to make in neuroradiology is *cortical vein thrombosis.* Clinical presentation may be simply that of a headache, with MRI showing a single cortical vein occluded. An unenhanced sagittal image may most conspicuously show a T1-weighted bright clot within a single cortical vein. If untreated, this may progress to a hemorrhagic venous infarct.

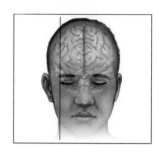

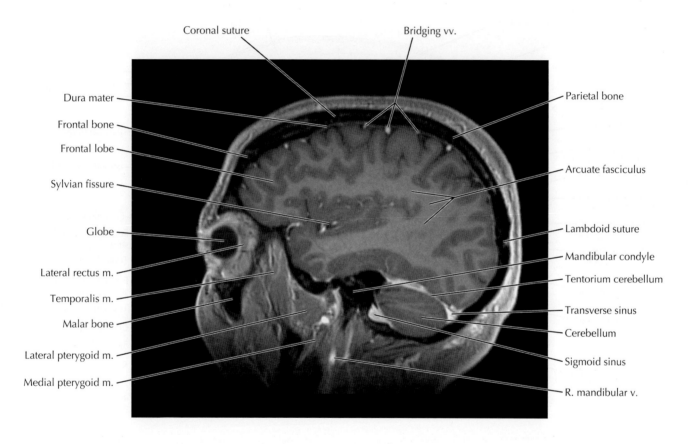

Coronal suture

Bridging vv.

Parietal bone

Dura mater

Frontal bone

Frontal lobe

Sylvian fissure

Globe

Lateral rectus m.

Temporalis m.

Malar bone

Lateral pterygoid m.

Medial pterygoid m.

Arcuate fasciculus

Lambdoid suture

Mandibular condyle

Tentorium cerebellum

Transverse sinus

Cerebellum

Sigmoid sinus

R. mandibular v.

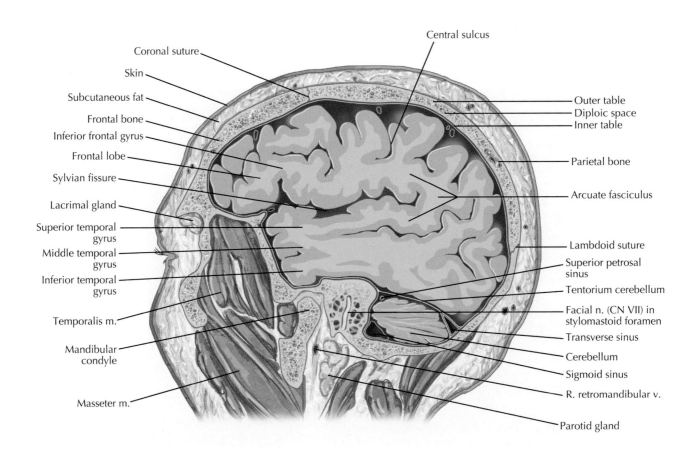

Central sulcus

Coronal suture

Skin

Subcutaneous fat

Frontal bone

Inferior frontal gyrus

Frontal lobe

Sylvian fissure

Lacrimal gland

Superior temporal gyrus

Middle temporal gyrus

Inferior temporal gyrus

Temporalis m.

Mandibular condyle

Masseter m.

Outer table

Diploic space

Inner table

Parietal bone

Arcuate fasciculus

Lambdoid suture

Superior petrosal sinus

Tentorium cerebellum

Facial n. (CN VII) in stylomastoid foramen

Transverse sinus

Cerebellum

Sigmoid sinus

R. retromandibular v.

Parotid gland

NORMAL ANATOMY

Note that this sagittal view shows the mastoid segment of the facial nerve (seventh cranial nerve, CN VII) as it descends through the mastoid bone and exits the stylomastiod foramen. Injury to the facial nerve (e.g., temporal bone fracture) can lead to hemifacial paralysis mimicking stroke, with life-altering effects on social interaction.

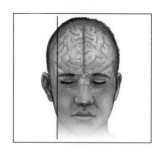

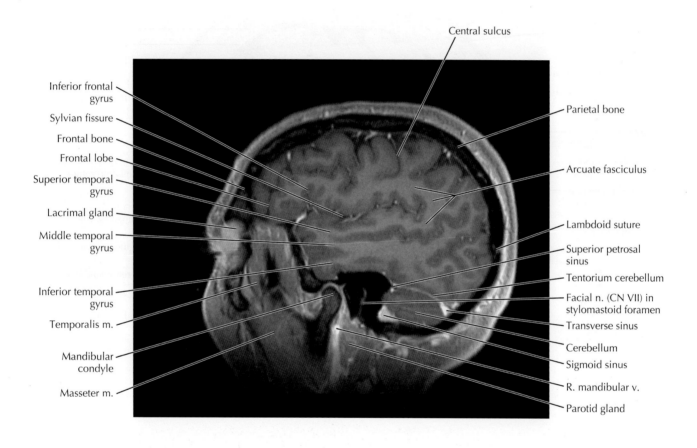

Central sulcus

Inferior frontal gyrus

Sylvian fissure

Frontal bone

Frontal lobe

Superior temporal gyrus

Lacrimal gland

Middle temporal gyrus

Inferior temporal gyrus

Temporalis m.

Mandibular condyle

Masseter m.

Parietal bone

Arcuate fasciculus

Lambdoid suture

Superior petrosal sinus

Tentorium cerebellum

Facial n. (CN VII) in stylomastoid foramen

Transverse sinus

Cerebellum

Sigmoid sinus

R. mandibular v.

Parotid gland

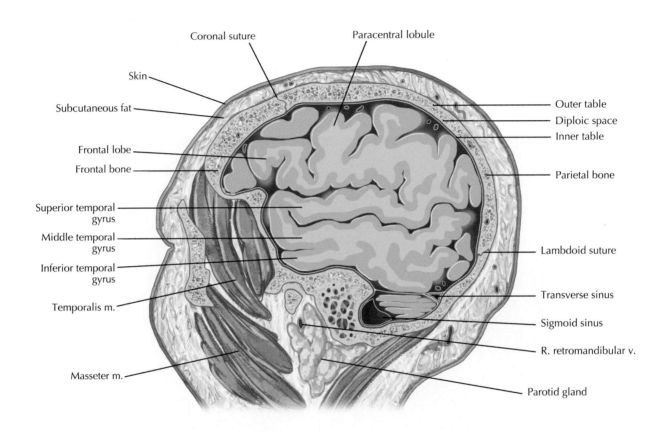

Coronal suture
Paracentral lobule
Skin
Subcutaneous fat
Outer table
Diploic space
Inner table
Frontal lobe
Frontal bone
Parietal bone
Superior temporal gyrus
Middle temporal gyrus
Inferior temporal gyrus
Lambdoid suture
Temporalis m.
Transverse sinus
Sigmoid sinus
R. retromandibular v.
Masseter m.
Parotid gland

IMAGING TECHNIQUE CONSIDERATION

Note that the vessels such as the transverse sinus and cortical vessels are bright because contrast has been given for this sagittal reformation of an axially acquired three-dimensional spoiled GRASS (3D SPGR) sequence. The advantage of 3D-acquired sequences is that the data can then be reformatted to thinner slices or any plane with minimal degradation of quality, unlike 2D-acquired spin-echo sequences. The disadvantage is that any motion will degrade the entire sequence rather than just one slice.

DIAGNOSTIC CONSIDERATION

The midline sagittal view is often recognized as important in assessing the pituitary gland, pineal gland, and cerebellar tonsils. Although the more laterally positioned sagittal views are often unappreciated in diagnostic evaluation because of the lack of symmetry, sagittal MR images are often valuable in assessing for lesions along the floor of the middle cranial fossa or at the vertex.

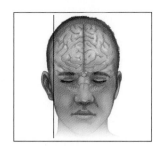

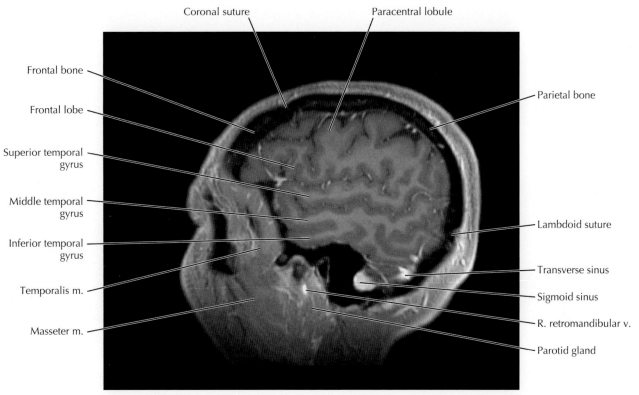

Coronal suture

Paracentral lobule

Frontal bone

Frontal lobe

Superior temporal gyrus

Middle temporal gyrus

Inferior temporal gyrus

Temporalis m.

Masseter m.

Parietal bone

Lambdoid suture

Transverse sinus

Sigmoid sinus

R. retromandibular v.

Parotid gland

Chapter 3 THALAMUS AND BASAL GANGLIA

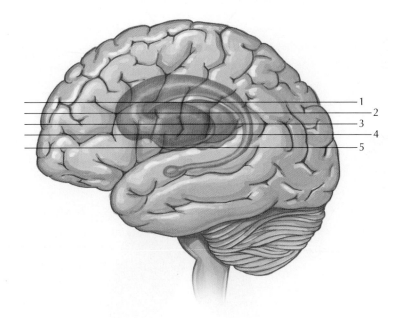

AXIAL   126

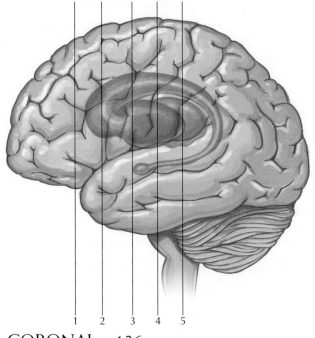

CORONAL   136

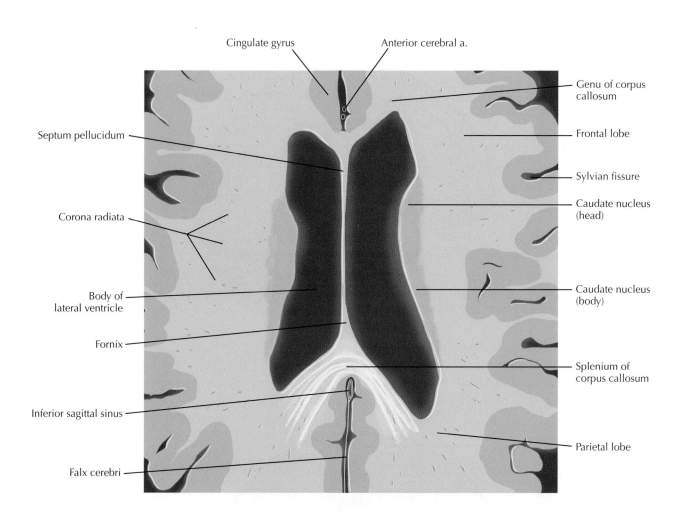

Cingulate gyrus

Anterior cerebral a.

Genu of corpus callosum

Septum pellucidum

Frontal lobe

Sylvian fissure

Caudate nucleus (head)

Corona radiata

Body of lateral ventricle

Caudate nucleus (body)

Fornix

Splenium of corpus callosum

Inferior sagittal sinus

Parietal lobe

Falx cerebri

NORMAL ANATOMY

The centrum semiovale, corona radiata, and internal capsules are all continuous white matter tracts. The *centrum semiovale* is the white matter deep to the gray matter on the surface of the brain and has an ovular shape. On axial imaging, it is generally a term used for white matter superior to the ventricles. The *corona radiata* (Latin: "sunburst") is the white matter connecting the centrum semiovale superiorly and the internal capsules inferiorly. On axial imaging the corona radiata can be seen with ventricles. The *internal capsule* connects the corona radiata superiorly with the pyramids of the medulla inferiorly. On axial imaging, the internal capsule is between the caudate and lentiform nucleus anteriorly and the thalamus and lentiform nucleus posteriorly.

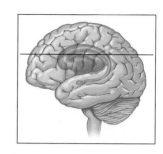

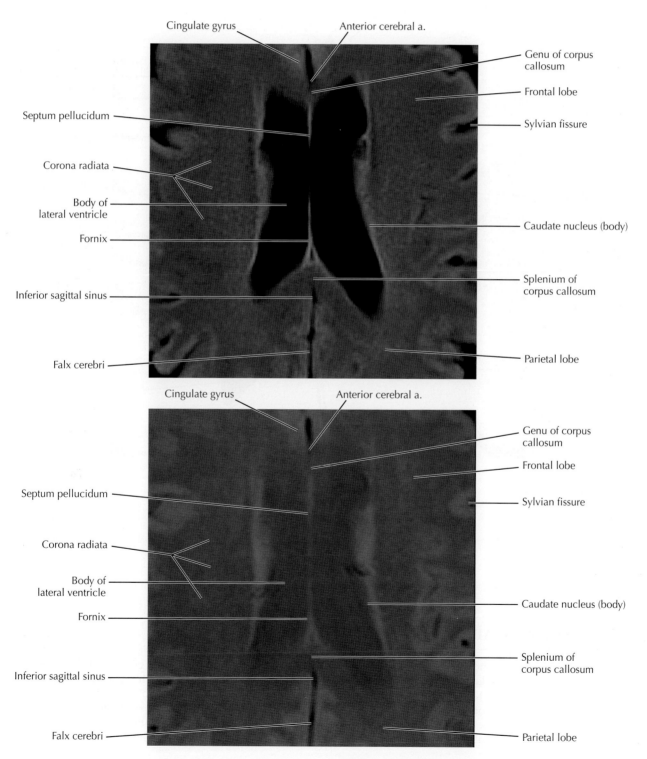

Cingulate gyrus

Anterior cerebral a.

Genu of corpus callosum

Frontal lobe

Sylvian fissure

Septum pellucidum

Corona radiata

Body of lateral ventricle

Caudate nucleus (body)

Fornix

Splenium of corpus callosum

Inferior sagittal sinus

Falx cerebri

Parietal lobe

Cingulate gyrus

Anterior cerebral a.

Genu of corpus callosum

Frontal lobe

Sylvian fissure

Septum pellucidum

Corona radiata

Body of lateral ventricle

Caudate nucleus (body)

Fornix

Splenium of corpus callosum

Inferior sagittal sinus

Falx cerebri

Parietal lobe

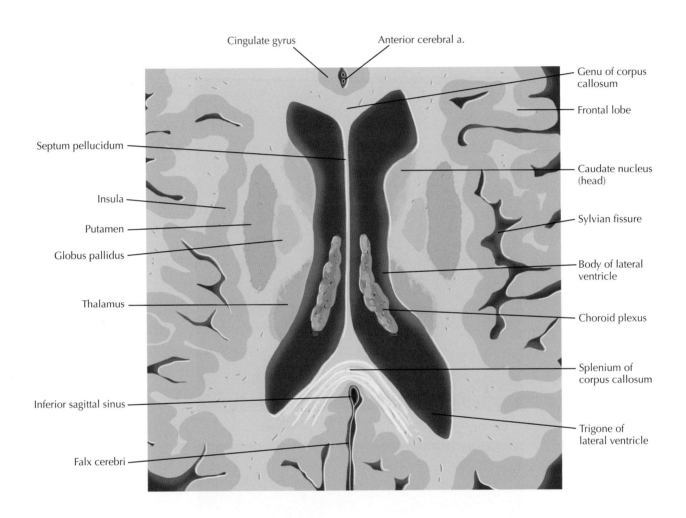

Cingulate gyrus

Anterior cerebral a.

Genu of corpus callosum

Frontal lobe

Septum pellucidum

Caudate nucleus (head)

Insula

Sylvian fissure

Putamen

Globus pallidus

Body of lateral ventricle

Thalamus

Choroid plexus

Splenium of corpus callosum

Inferior sagittal sinus

Falx cerebri

Trigone of lateral ventricle

NORMAL ANATOMY

The *lentiform nucleus*, a triangular-shaped structure on axial imaging, consists of the globus pallidus medially and the putamen laterally. The lentiform nucleus with the caudate nucleus constitutes the basal ganglia. The *basal ganglia* represent a large collection of nuclei that constantly modifies movement along with the cerebellum. The motor cortex sends information to both the cerebellum and basal ganglia, and both structures send information back to cortex via the thalamus (i.e., to gain access to the cortex, signals must pass through the thalamus).

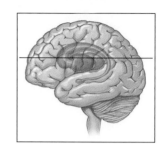

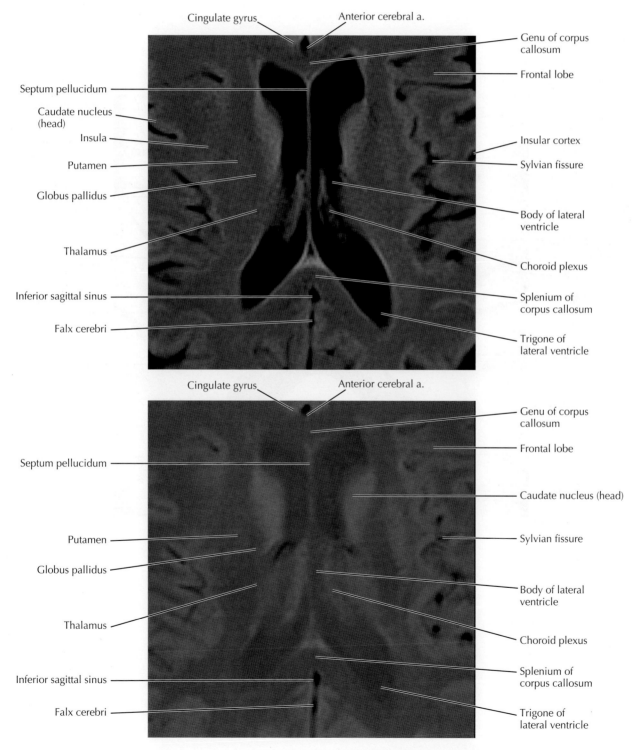

Cingulate gyrus

Anterior cerebral a.

Genu of corpus callosum

Frontal lobe

Septum pellucidum

Caudate nucleus (head)

Insula

Putamen

Globus pallidus

Thalamus

Inferior sagittal sinus

Falx cerebri

Insular cortex

Sylvian fissure

Body of lateral ventricle

Choroid plexus

Splenium of corpus callosum

Trigone of lateral ventricle

Cingulate gyrus

Anterior cerebral a.

Genu of corpus callosum

Frontal lobe

Septum pellucidum

Caudate nucleus (head)

Sylvian fissure

Putamen

Globus pallidus

Thalamus

Inferior sagittal sinus

Falx cerebri

Body of lateral ventricle

Choroid plexus

Splenium of corpus callosum

Trigone of lateral ventricle

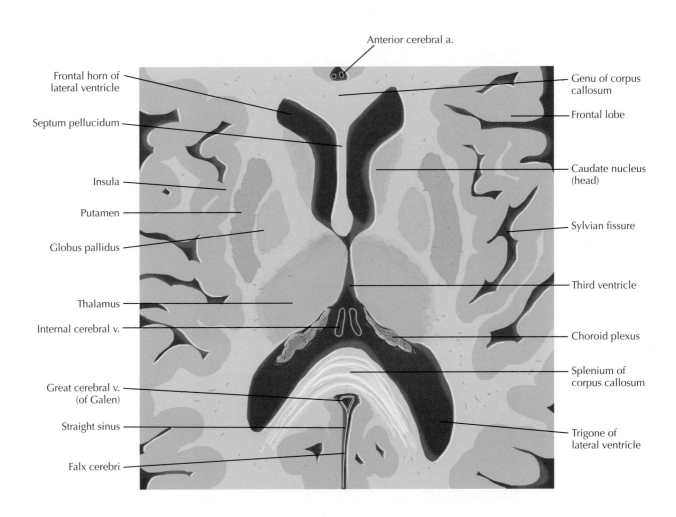

Anterior cerebral a.

Frontal horn of
lateral ventricle

Septum pellucidum

Insula

Putamen

Globus pallidus

Thalamus

Internal cerebral v.

Great cerebral v.
(of Galen)

Straight sinus

Falx cerebri

Genu of corpus
callosum

Frontal lobe

Caudate nucleus
(head)

Sylvian fissure

Third ventricle

Choroid plexus

Splenium of
corpus callosum

Trigone of
lateral ventricle

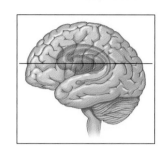

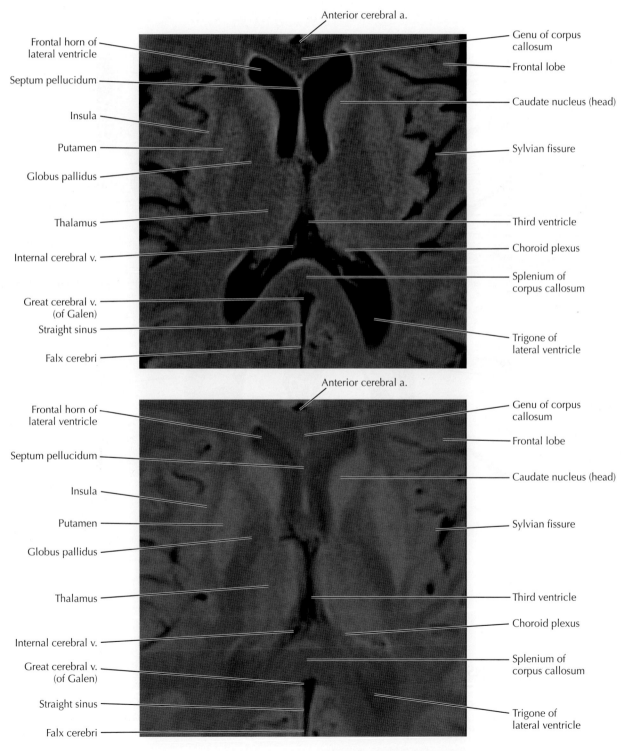

Anterior cerebral a.

Frontal horn of lateral ventricle

Septum pellucidum

Insula

Putamen

Globus pallidus

Thalamus

Internal cerebral v.

Great cerebral v. (of Galen)

Straight sinus

Falx cerebri

Genu of corpus callosum

Frontal lobe

Caudate nucleus (head)

Sylvian fissure

Third ventricle

Choroid plexus

Splenium of corpus callosum

Trigone of lateral ventricle

Anterior cerebral a.

Frontal horn of lateral ventricle

Septum pellucidum

Insula

Putamen

Globus pallidus

Thalamus

Internal cerebral v.

Great cerebral v. (of Galen)

Straight sinus

Falx cerebri

Genu of corpus callosum

Frontal lobe

Caudate nucleus (head)

Sylvian fissure

Third ventricle

Choroid plexus

Splenium of corpus callosum

Trigone of lateral ventricle

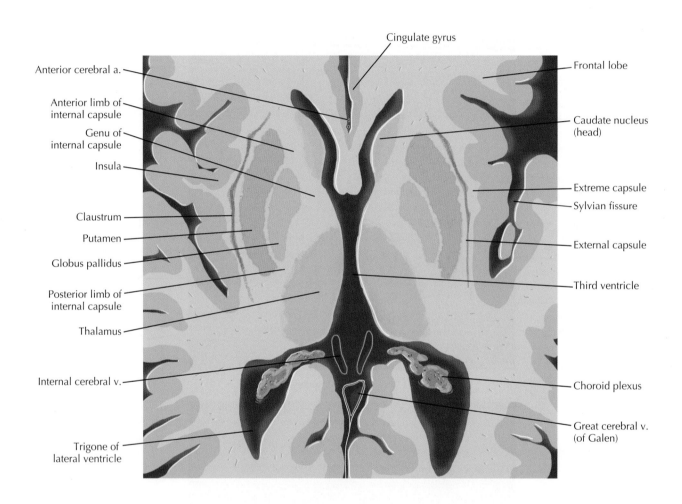

Cingulate gyrus

Anterior cerebral a.

Anterior limb of internal capsule

Genu of internal capsule

Insula

Claustrum

Putamen

Globus pallidus

Posterior limb of internal capsule

Thalamus

Internal cerebral v.

Trigone of lateral ventricle

Frontal lobe

Caudate nucleus (head)

Extreme capsule

Sylvian fissure

External capsule

Third ventricle

Choroid plexus

Great cerebral v. (of Galen)

DIAGNOSTIC CONSIDERATION

Proton-density (PD) sequence is used instead of the more routine T1-weighted sequence to accentuate the signal in the basal ganglia and thalami (compare with T1-weighted images in chapter 4).

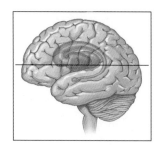

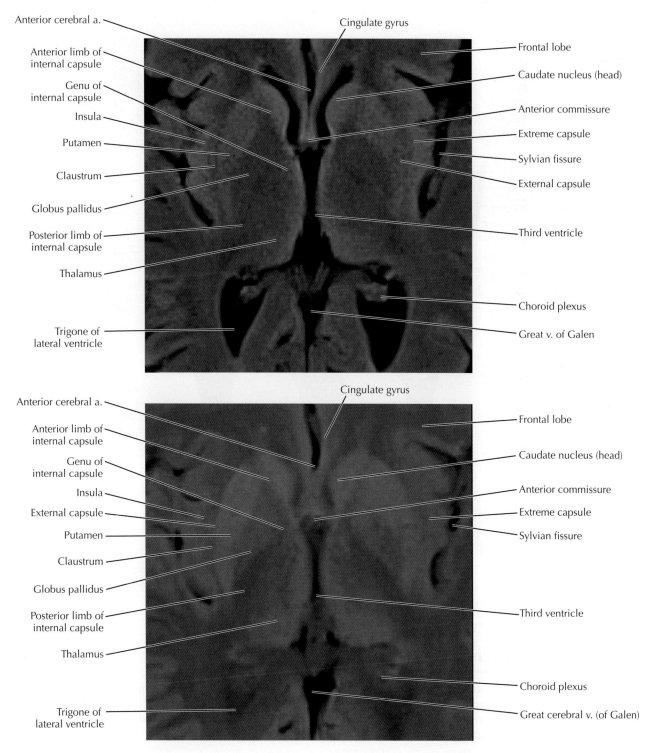

Anterior cerebral a.

Anterior limb of internal capsule

Genu of internal capsule

Insula

Putamen

Claustrum

Globus pallidus

Posterior limb of internal capsule

Thalamus

Trigone of lateral ventricle

Cingulate gyrus

Frontal lobe

Caudate nucleus (head)

Anterior commissure

Extreme capsule

Sylvian fissure

External capsule

Third ventricle

Choroid plexus

Great v. of Galen

Anterior cerebral a.

Anterior limb of internal capsule

Genu of internal capsule

Insula

External capsule

Putamen

Claustrum

Globus pallidus

Posterior limb of internal capsule

Thalamus

Trigone of lateral ventricle

Cingulate gyrus

Frontal lobe

Caudate nucleus (head)

Anterior commissure

Extreme capsule

Sylvian fissure

Third ventricle

Choroid plexus

Great cerebral v. (of Galen)

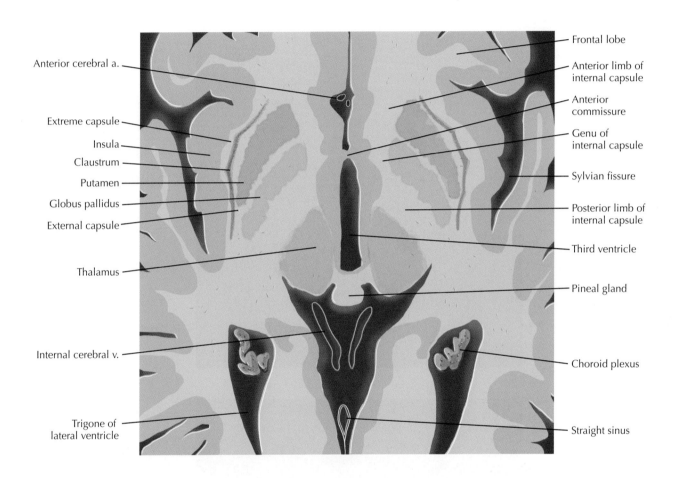

Anterior cerebral a.

Extreme capsule

Insula

Claustrum

Putamen

Globus pallidus

External capsule

Thalamus

Internal cerebral v.

Trigone of
lateral ventricle

Frontal lobe

Anterior limb of
internal capsule

Anterior
commissure

Genu of
internal capsule

Sylvian fissure

Posterior limb of
internal capsule

Third ventricle

Pineal gland

Choroid plexus

Straight sinus

NORMAL ANATOMY

The vein of Galen (great cerebral vein) is a triangular-shaped structure on axial imaging, larger than the paired internal cerebral veins that feed into it, and larger than the inferior sagittal sinus that joins the vein of Galen to feed into the straight sinus. Loss of the normal dark flow void on T2-weighted or PD-weighted images is seen with venous sinus thrombosis.

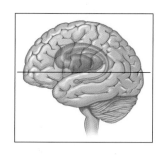

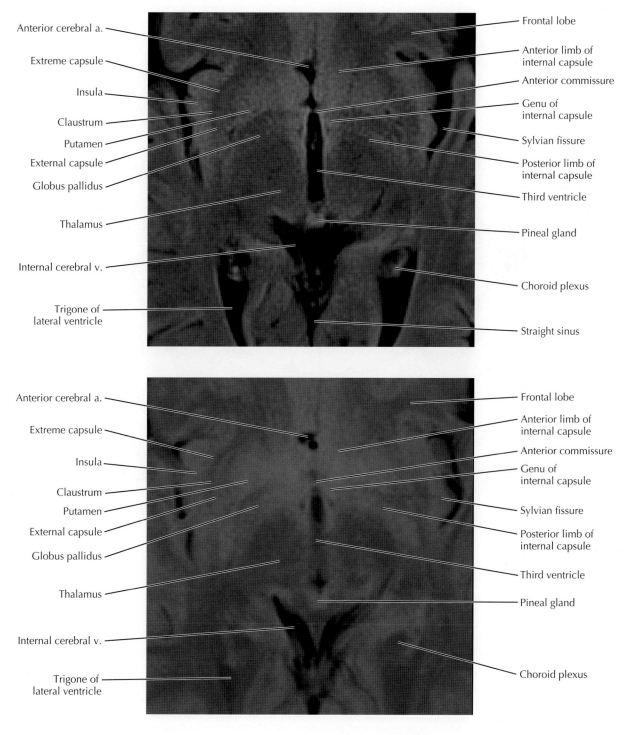

Anterior cerebral a.

Extreme capsule

Insula

Claustrum

Putamen

External capsule

Globus pallidus

Thalamus

Internal cerebral v.

Trigone of
lateral ventricle

Frontal lobe

Anterior limb of
internal capsule

Anterior commissure

Genu of
internal capsule

Sylvian fissure

Posterior limb of
internal capsule

Third ventricle

Pineal gland

Choroid plexus

Straight sinus

Anterior cerebral a.

Extreme capsule

Insula

Claustrum

Putamen

External capsule

Globus pallidus

Thalamus

Internal cerebral v.

Trigone of
lateral ventricle

Frontal lobe

Anterior limb of
internal capsule

Anterior commissure

Genu of
internal capsule

Sylvian fissure

Posterior limb of
internal capsule

Third ventricle

Pineal gland

Choroid plexus

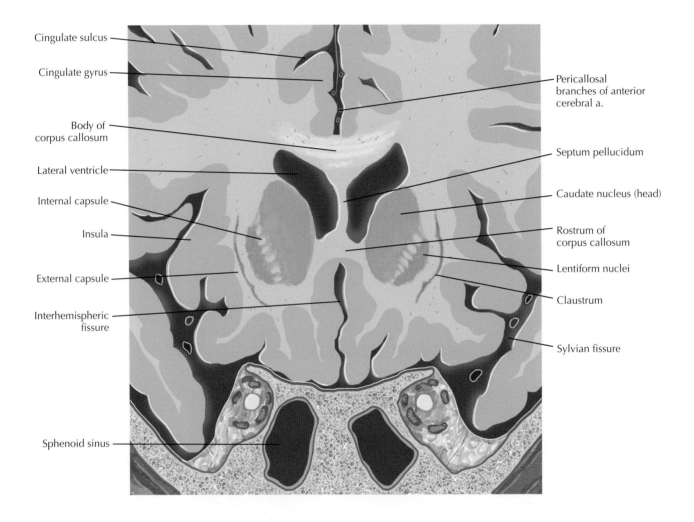

Cingulate sulcus

Cingulate gyrus

Body of corpus callosum

Lateral ventricle

Internal capsule

Insula

External capsule

Interhemispheric fissure

Sphenoid sinus

Pericallosal branches of anterior cerebral a.

Septum pellucidum

Caudate nucleus (head)

Rostrum of corpus callosum

Lentiform nuclei

Claustrum

Sylvian fissure

NORMAL ANATOMY

Note that from medial to lateral on this coronal MR image, the structures are septum pellucidum, lateral ventricle, caudate nucleus, internal capsule, lentiform nucleus, external capsule, claustrum, extreme capsule (difficult to see on most images), and insular cortex.

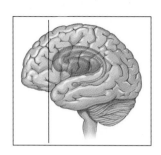

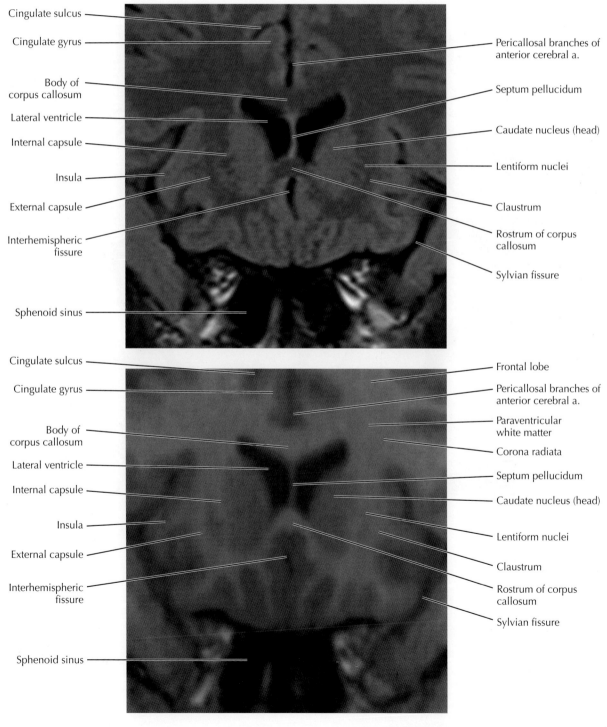

Cingulate sulcus

Cingulate gyrus

Body of corpus callosum

Lateral ventricle

Internal capsule

Insula

External capsule

Interhemispheric fissure

Sphenoid sinus

Pericallosal branches of anterior cerebral a.

Septum pellucidum

Caudate nucleus (head)

Lentiform nuclei

Claustrum

Rostrum of corpus callosum

Sylvian fissure

Cingulate sulcus

Cingulate gyrus

Body of corpus callosum

Lateral ventricle

Internal capsule

Insula

External capsule

Interhemispheric fissure

Sphenoid sinus

Frontal lobe

Pericallosal branches of anterior cerebral a.

Paraventricular white matter

Corona radiata

Septum pellucidum

Caudate nucleus (head)

Lentiform nuclei

Claustrum

Rostrum of corpus callosum

Sylvian fissure

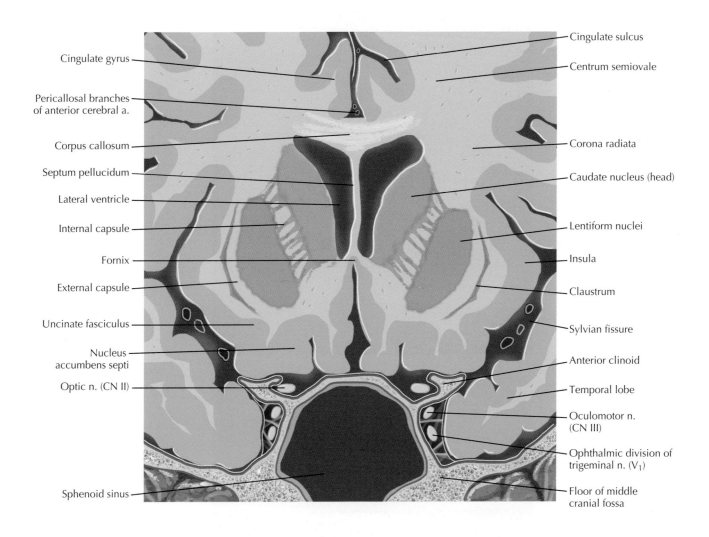

Cingulate gyrus

Pericallosal branches of anterior cerebral a.

Corpus callosum

Septum pellucidum

Lateral ventricle

Internal capsule

Fornix

External capsule

Uncinate fasciculus

Nucleus accumbens septi

Optic n. (CN II)

Sphenoid sinus

Cingulate sulcus

Centrum semiovale

Corona radiata

Caudate nucleus (head)

Lentiform nuclei

Insula

Claustrum

Sylvian fissure

Anterior clinoid

Temporal lobe

Oculomotor n. (CN III)

Ophthalmic division of trigeminal n. (V₁)

Floor of middle cranial fossa

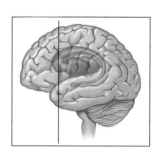

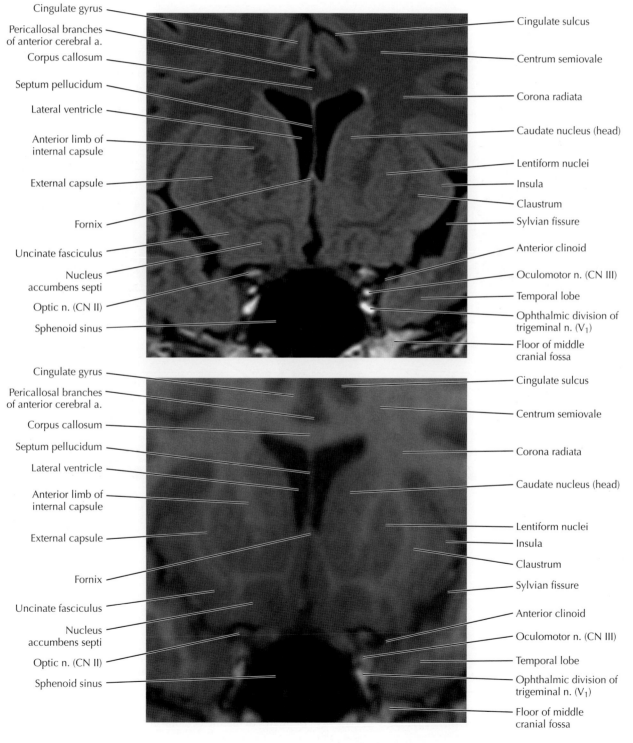

Cingulate gyrus

Pericallosal branches of anterior cerebral a.

Corpus callosum

Septum pellucidum

Lateral ventricle

Anterior limb of internal capsule

External capsule

Fornix

Uncinate fasciculus

Nucleus accumbens septi

Optic n. (CN II)

Sphenoid sinus

Cingulate sulcus

Centrum semiovale

Corona radiata

Caudate nucleus (head)

Lentiform nuclei

Insula

Claustrum

Sylvian fissure

Anterior clinoid

Oculomotor n. (CN III)

Temporal lobe

Ophthalmic division of trigeminal n. (V$_1$)

Floor of middle cranial fossa

Cingulate gyrus

Pericallosal branches of anterior cerebral a.

Corpus callosum

Septum pellucidum

Lateral ventricle

Anterior limb of internal capsule

External capsule

Fornix

Uncinate fasciculus

Nucleus accumbens septi

Optic n. (CN II)

Sphenoid sinus

Cingulate sulcus

Centrum semiovale

Corona radiata

Caudate nucleus (head)

Lentiform nuclei

Insula

Claustrum

Sylvian fissure

Anterior clinoid

Oculomotor n. (CN III)

Temporal lobe

Ophthalmic division of trigeminal n. (V$_1$)

Floor of middle cranial fossa

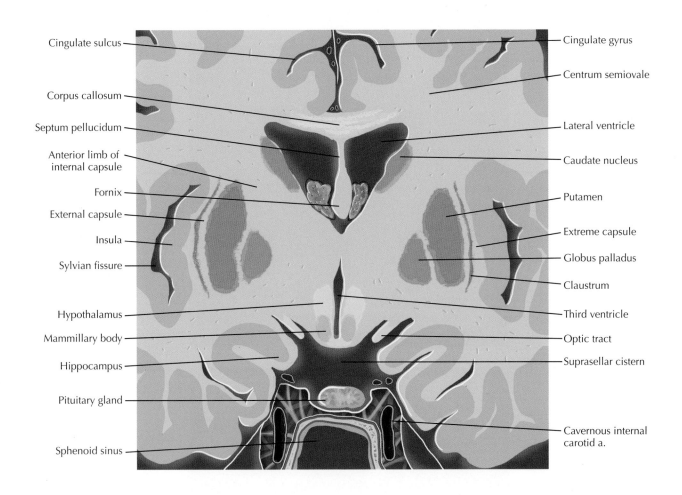

Cingulate sulcus

Corpus callosum

Septum pellucidum

Anterior limb of
internal capsule

Fornix

External capsule

Insula

Sylvian fissure

Hypothalamus

Mammillary body

Hippocampus

Pituitary gland

Sphenoid sinus

Cingulate gyrus

Centrum semiovale

Lateral ventricle

Caudate nucleus

Putamen

Extreme capsule

Globus palladus

Claustrum

Third ventricle

Optic tract

Suprasellar cistern

Cavernous internal
carotid a.

DIAGNOSTIC CONSIDERATION

Loss of differentiation between the insular cortex and the subjacent white matter (extreme and external capsules) is an early sign of infarct in middle cerebral artery territory.

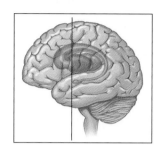

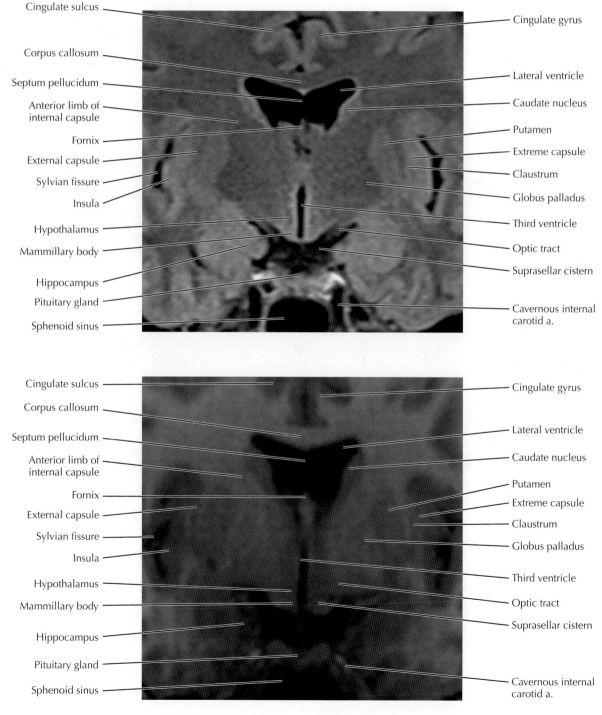

Cingulate sulcus

Corpus callosum

Septum pellucidum

Anterior limb of internal capsule

Fornix

External capsule

Sylvian fissure

Insula

Hypothalamus

Mammillary body

Hippocampus

Pituitary gland

Sphenoid sinus

Cingulate gyrus

Lateral ventricle

Caudate nucleus

Putamen

Extreme capsule

Claustrum

Globus palladus

Third ventricle

Optic tract

Suprasellar cistern

Cavernous internal carotid a.

Cingulate sulcus

Corpus callosum

Septum pellucidum

Anterior limb of internal capsule

Fornix

External capsule

Sylvian fissure

Insula

Hypothalamus

Mammillary body

Hippocampus

Pituitary gland

Sphenoid sinus

Cingulate gyrus

Lateral ventricle

Caudate nucleus

Putamen

Extreme capsule

Claustrum

Globus palladus

Third ventricle

Optic tract

Suprasellar cistern

Cavernous internal carotid a.

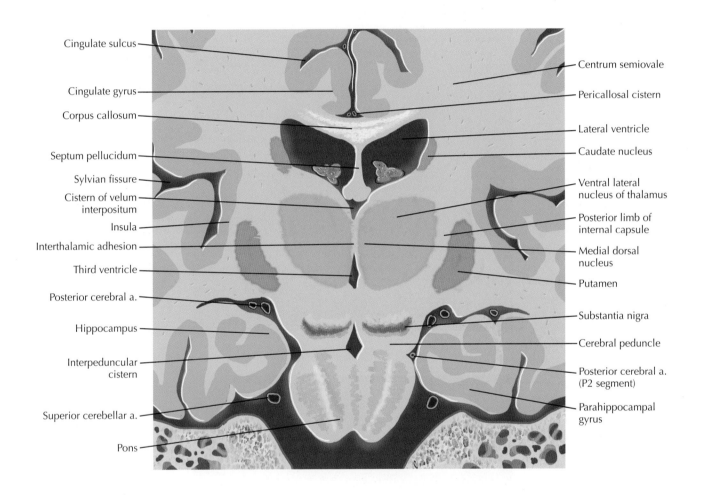

Cingulate sulcus

Cingulate gyrus

Corpus callosum

Septum pellucidum

Sylvian fissure

Cistern of velum interpositum

Insula

Interthalamic adhesion

Third ventricle

Posterior cerebral a.

Hippocampus

Interpeduncular cistern

Superior cerebellar a.

Pons

Centrum semiovale

Pericallosal cistern

Lateral ventricle

Caudate nucleus

Ventral lateral nucleus of thalamus

Posterior limb of internal capsule

Medial dorsal nucleus

Putamen

Substantia nigra

Cerebral peduncle

Posterior cerebral a. (P2 segment)

Parahippocampal gyrus

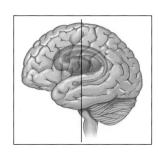

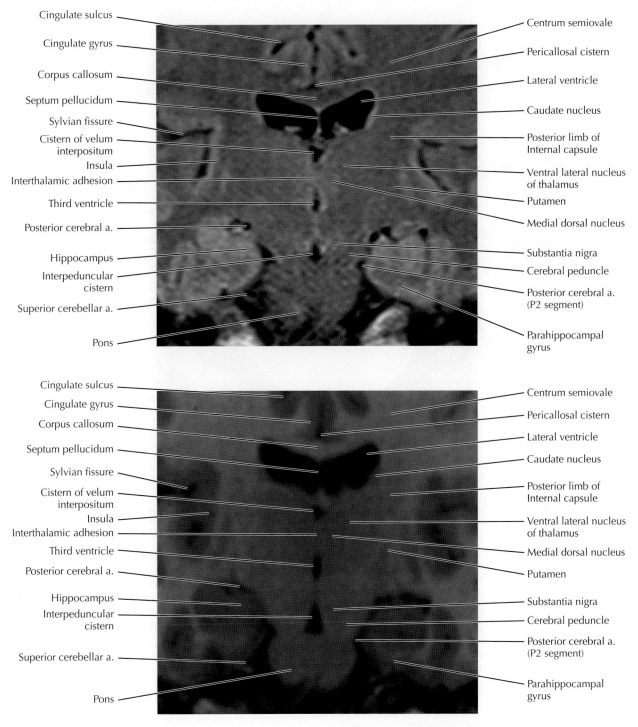

Cingulate sulcus

Cingulate gyrus

Corpus callosum

Septum pellucidum

Sylvian fissure

Cistern of velum interpositum

Insula

Interthalamic adhesion

Third ventricle

Posterior cerebral a.

Hippocampus

Interpeduncular cistern

Superior cerebellar a.

Pons

Centrum semiovale

Pericallosal cistern

Lateral ventricle

Caudate nucleus

Posterior limb of Internal capsule

Ventral lateral nucleus of thalamus

Putamen

Medial dorsal nucleus

Substantia nigra

Cerebral peduncle

Posterior cerebral a. (P2 segment)

Parahippocampal gyrus

Cingulate sulcus

Cingulate gyrus

Corpus callosum

Septum pellucidum

Sylvian fissure

Cistern of velum interpositum

Insula

Interthalamic adhesion

Third ventricle

Posterior cerebral a.

Hippocampus

Interpeduncular cistern

Superior cerebellar a.

Pons

Centrum semiovale

Pericallosal cistern

Lateral ventricle

Caudate nucleus

Posterior limb of Internal capsule

Ventral lateral nucleus of thalamus

Medial dorsal nucleus

Putamen

Substantia nigra

Cerebral peduncle

Posterior cerebral a. (P2 segment)

Parahippocampal gyrus

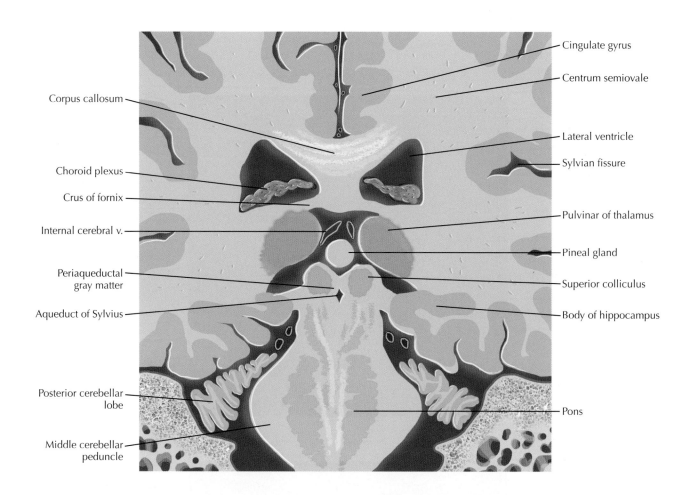

Cingulate gyrus

Centrum semiovale

Corpus callosum

Lateral ventricle

Sylvian fissure

Choroid plexus

Crus of fornix

Pulvinar of thalamus

Internal cerebral v.

Pineal gland

Periaqueductal
gray matter

Superior colliculus

Aqueduct of Sylvius

Body of hippocampus

Posterior cerebellar
lobe

Pons

Middle cerebellar
peduncle

IMAGING TECHNIQUE CONSIDERATION

The white matter is "white" on T1-weighted MRI. One simple mnemonic to remember this fact is to think of myelin sheaths as "fatty," with fat typically bright on T1-weighted images. Fat is not bright on standard T2-weighted images; however, most T2-weighted images are now done with multiple spin-echo pulses (e.g., Turbo-SE), which breaks the strong homonuclear forces (molecules with identical nuclei), called *J-coupling*, between the hydrogen (H) atoms on the long hydrocarbon chains of fat. This allows the H atoms to precess more freely, similar to the two hydrogen atoms on an H_2O molecule, making the appearance of fat bright, like water.

Note that on the superior radiology image, T2-weighted fluid-attenuated inversion recovery (FLAIR) images, the white matter is darker than the cortex.

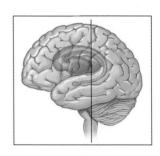

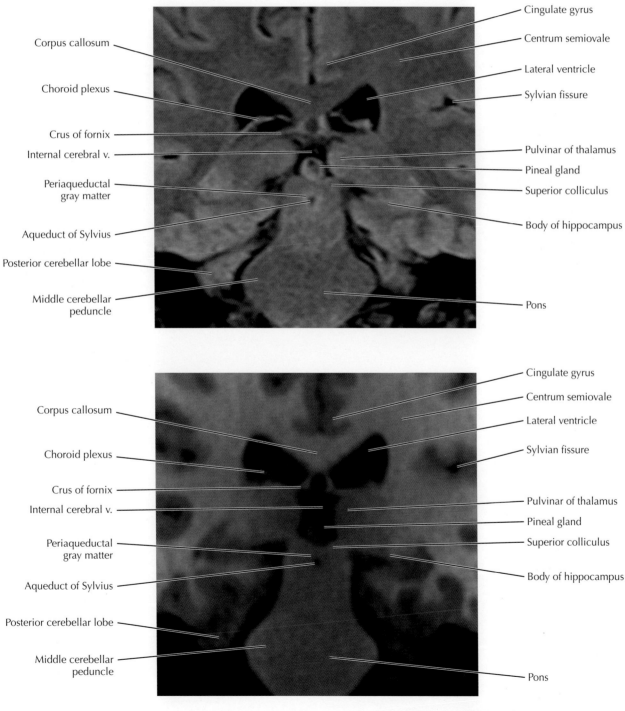

Corpus callosum

Choroid plexus

Crus of fornix

Internal cerebral v.

Periaqueductal gray matter

Aqueduct of Sylvius

Posterior cerebellar lobe

Middle cerebellar peduncle

Cingulate gyrus

Centrum semiovale

Lateral ventricle

Sylvian fissure

Pulvinar of thalamus

Pineal gland

Superior colliculus

Body of hippocampus

Pons

Corpus callosum

Choroid plexus

Crus of fornix

Internal cerebral v.

Periaqueductal gray matter

Aqueduct of Sylvius

Posterior cerebellar lobe

Middle cerebellar peduncle

Cingulate gyrus

Centrum semiovale

Lateral ventricle

Sylvian fissure

Pulvinar of thalamus

Pineal gland

Superior colliculus

Body of hippocampus

Pons

Chapter 4 LIMBIC SYSTEM

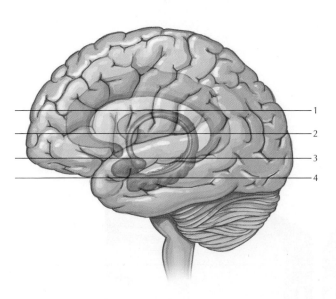

AXIAL 148

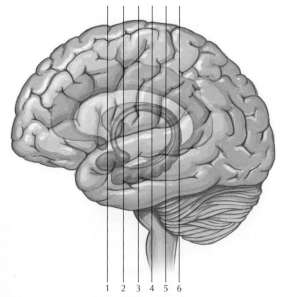

CORONAL 156

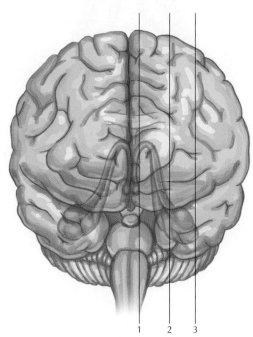

SAGITTAL 168

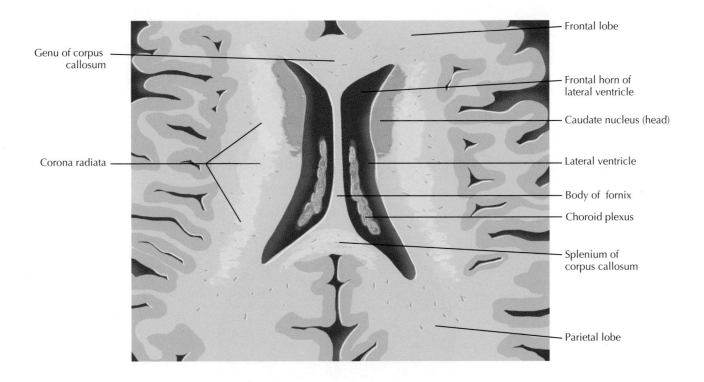

Genu of corpus callosum

Corona radiata

Frontal lobe

Frontal horn of lateral ventricle

Caudate nucleus (head)

Lateral ventricle

Body of fornix

Choroid plexus

Splenium of corpus callosum

Parietal lobe

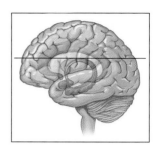

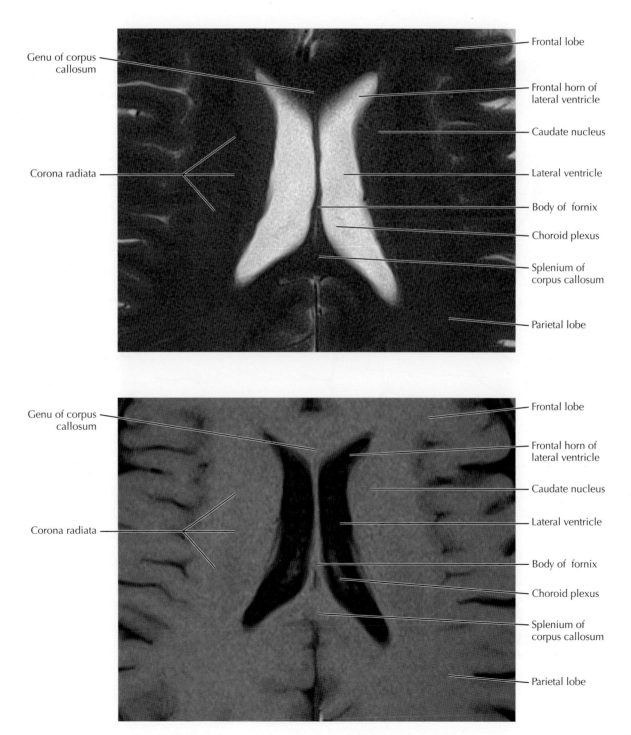

Genu of corpus callosum

Corona radiata

Frontal lobe

Frontal horn of lateral ventricle

Caudate nucleus

Lateral ventricle

Body of fornix

Choroid plexus

Splenium of corpus callosum

Parietal lobe

Genu of corpus callosum

Corona radiata

Frontal lobe

Frontal horn of lateral ventricle

Caudate nucleus

Lateral ventricle

Body of fornix

Choroid plexus

Splenium of corpus callosum

Parietal lobe

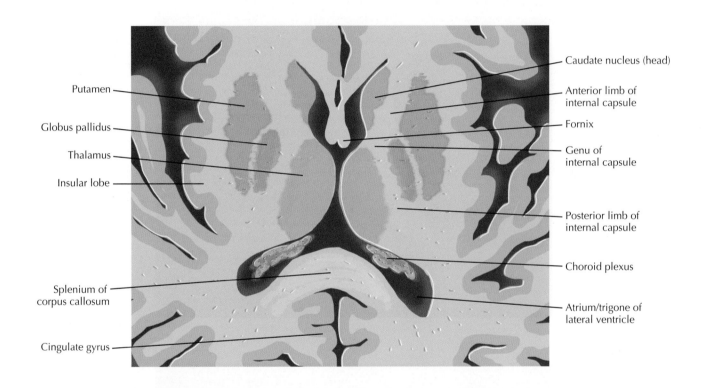

Putamen

Globus pallidus

Thalamus

Insular lobe

Splenium of
corpus callosum

Cingulate gyrus

Caudate nucleus (head)

Anterior limb of
internal capsule

Fornix

Genu of
internal capsule

Posterior limb of
internal capsule

Choroid plexus

Atrium/trigone of
lateral ventricle

NORMAL ANATOMY

Note how the *fornix* (Latin, "arch" or "vault") is more easily seen as a paired structure on the T2-weighted axial magnetic resonance image (upper radiology image), compared with the fornix as seen in the Chapter 3 images focusing on the basal ganglia and thalami. The fornix is a **C**-shaped bundle of axons in the brain and carries signals from the hippocampus to the hypothalamus.

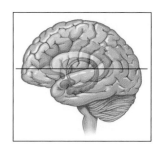

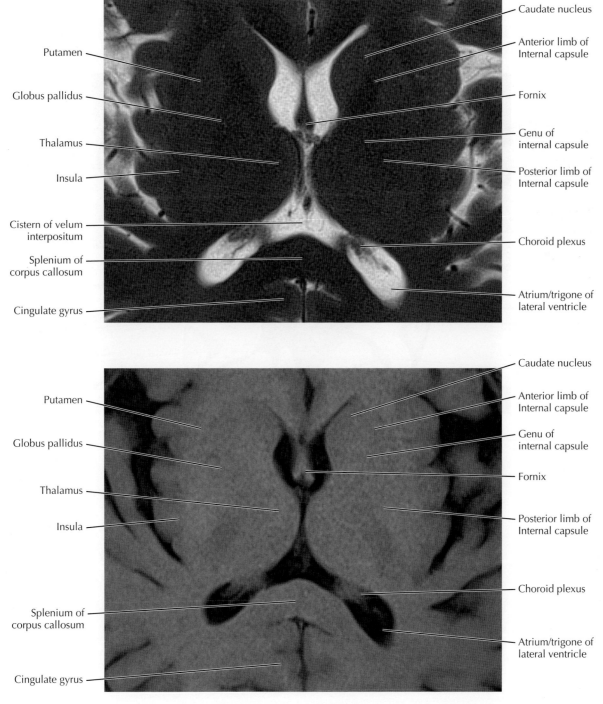

Caudate nucleus

Putamen

Anterior limb of
Internal capsule

Globus pallidus

Fornix

Genu of
internal capsule

Thalamus

Insula

Posterior limb of
Internal capsule

Cistern of velum
interpositum

Splenium of
corpus callosum

Choroid plexus

Cingulate gyrus

Atrium/trigone of
lateral ventricle

Caudate nucleus

Putamen

Anterior limb of
Internal capsule

Genu of
internal capsule

Globus pallidus

Thalamus

Fornix

Insula

Posterior limb of
Internal capsule

Splenium of
corpus callosum

Choroid plexus

Atrium/trigone of
lateral ventricle

Cingulate gyrus

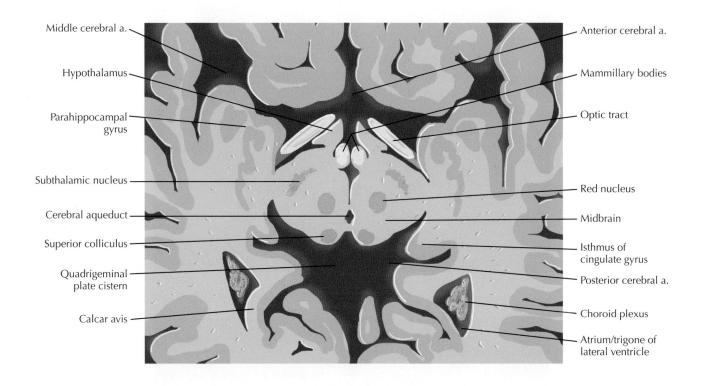

Middle cerebral a.

Hypothalamus

Parahippocampal gyrus

Subthalamic nucleus

Cerebral aqueduct

Superior colliculus

Quadrigeminal plate cistern

Calcar avis

Anterior cerebral a.

Mammillary bodies

Optic tract

Red nucleus

Midbrain

Isthmus of cingulate gyrus

Posterior cerebral a.

Choroid plexus

Atrium/trigone of lateral ventricle

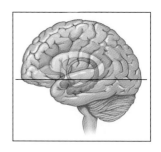

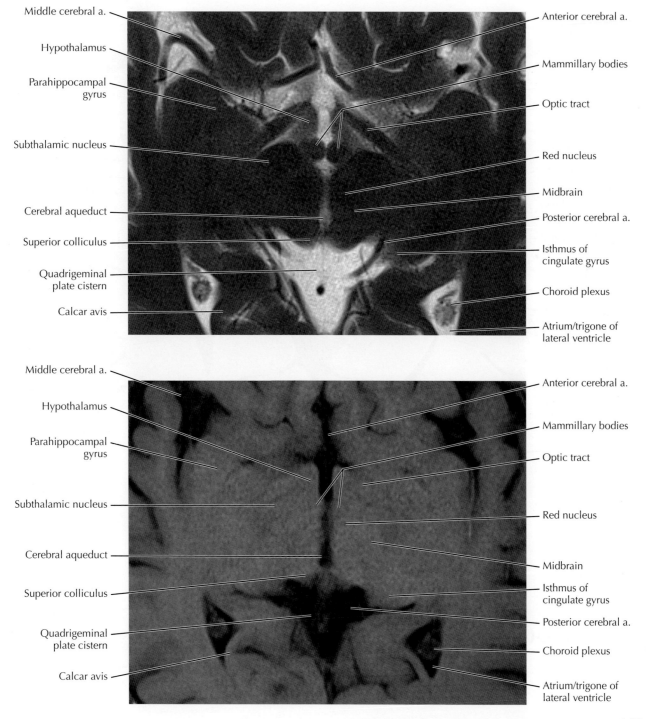

Middle cerebral a.

Hypothalamus

Parahippocampal gyrus

Subthalamic nucleus

Cerebral aqueduct

Superior colliculus

Quadrigeminal plate cistern

Calcar avis

Anterior cerebral a.

Mammillary bodies

Optic tract

Red nucleus

Midbrain

Posterior cerebral a.

Isthmus of cingulate gyrus

Choroid plexus

Atrium/trigone of lateral ventricle

Middle cerebral a.

Hypothalamus

Parahippocampal gyrus

Subthalamic nucleus

Cerebral aqueduct

Superior colliculus

Quadrigeminal plate cistern

Calcar avis

Anterior cerebral a.

Mammillary bodies

Optic tract

Red nucleus

Midbrain

Isthmus of cingulate gyrus

Posterior cerebral a.

Choroid plexus

Atrium/trigone of lateral ventricle

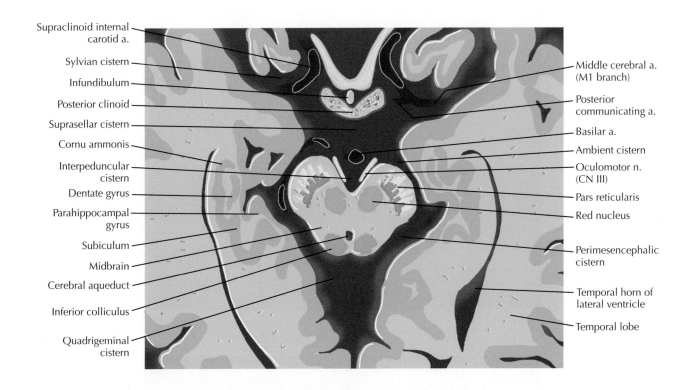

Supraclinoid internal carotid a.
Sylvian cistern
Infundibulum
Posterior clinoid
Suprasellar cistern
Cornu ammonis
Interpeduncular cistern
Dentate gyrus
Parahippocampal gyrus
Subiculum
Midbrain
Cerebral aqueduct
Inferior colliculus
Quadrigeminal cistern

Middle cerebral a. (M1 branch)
Posterior communicating a.
Basilar a.
Ambient cistern
Oculomotor n. (CN III)
Pars reticularis
Red nucleus
Perimesencephalic cistern
Temporal horn of lateral ventricle
Temporal lobe

NORMAL ANATOMY

The architecture of the dentate nucleus and cornu ammonis (hippocampus) is not well defined on axial magnetic resonance imaging. Asymmetry and abnormal signal are much better appreciated on coronal MR images.

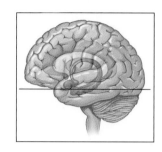

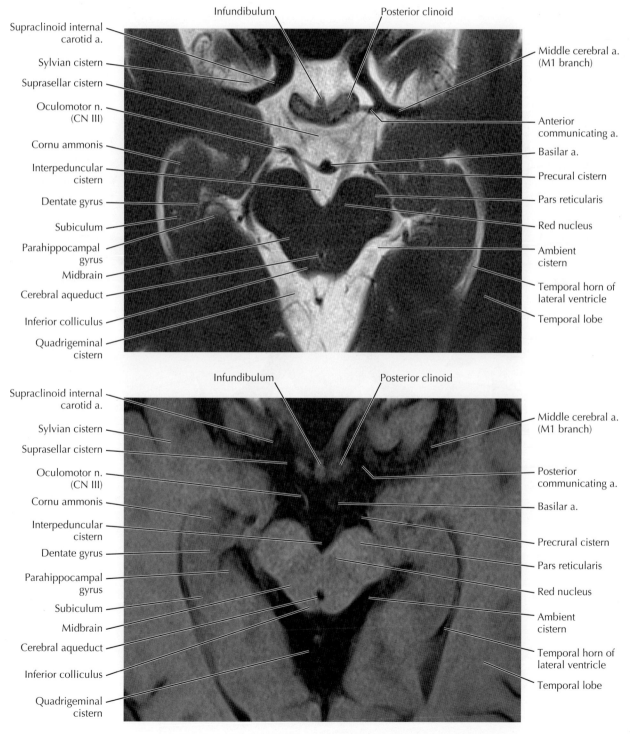

Infundibulum   Posterior clinoid

Supraclinoid internal carotid a.

Sylvian cistern

Suprasellar cistern

Oculomotor n. (CN III)

Cornu ammonis

Interpeduncular cistern

Dentate gyrus

Subiculum

Parahippocampal gyrus

Midbrain

Cerebral aqueduct

Inferior colliculus

Quadrigeminal cistern

Middle cerebral a. (M1 branch)

Anterior communicating a.

Basilar a.

Precural cistern

Pars reticularis

Red nucleus

Ambient cistern

Temporal horn of lateral ventricle

Temporal lobe

Infundibulum   Posterior clinoid

Supraclinoid internal carotid a.

Sylvian cistern

Suprasellar cistern

Oculomotor n. (CN III)

Cornu ammonis

Interpeduncular cistern

Dentate gyrus

Parahippocampal gyrus

Subiculum

Midbrain

Cerebral aqueduct

Inferior colliculus

Quadrigeminal cistern

Middle cerebral a. (M1 branch)

Posterior communicating a.

Basilar a.

Precrural cistern

Pars reticularis

Red nucleus

Ambient cistern

Temporal horn of lateral ventricle

Temporal lobe

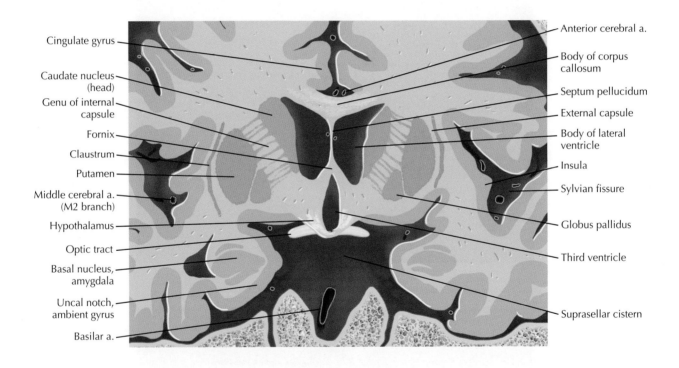

Cingulate gyrus

Caudate nucleus (head)

Genu of internal capsule

Fornix

Claustrum

Putamen

Middle cerebral a. (M2 branch)

Hypothalamus

Optic tract

Basal nucleus, amygdala

Uncal notch, ambient gyrus

Basilar a.

Anterior cerebral a.

Body of corpus callosum

Septum pellucidum

External capsule

Body of lateral ventricle

Insula

Sylvian fissure

Globus pallidus

Third ventricle

Suprasellar cistern

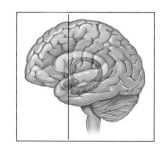

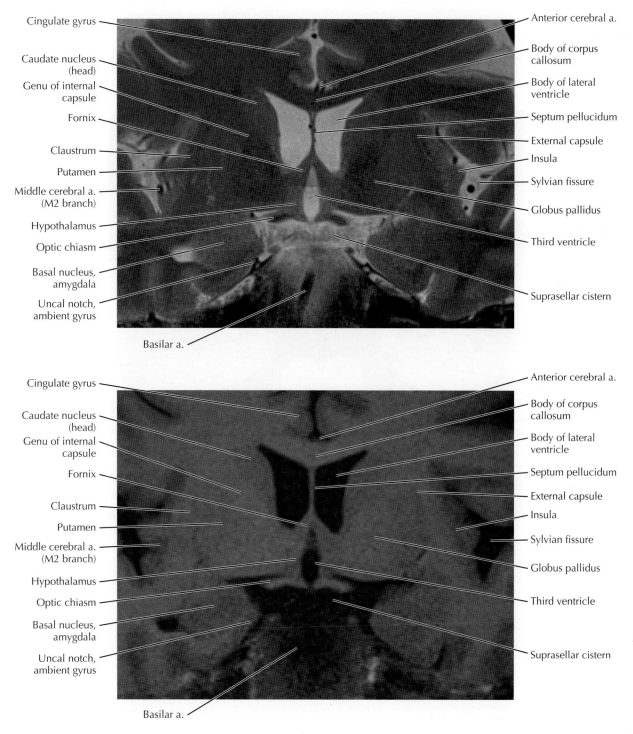

Cingulate gyrus

Caudate nucleus (head)

Genu of internal capsule

Fornix

Claustrum

Putamen

Middle cerebral a. (M2 branch)

Hypothalamus

Optic chiasm

Basal nucleus, amygdala

Uncal notch, ambient gyrus

Basilar a.

Anterior cerebral a.

Body of corpus callosum

Body of lateral ventricle

Septum pellucidum

External capsule

Insula

Sylvian fissure

Globus pallidus

Third ventricle

Suprasellar cistern

Cingulate gyrus

Caudate nucleus (head)

Genu of internal capsule

Fornix

Claustrum

Putamen

Middle cerebral a. (M2 branch)

Hypothalamus

Optic chiasm

Basal nucleus, amygdala

Uncal notch, ambient gyrus

Basilar a.

Anterior cerebral a.

Body of corpus callosum

Body of lateral ventricle

Septum pellucidum

External capsule

Insula

Sylvian fissure

Globus pallidus

Third ventricle

Suprasellar cistern

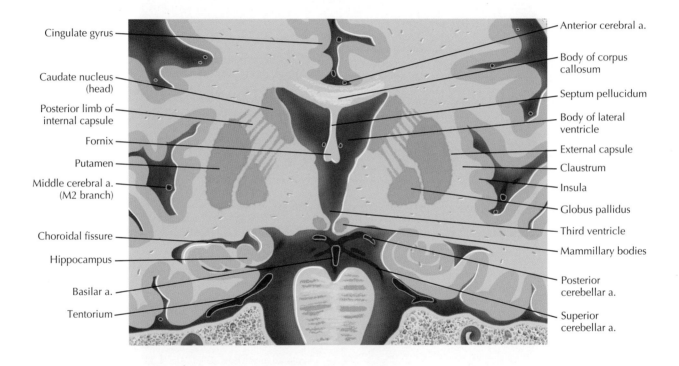

Cingulate gyrus

Caudate nucleus
(head)

Posterior limb of
internal capsule

Fornix

Putamen

Middle cerebral a.
(M2 branch)

Choroidal fissure

Hippocampus

Basilar a.

Tentorium

Anterior cerebral a.

Body of corpus
callosum

Septum pellucidum

Body of lateral
ventricle

External capsule

Claustrum

Insula

Globus pallidus

Third ventricle

Mammillary bodies

Posterior
cerebellar a.

Superior
cerebellar a.

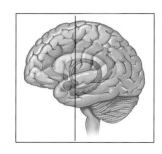

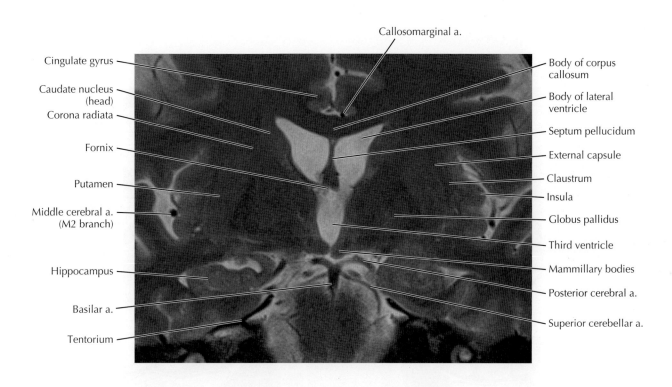

Callosomarginal a.

Cingulate gyrus

Caudate nucleus (head)

Corona radiata

Fornix

Putamen

Middle cerebral a. (M2 branch)

Hippocampus

Basilar a.

Tentorium

Body of corpus callosum

Body of lateral ventricle

Septum pellucidum

External capsule

Claustrum

Insula

Globus pallidus

Third ventricle

Mammillary bodies

Posterior cerebral a.

Superior cerebellar a.

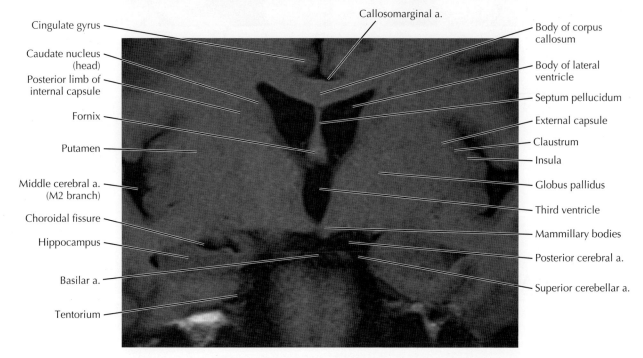

Callosomarginal a.

Cingulate gyrus

Caudate nucleus (head)

Posterior limb of internal capsule

Fornix

Putamen

Middle cerebral a. (M2 branch)

Choroidal fissure

Hippocampus

Basilar a.

Tentorium

Body of corpus callosum

Body of lateral ventricle

Septum pellucidum

External capsule

Claustrum

Insula

Globus pallidus

Third ventricle

Mammillary bodies

Posterior cerebral a.

Superior cerebellar a.

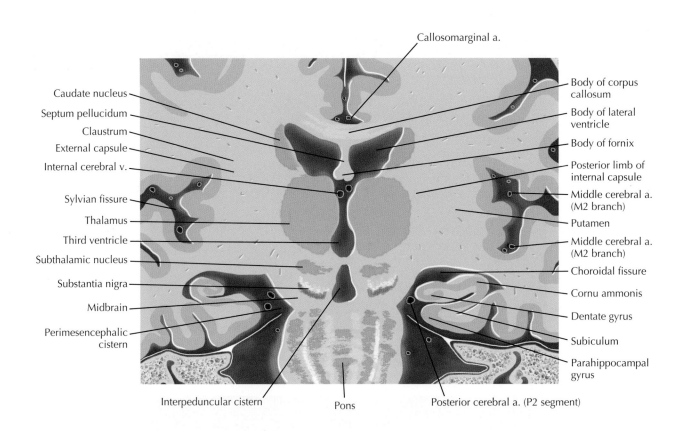

Callosomarginal a.

Caudate nucleus

Septum pellucidum

Claustrum

External capsule

Internal cerebral v.

Sylvian fissure

Thalamus

Third ventricle

Subthalamic nucleus

Substantia nigra

Midbrain

Perimesencephalic cistern

Body of corpus callosum

Body of lateral ventricle

Body of fornix

Posterior limb of internal capsule

Middle cerebral a. (M2 branch)

Putamen

Middle cerebral a. (M2 branch)

Choroidal fissure

Cornu ammonis

Dentate gyrus

Subiculum

Parahippocampal gyrus

Interpeduncular cistern   Pons   Posterior cerebral a. (P2 segment)

NORMAL ANATOMY

The normal appearance of the hippocampus on coronal MRI is that of a jelly roll, with the dentate gyrus in the center and the four segments of the cornu ammonis wrapped around it (see Axial 4).

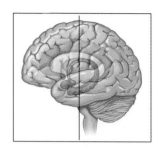

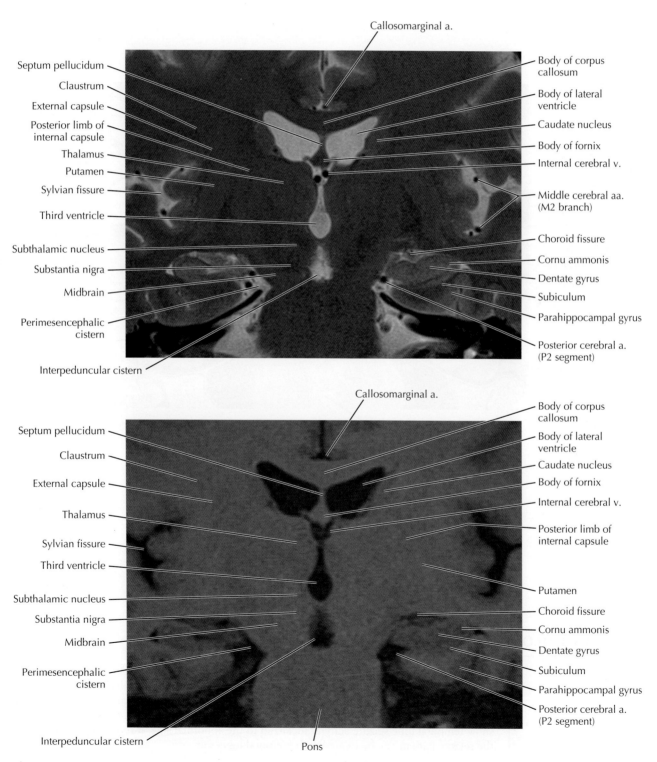

Callosomarginal a.

Septum pellucidum

Claustrum

External capsule

Posterior limb of
internal capsule

Thalamus

Putamen

Sylvian fissure

Third ventricle

Subthalamic nucleus

Substantia nigra

Midbrain

Perimesencephalic
cistern

Interpeduncular cistern

Body of corpus
callosum

Body of lateral
ventricle

Caudate nucleus

Body of fornix

Internal cerebral v.

Middle cerebral aa.
(M2 branch)

Choroid fissure

Cornu ammonis

Dentate gyrus

Subiculum

Parahippocampal gyrus

Posterior cerebral a.
(P2 segment)

Callosomarginal a.

Septum pellucidum

Claustrum

External capsule

Thalamus

Sylvian fissure

Third ventricle

Subthalamic nucleus

Substantia nigra

Midbrain

Perimesencephalic
cistern

Interpeduncular cistern

Pons

Body of corpus
callosum

Body of lateral
ventricle

Caudate nucleus

Body of fornix

Internal cerebral v.

Posterior limb of
internal capsule

Putamen

Choroid fissure

Cornu ammonis

Dentate gyrus

Subiculum

Parahippocampal gyrus

Posterior cerebral a.
(P2 segment)

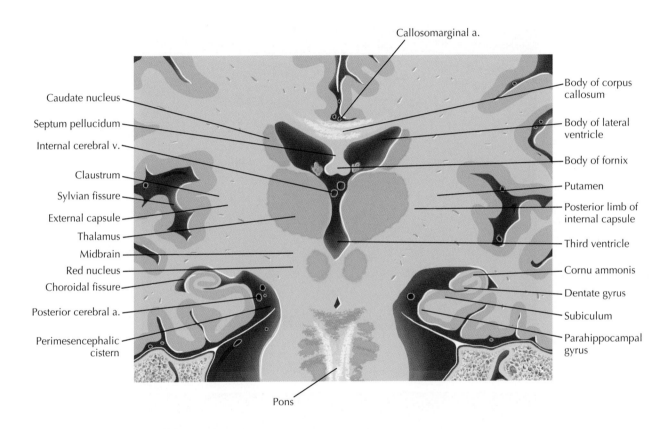

Callosomarginal a.

Caudate nucleus

Septum pellucidum

Internal cerebral v.

Claustrum

Sylvian fissure

External capsule

Thalamus

Midbrain

Red nucleus

Choroidal fissure

Posterior cerebral a.

Perimesencephalic cistern

Body of corpus callosum

Body of lateral ventricle

Body of fornix

Putamen

Posterior limb of internal capsule

Third ventricle

Cornu ammonis

Dentate gyrus

Subiculum

Parahippocampal gyrus

Pons

PATHOLOGIC PROCESS

Coronal imaging through the hippocampus and amygdala is not part of routine brain MRI. However, coronal images are helpful for evaluation of temporal lobe epilepsy, which may show findings of *mesial temporal sclerosis*, typically seen as an asymmetrically small hippocampus and amygdala with increased T2-weighted signal. Electroencephalography (EEG) will typically show temporal lobe seizure activity localized to the abnormal side. If refractory to medication, the seizure patient can be treated with temporal lobectomy.

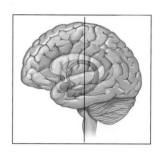

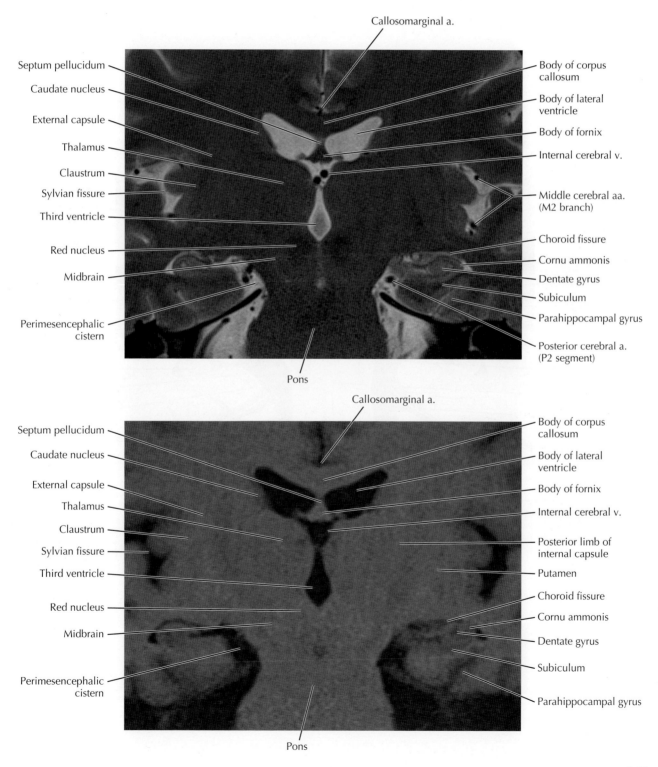

Callosomarginal a.

Septum pellucidum

Caudate nucleus

External capsule

Thalamus

Claustrum

Sylvian fissure

Third ventricle

Red nucleus

Midbrain

Perimesencephalic cistern

Body of corpus callosum

Body of lateral ventricle

Body of fornix

Internal cerebral v.

Middle cerebral aa. (M2 branch)

Choroid fissure

Cornu ammonis

Dentate gyrus

Subiculum

Parahippocampal gyrus

Posterior cerebral a. (P2 segment)

Pons

Callosomarginal a.

Septum pellucidum

Caudate nucleus

External capsule

Thalamus

Claustrum

Sylvian fissure

Third ventricle

Red nucleus

Midbrain

Perimesencephalic cistern

Body of corpus callosum

Body of lateral ventricle

Body of fornix

Internal cerebral v.

Posterior limb of internal capsule

Putamen

Choroid fissure

Cornu ammonis

Dentate gyrus

Subiculum

Parahippocampal gyrus

Pons

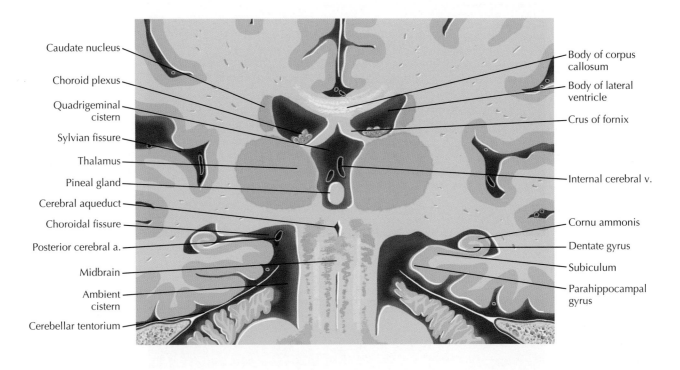

Caudate nucleus

Choroid plexus

Quadrigeminal cistern

Sylvian fissure

Thalamus

Pineal gland

Cerebral aqueduct

Choroidal fissure

Posterior cerebral a.

Midbrain

Ambient cistern

Cerebellar tentorium

Body of corpus callosum

Body of lateral ventricle

Crus of fornix

Internal cerebral v.

Cornu ammonis

Dentate gyrus

Subiculum

Parahippocampal gyrus

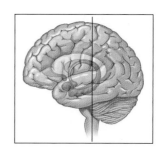

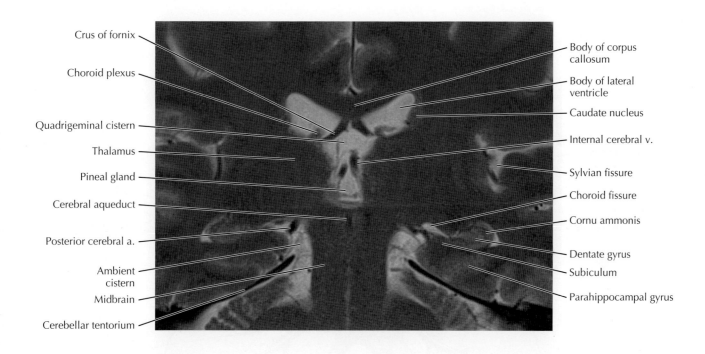

Crus of fornix

Choroid plexus

Quadrigeminal cistern

Thalamus

Pineal gland

Cerebral aqueduct

Posterior cerebral a.

Ambient cistern

Midbrain

Cerebellar tentorium

Body of corpus callosum

Body of lateral ventricle

Caudate nucleus

Internal cerebral v.

Sylvian fissure

Choroid fissure

Cornu ammonis

Dentate gyrus

Subiculum

Parahippocampal gyrus

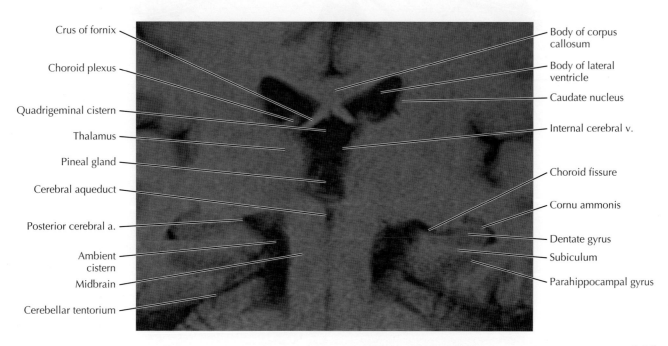

Crus of fornix

Choroid plexus

Quadrigeminal cistern

Thalamus

Pineal gland

Cerebral aqueduct

Posterior cerebral a.

Ambient cistern

Midbrain

Cerebellar tentorium

Body of corpus callosum

Body of lateral ventricle

Caudate nucleus

Internal cerebral v.

Choroid fissure

Cornu ammonis

Dentate gyrus

Subiculum

Parahippocampal gyrus

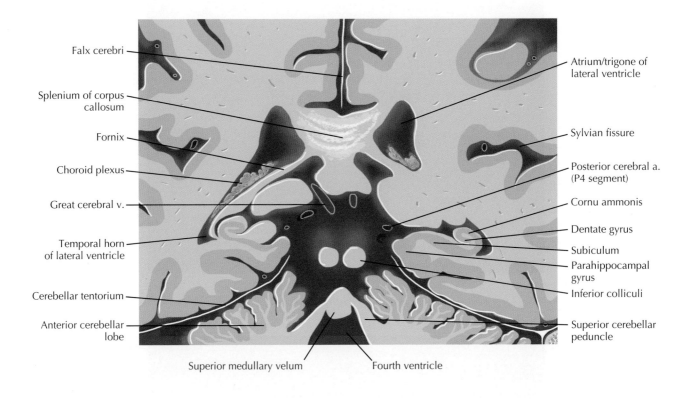

Falx cerebri

Splenium of corpus callosum

Fornix

Choroid plexus

Great cerebral v.

Temporal horn of lateral ventricle

Cerebellar tentorium

Anterior cerebellar lobe

Superior medullary velum

Fourth ventricle

Atrium/trigone of lateral ventricle

Sylvian fissure

Posterior cerebral a. (P4 segment)

Cornu ammonis

Dentate gyrus

Subiculum

Parahippocampal gyrus

Inferior colliculi

Superior cerebellar peduncle

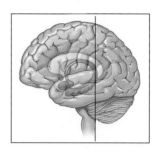

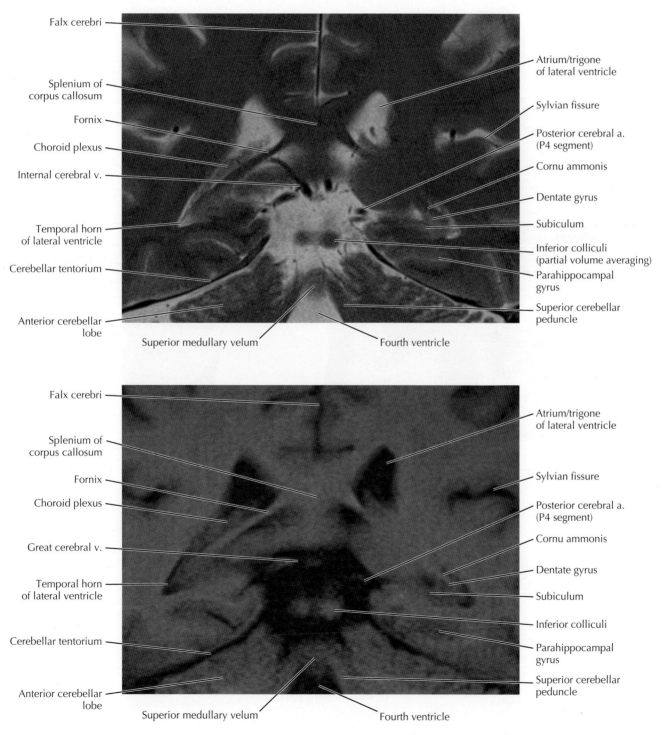

Falx cerebri

Splenium of
corpus callosum

Fornix

Choroid plexus

Internal cerebral v.

Temporal horn
of lateral ventricle

Cerebellar tentorium

Anterior cerebellar
lobe

Superior medullary velum

Atrium/trigone
of lateral ventricle

Sylvian fissure

Posterior cerebral a.
(P4 segment)

Cornu ammonis

Dentate gyrus

Subiculum

Inferior colliculi
(partial volume averaging)

Parahippocampal
gyrus

Superior cerebellar
peduncle

Fourth ventricle

Falx cerebri

Splenium of
corpus callosum

Fornix

Choroid plexus

Great cerebral v.

Temporal horn
of lateral ventricle

Cerebellar tentorium

Anterior cerebellar
lobe

Superior medullary velum

Atrium/trigone
of lateral ventricle

Sylvian fissure

Posterior cerebral a.
(P4 segment)

Cornu ammonis

Dentate gyrus

Subiculum

Inferior colliculi

Parahippocampal
gyrus

Superior cerebellar
peduncle

Fourth ventricle

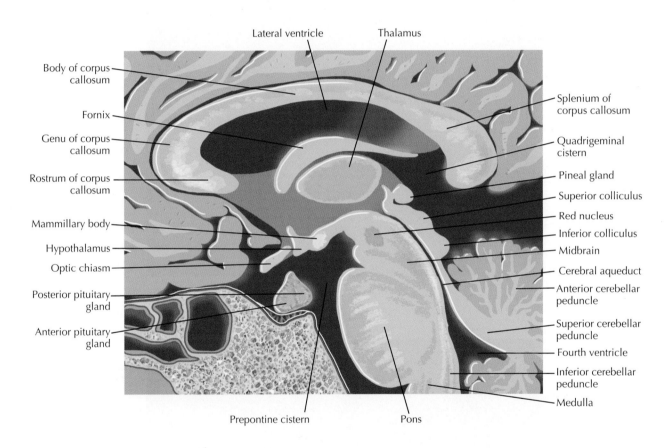

Body of corpus callosum

Fornix

Genu of corpus callosum

Rostrum of corpus callosum

Mammillary body

Hypothalamus

Optic chiasm

Posterior pituitary gland

Anterior pituitary gland

Lateral ventricle

Thalamus

Splenium of corpus callosum

Quadrigeminal cistern

Pineal gland

Superior colliculus

Red nucleus

Inferior colliculus

Midbrain

Cerebral aqueduct

Anterior cerebellar peduncle

Superior cerebellar peduncle

Fourth ventricle

Inferior cerebellar peduncle

Medulla

Prepontine cistern

Pons

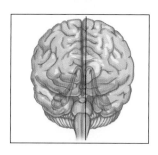

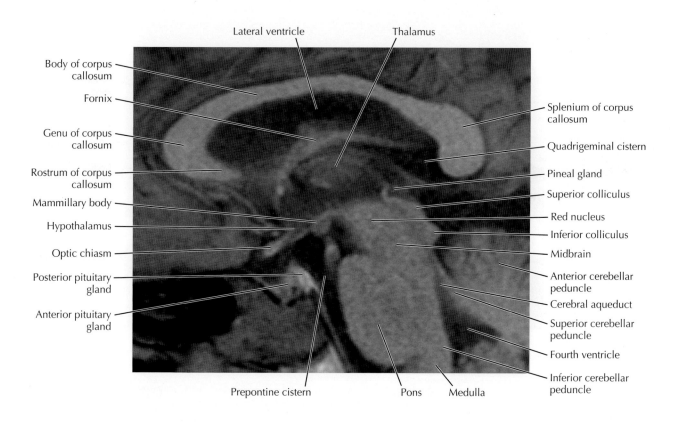

Lateral ventricle

Thalamus

Body of corpus callosum

Fornix

Genu of corpus callosum

Rostrum of corpus callosum

Mammillary body

Hypothalamus

Optic chiasm

Posterior pituitary gland

Anterior pituitary gland

Splenium of corpus callosum

Quadrigeminal cistern

Pineal gland

Superior colliculus

Red nucleus

Inferior colliculus

Midbrain

Anterior cerebellar peduncle

Cerebral aqueduct

Superior cerebellar peduncle

Fourth ventricle

Inferior cerebellar peduncle

Prepontine cistern

Pons

Medulla

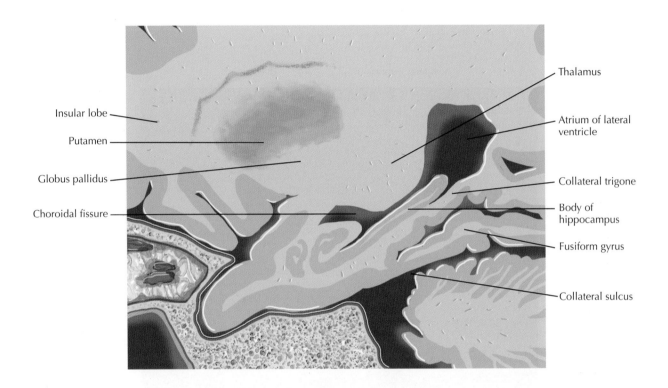

Insular lobe

Putamen

Globus pallidus

Choroidal fissure

Thalamus

Atrium of lateral ventricle

Collateral trigone

Body of hippocampus

Fusiform gyrus

Collateral sulcus

NORMAL ANATOMY

The hippocampus is a ridge running along the floor of the temporal horn of the lateral ventricle. Venetian anatomist Aranzi (1578) first described its seahorse appearance using the Latin term *hippocampus* (Greek *hippokampos*). In 1832, Parisian surgeon de Garengeot used the term *cornu ammonis* ("horn of Ammon").

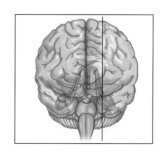

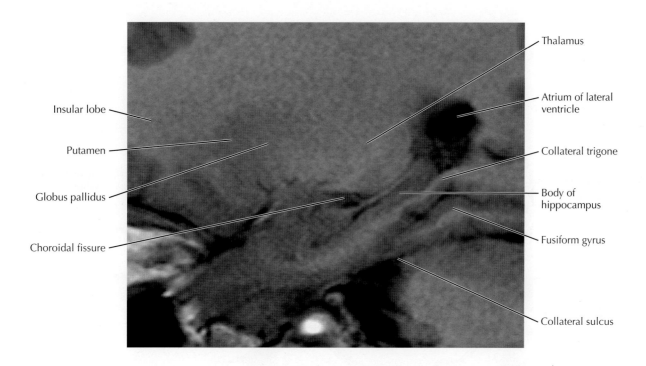

Thalamus

Atrium of lateral ventricle

Insular lobe

Collateral trigone

Putamen

Body of hippocampus

Globus pallidus

Fusiform gyrus

Choroidal fissure

Collateral sulcus

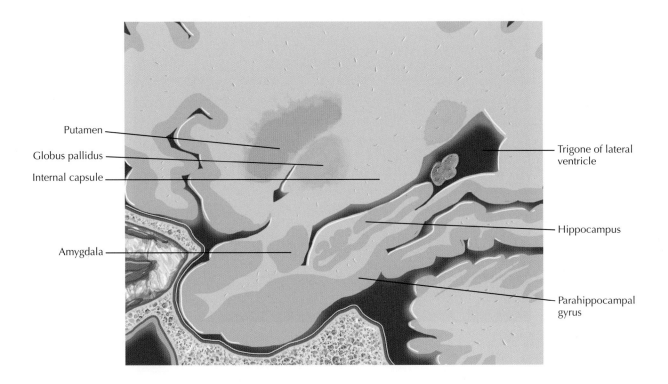

Putamen

Globus pallidus

Internal capsule

Amygdala

Trigone of lateral
ventricle

Hippocampus

Parahippocampal
gyrus

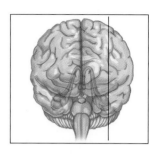

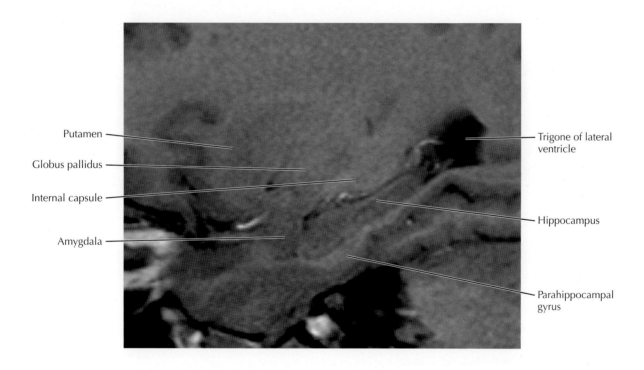

Putamen

Globus pallidus

Internal capsule

Amygdala

Trigone of lateral
ventricle

Hippocampus

Parahippocampal
gyrus

Chapter 5 BRAINSTEM AND CRANIAL NERVES

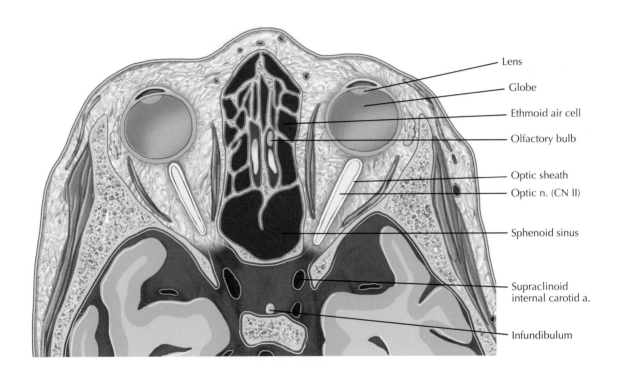

Lens

Globe

Ethmoid air cell

Olfactory bulb

Optic sheath

Optic n. (CN II)

Sphenoid sinus

Supraclinoid
internal carotid a.

Infundibulum

NORMAL ANATOMY

The olfactory nerve, or cranial nerve (CN) I, is the first of 12 cranial nerves and provides innervation for the sense of smell. CN I can often be seen on axial magnetic resonance imaging of the brain at the level of the temporal lobes. Nerve fibers from the olfactory mucosa in the anterosuperior nasal cavity join with the olfactory bulb, from which signals pass through nerves running within olfactory foramina in the cribriform plate in the superior nasal cavity.

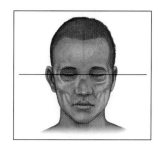

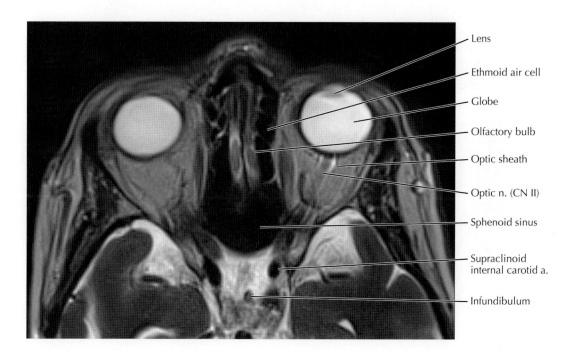

Lens

Ethmoid air cell

Globe

Olfactory bulb

Optic sheath

Optic n. (CN II)

Sphenoid sinus

Supraclinoid
internal carotid a.

Infundibulum

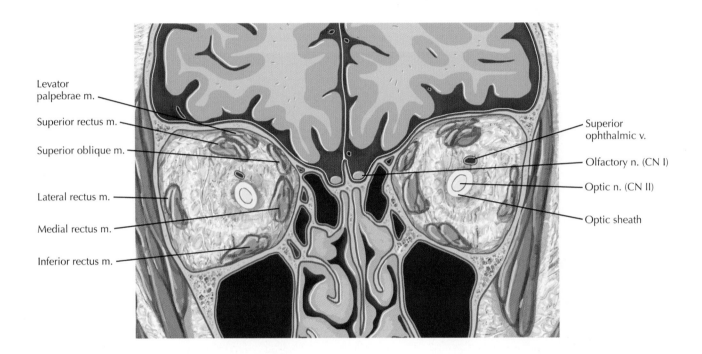

Levator palpebrae m.

Superior rectus m.

Superior oblique m.

Lateral rectus m.

Medial rectus m.

Inferior rectus m.

Superior ophthalmic v.

Olfactory n. (CN I)

Optic n. (CN II)

Optic sheath

IMAGING TECHNIQUE CONSIDERATION

Clinicians should always approach loss of smell as a serious symptom and explore anatomic causes. The best imaging plane to assess the olfactory nerves is coronal, perpendicular to the long axis of the nerves. T2-weighted MR coronal images help to delineate the olfactory nerves, with surrounding cerebrospinal fluid (CSF) between the nerves and the bony walls of the olfactory grooves. In some patients, one olfactory groove may be asymmetrically lower than the other, an important consideration if the patient may be undergoing functional endoscopic sinus surgery (FES). One notable tumor centered on the olfactory nerves is *esthesioneuroblastoma* (olfactory neuroblastoma).

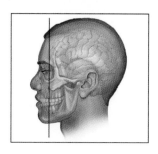

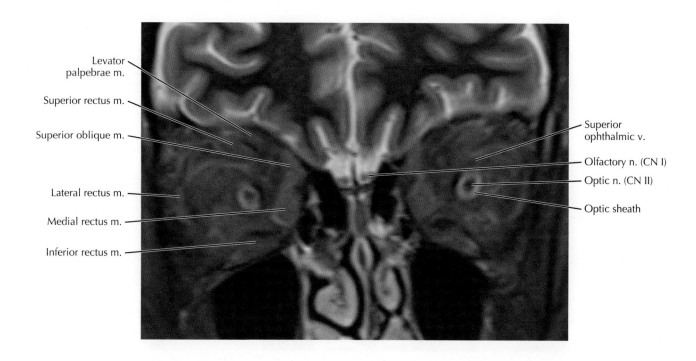

Levator palpebrae m.

Superior rectus m.

Superior oblique m.

Lateral rectus m.

Medial rectus m.

Inferior rectus m.

Superior ophthalmic v.

Olfactory n. (CN I)

Optic n. (CN II)

Optic sheath

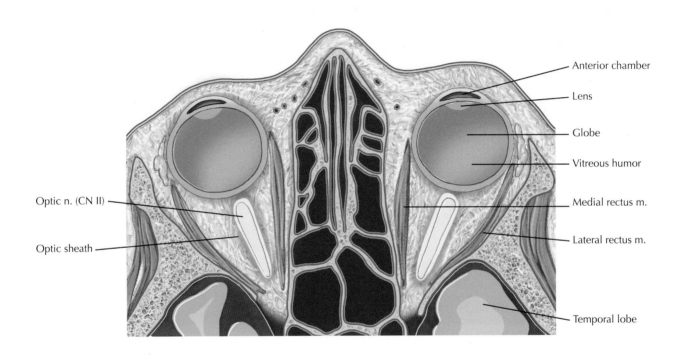

Anterior chamber

Lens

Globe

Vitreous humor

Medial rectus m.

Lateral rectus m.

Temporal lobe

Optic n. (CN II)

Optic sheath

DIAGNOSTIC CONSIDERATION

The optic nerve (second cranial, CN II) is the only cranial nerve that is part of the central nervous system. CN II is a direct extension of the brain and thus is surrounded by CSF and a dural sheath. Ophthalmoscopic (funduscopic) examination of the eyes can reveal papilledema when intracranial pressure is increased. On axial imaging, flattening of the posterior aspect of the globes has been described as the most specific sign of *idiopathic intracranial hypertension,* also called benign intracranial hypertension or pseudotumor cerebri.

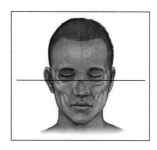

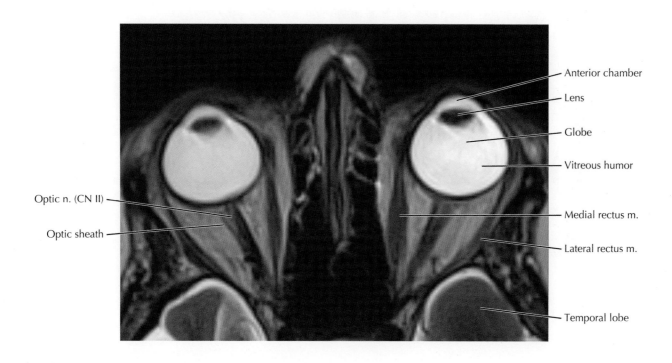

Anterior chamber

Lens

Globe

Vitreous humor

Optic n. (CN II)

Optic sheath

Medial rectus m.

Lateral rectus m.

Temporal lobe

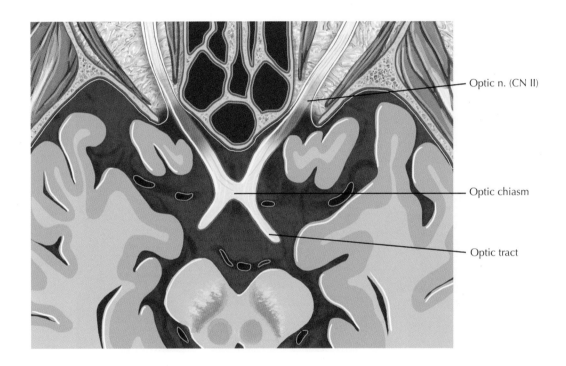

Optic n. (CN II)

Optic chiasm

Optic tract

NORMAL ANATOMY AND PATHOLOGIC CONSIDERATION

Sensory signals from the retina transmit posteriorly along the optic nerves until the signals join at the optic chiasm, where the medial fibers of each nerve cross to the other side. The optic chiasm is immediately superior to the pituitary gland (hypophysis) and suprasellar cistern. A large pituitary adenoma therefore can compress the crossing fibers, leading to *bitemporal hemanopia* (or hemianopsia), with defects in the temporal, or lateral, half of the visual field in each eye. A light object in the temporal (lateral) field of view sends light through the lens to the nasal (medial) retina, which then sends signals through the medial fibers of the optic nerves, which in turn cross midline at the optic chiasm.

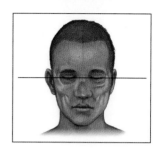

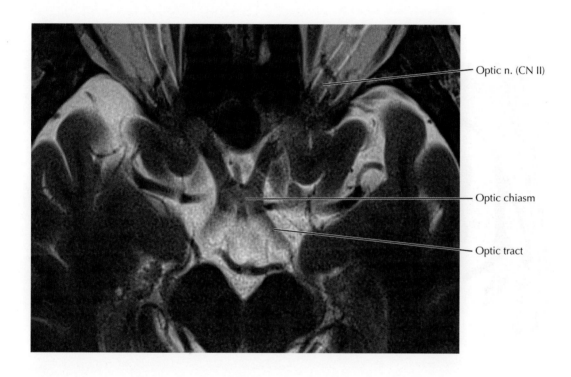

Optic n. (CN II)

Optic chiasm

Optic tract

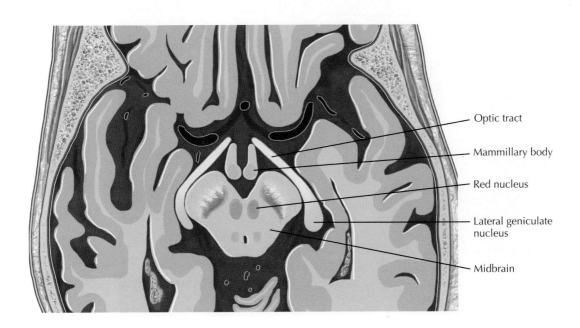

Optic tract

Mammillary body

Red nucleus

Lateral geniculate
nucleus

Midbrain

NORMAL ANATOMY

The optic tract contains the lateral, or temporal, nerves of the ipsilateral optic nerve and the medial, or nasal, nerves of the contralateral optic nerve. The optic tract joins the optic chiasm to the lateral geniculate nucleus (LGN). The LGN is located within the thalamus and is the primary relay center for visual information received from the retina. A mass along the optic tract can cause contralateral hemianopia, with blocked signals at the right optic tract causing a left-sided hemianopia.

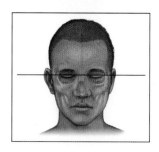

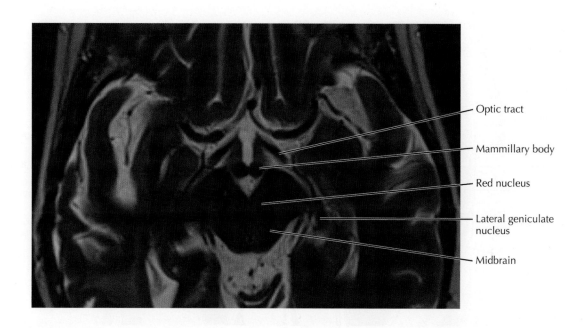

Optic tract

Mammillary body

Red nucleus

Lateral geniculate
nucleus

Midbrain

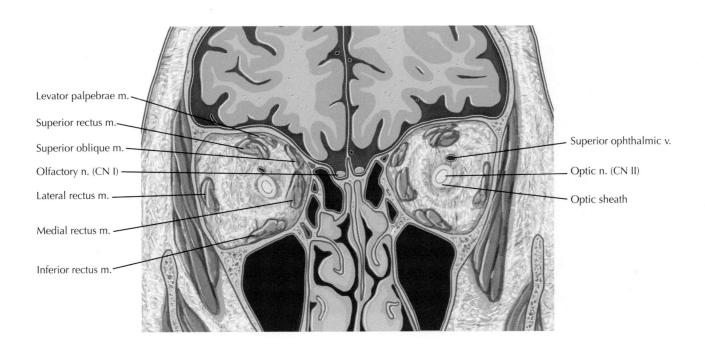

Levator palpebrae m.

Superior rectus m.

Superior oblique m.

Olfactory n. (CN I)

Lateral rectus m.

Medial rectus m.

Inferior rectus m.

Superior ophthalmic v.

Optic n. (CN II)

Optic sheath

DIAGNOSTIC CONSIDERATION

The coronal plane is often the best imaging plane to assess the optic nerve (CN II). Note the ring of cerebrospinal fluid around the optic nerves. As an extension of the brain and dura, the optic nerve sheath complex is subject to the same pathology, such as a glioma of the optic nerves or meningioma of the surrounding dural sheath. This coronal plane is often the best plane to identify a mass arising from the sheath and compressing the optic nerve, versus an expansion of the optic nerve.

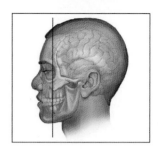

Levator palpebrae m.

Superior rectus m.

Superior oblique m.

Olfactory n. (CN I)

Lateral rectus m.

Medial rectus m.

Inferior rectus m.

Superior
ophthalmic v.

Optic n. (CN II)

Optic sheath

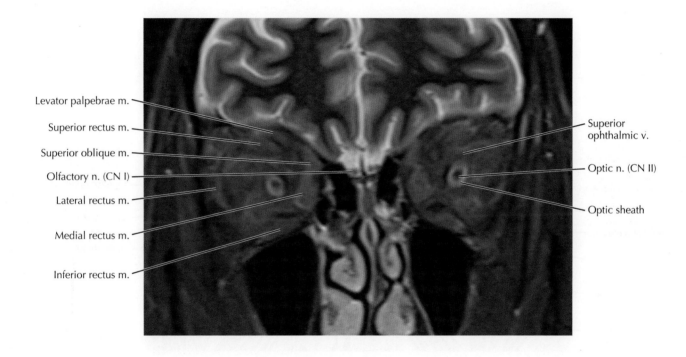

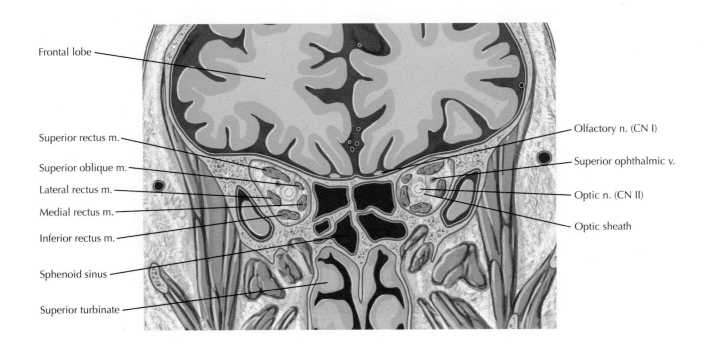

Frontal lobe

Superior rectus m.

Superior oblique m.

Lateral rectus m.

Medial rectus m.

Inferior rectus m.

Sphenoid sinus

Superior turbinate

Olfactory n. (CN I)

Superior ophthalmic v.

Optic n. (CN II)

Optic sheath

NORMAL ANATOMY

Note the superior ophthalmic vein above the optic nerve. Abnormal shunting of arterial blood into the cavernous sinus, as in a post-traumatic carotid cavernous fistula (CCF), will cause enlargement of the superior ophthalmic vein.

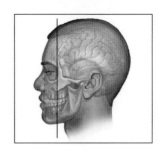

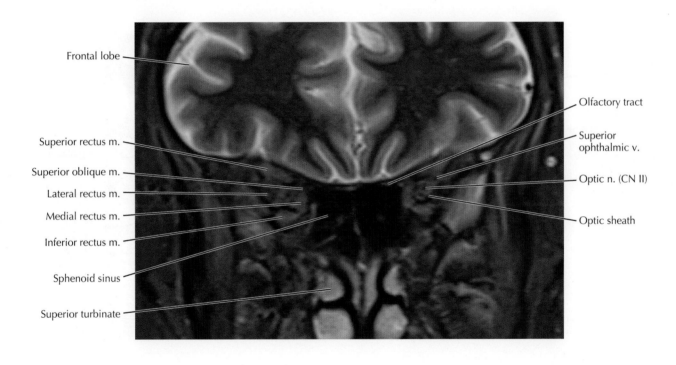

Frontal lobe

Superior rectus m.

Superior oblique m.

Lateral rectus m.

Medial rectus m.

Inferior rectus m.

Sphenoid sinus

Superior turbinate

Olfactory tract

Superior ophthalmic v.

Optic n. (CN II)

Optic sheath

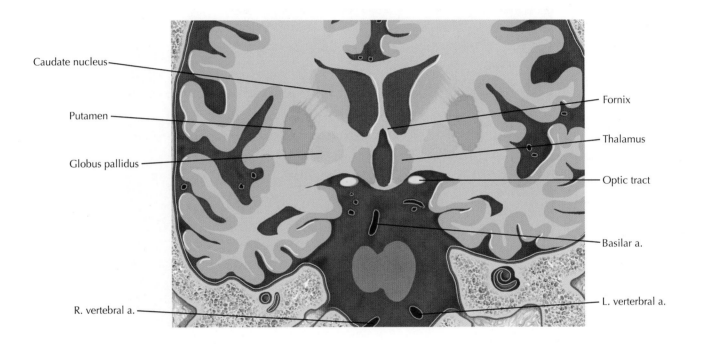

Caudate nucleus

Putamen

Globus pallidus

Fornix

Thalamus

Optic tract

Basilar a.

R. vertebral a.

L. verterbral a.

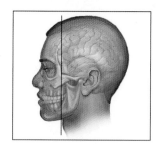

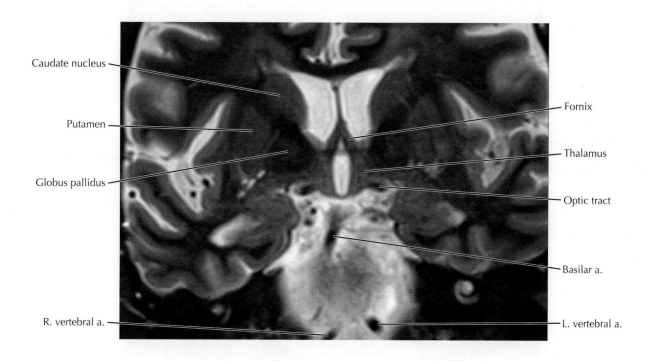

Caudate nucleus

Putamen

Globus pallidus

Fornix

Thalamus

Optic tract

Basilar a.

R. vertebral a.

L. vertebral a.

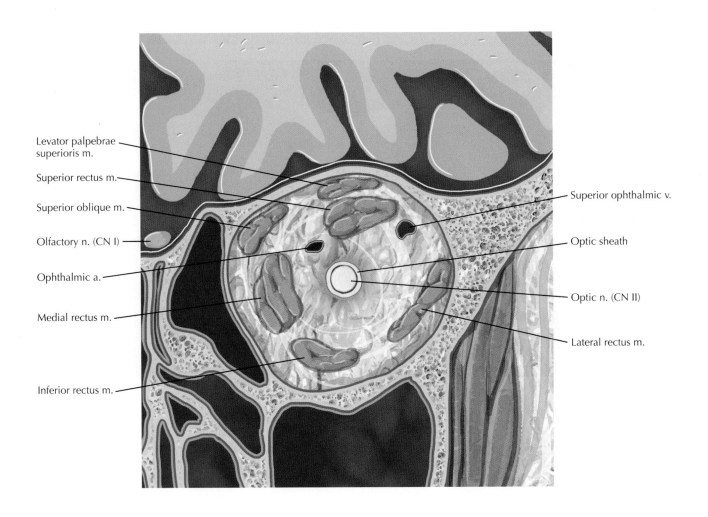

Levator palpebrae superioris m.

Superior rectus m.

Superior oblique m.

Olfactory n. (CN I)

Ophthalmic a.

Medial rectus m.

Inferior rectus m.

Superior ophthalmic v.

Optic sheath

Optic n. (CN II)

Lateral rectus m.

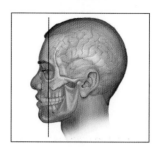

Levator palpebrae
superioris m.

Superior rectus m.

Superior oblique m.

Ophthalmic a.

Medial rectus m.

Inferior rectus m.

Superior ophthalmic v.

Optic sheath

Optic n. (CN II)

Lateral rectus m.

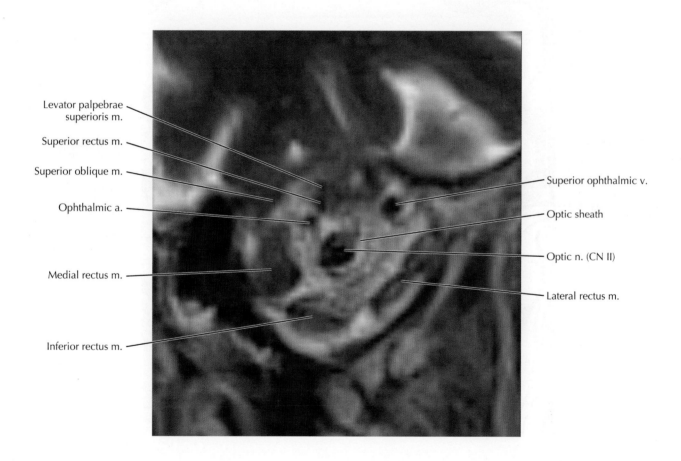

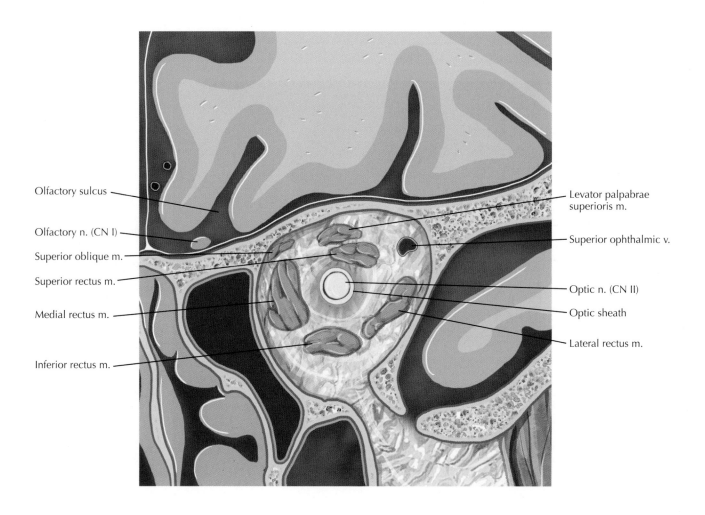

Olfactory sulcus

Olfactory n. (CN I)

Superior oblique m.

Superior rectus m.

Medial rectus m.

Inferior rectus m.

Levator palpabrae superioris m.

Superior ophthalmic v.

Optic n. (CN II)

Optic sheath

Lateral rectus m.

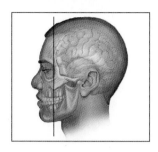

Olfactory sulcus

Olfactory n. (CN I)

Superior oblique m.

Superior rectus m.

Medial rectus m.

Inferior rectus m.

Levator palpabrae superioris m.

Superior ophthalmic v.

Optic n. (CN II)

Optic sheath

Lateral rectus m.

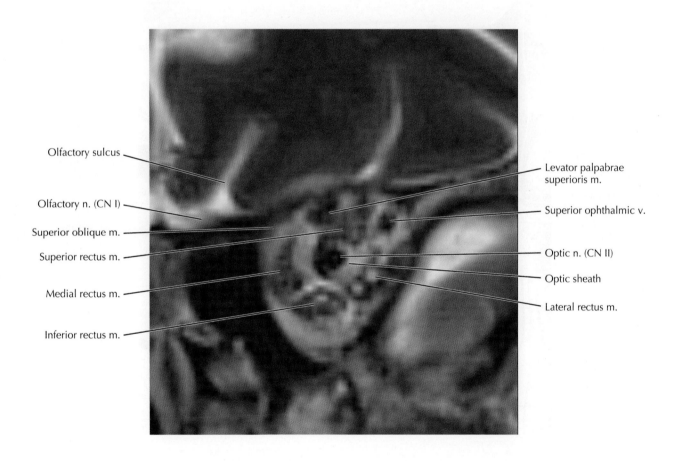

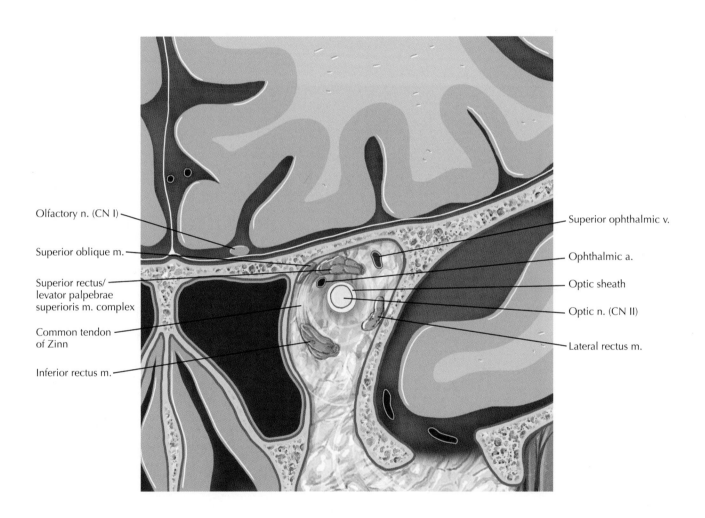

Olfactory n. (CN I)

Superior oblique m.

Superior rectus/
levator palpebrae
superioris m. complex

Common tendon
of Zinn

Inferior rectus m.

Superior ophthalmic v.

Ophthalmic a.

Optic sheath

Optic n. (CN II)

Lateral rectus m.

DIAGNOSTIC CONSIDERATION

As the optic nerve passes posteriorly in the orbit toward the apex, it is often difficult to separate the nerve from the surrounding orbital muscles and bony walls of the apex. Subtle lesions may be detected best on a coronal oblique image aligned perpendicular to the optic nerve, as seen in this image.

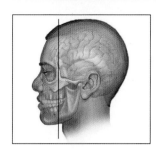

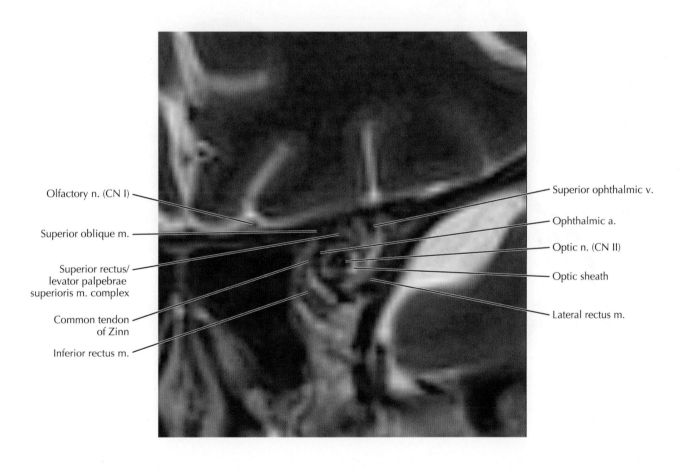

Olfactory n. (CN I)

Superior oblique m.

Superior rectus/
levator palpebrae
superioris m. complex

Common tendon
of Zinn

Inferior rectus m.

Superior ophthalmic v.

Ophthalmic a.

Optic n. (CN II)

Optic sheath

Lateral rectus m.

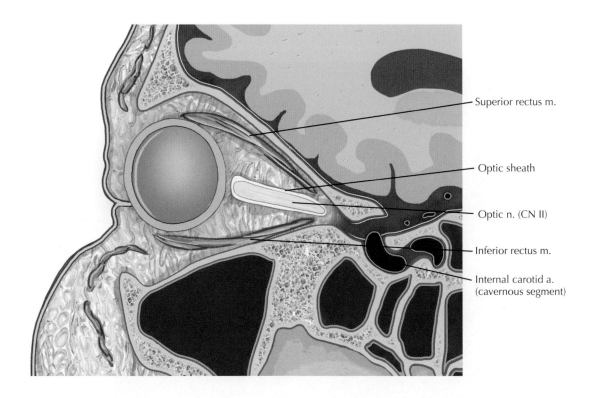

Superior rectus m.

Optic sheath

Optic n. (CN II)

Inferior rectus m.

Internal carotid a.
(cavernous segment)

NORMAL ANATOMY

Pathology, such as a posterior cerebral infarct involving the left occipital lobe, may result in a right-sided visual field deficit in each eye.

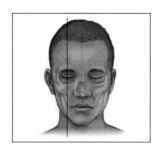

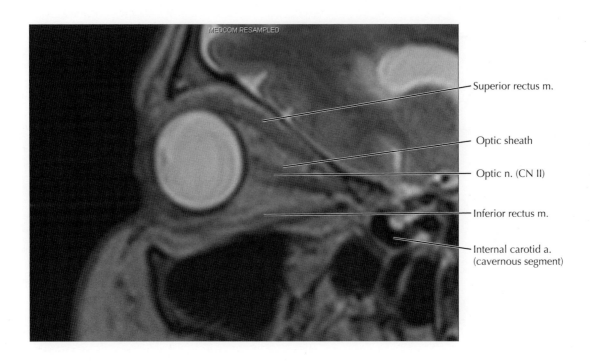

- Superior rectus m.

- Optic sheath

- Optic n. (CN II)

- Inferior rectus m.

- Internal carotid a. (cavernous segment)

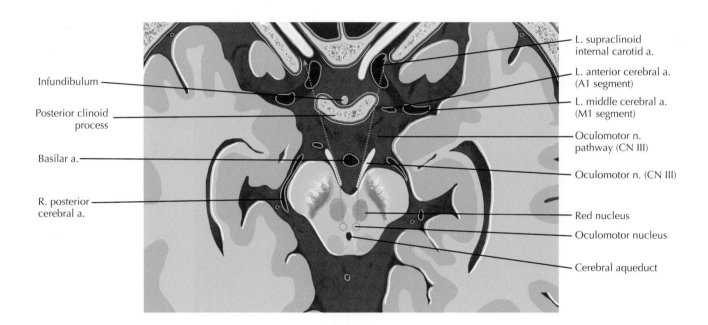

Infundibulum

Posterior clinoid process

Basilar a.

R. posterior cerebral a.

L. supraclinoid internal carotid a.

L. anterior cerebral a. (A1 segment)

L. middle cerebral a. (M1 segment)

Oculomotor n. pathway (CN III)

Oculomotor n. (CN III)

Red nucleus

Oculomotor nucleus

Cerebral aqueduct

NORMAL ANATOMY

The oculomotor nerve (CN III) is the third of the 12 pairs of cranial nerves. CN III arises from two nuclei. The *oculomotor nucleus* originates at the level of the superior colliculus and controls the striated muscle in the levator palpebrae superioris and all extraocular muscles, except the superior oblique and lateral rectus muscles (see also Optic Coronal 6). *Edinger-Westphal (accessory oculomotor) nuclei* supply parasympathetic fibers to the eye through the ciliary ganglia and control the sphincter pupillae muscle for pupil constriction and the ciliary muscle for accommodation.

Fibers for the oculomotor nerve pass anteriorly from the oculomotor nucleus through the red nucleus and substantia nigra and exit the brainstem at the interpeduncular fossa.

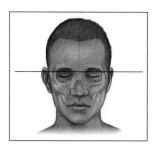

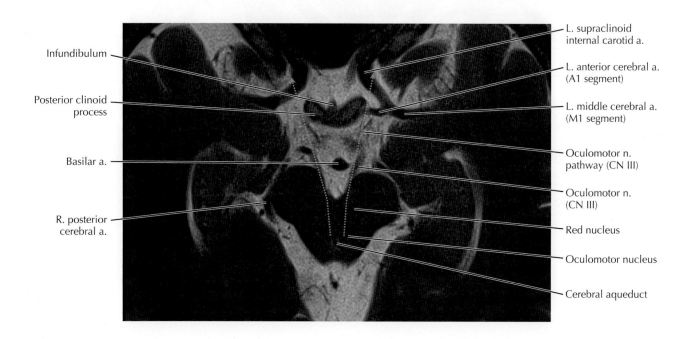

Infundibulum

Posterior clinoid process

Basilar a.

R. posterior cerebral a.

L. supraclinoid internal carotid a.

L. anterior cerebral a. (A1 segment)

L. middle cerebral a. (M1 segment)

Oculomotor n. pathway (CN III)

Oculomotor n. (CN III)

Red nucleus

Oculomotor nucleus

Cerebral aqueduct

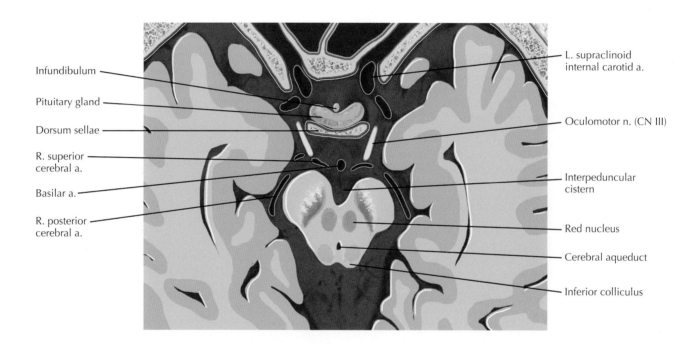

Infundibulum

Pituitary gland

Dorsum sellae

R. superior
cerebral a.

Basilar a.

R. posterior
cerebral a.

L. supraclinoid
internal carotid a.

Oculomotor n. (CN III)

Interpeduncular
cistern

Red nucleus

Cerebral aqueduct

Inferior colliculus

PATHOLOGIC PROCESS

The cisternal segment of the oculomotor nerve is intimately associated with blood vessels of the circle of Willis. After exiting the brainstem, CN III passes anteriorly between the posterior cerebral and superior cerebellar arteries and parallels the posterior communicating artery before entering the cavernous sinus. An aneurysm arising from the origin of the posterior communicating artery off the internal carotid artery classically causes compression of CN III, leading to oculomotor nerve palsy.

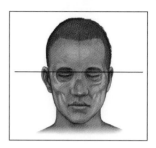

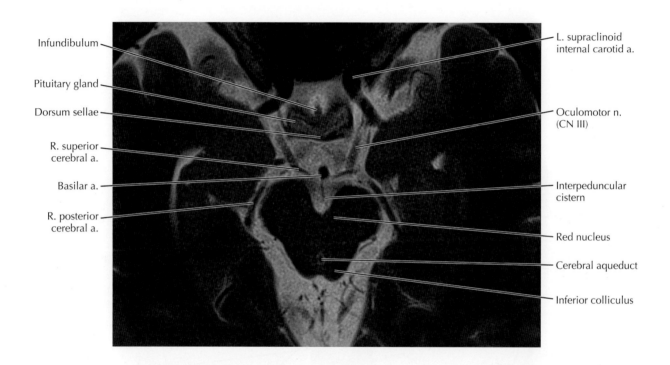

Infundibulum

Pituitary gland

Dorsum sellae

R. superior
cerebral a.

Basilar a.

R. posterior
cerebral a.

L. supraclinoid
internal carotid a.

Oculomotor n.
(CN III)

Interpeduncular
cistern

Red nucleus

Cerebral aqueduct

Inferior colliculus

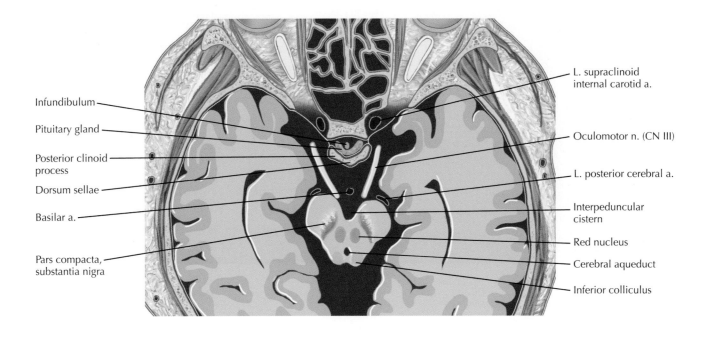

Infundibulum

Pituitary gland

Posterior clinoid process

Dorsum sellae

Basilar a.

Pars compacta, substantia nigra

L. supraclinoid internal carotid a.

Oculomotor n. (CN III)

L. posterior cerebral a.

Interpeduncular cistern

Red nucleus

Cerebral aqueduct

Inferior colliculus

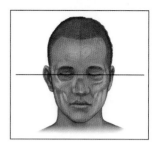

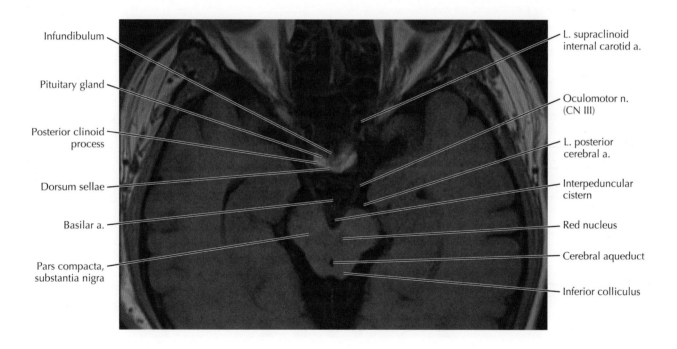

Infundibulum

Pituitary gland

Posterior clinoid process

Dorsum sellae

Basilar a.

Pars compacta, substantia nigra

L. supraclinoid internal carotid a.

Oculomotor n. (CN III)

L. posterior cerebral a.

Interpeduncular cistern

Red nucleus

Cerebral aqueduct

Inferior colliculus

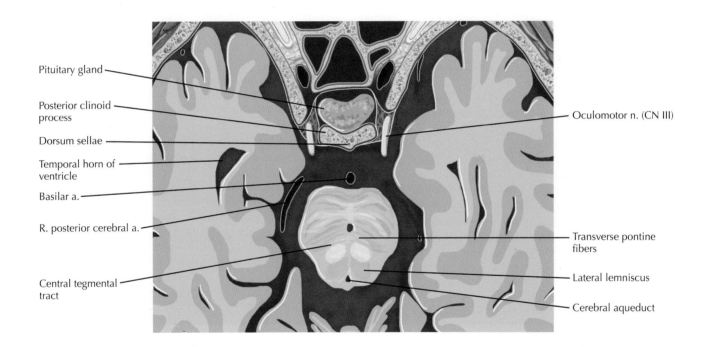

Pituitary gland

Posterior clinoid process

Dorsum sellae

Temporal horn of ventricle

Basilar a.

R. posterior cerebral a.

Central tegmental tract

Oculomotor n. (CN III)

Transverse pontine fibers

Lateral lemniscus

Cerebral aqueduct

NORMAL ANATOMY

Note there is an incidental tiny cyst in the middle of the pons on this image. The aqueduct is located more posteriorly.

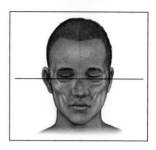

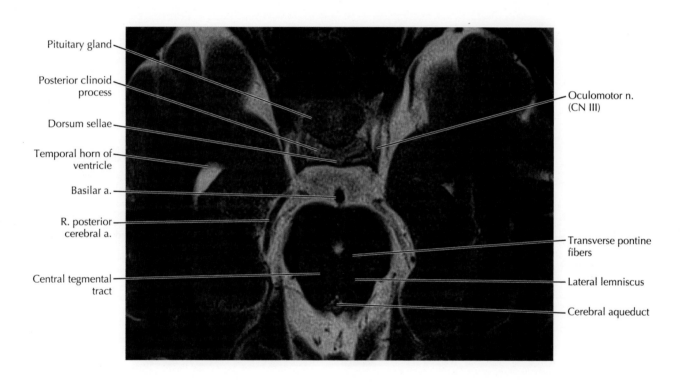

Pituitary gland

Posterior clinoid process

Dorsum sellae

Temporal horn of ventricle

Basilar a.

R. posterior cerebral a.

Central tegmental tract

Oculomotor n. (CN III)

Transverse pontine fibers

Lateral lemniscus

Cerebral aqueduct

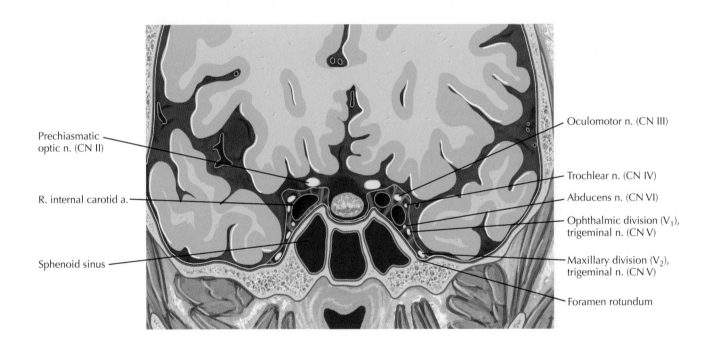

Prechiasmatic optic n. (CN II)

R. internal carotid a.

Sphenoid sinus

Oculomotor n. (CN III)

Trochlear n. (CN IV)

Abducens n. (CN VI)

Ophthalmic division (V₁), trigeminal n. (CN V)

Maxillary division (V₂), trigeminal n. (CN V)

Foramen rotundum

NORMAL ANATOMY

The oculomotor nerve (CN III) is the most superior of the cranial nerves in the cavernous sinus.

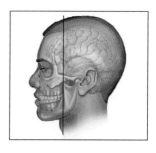

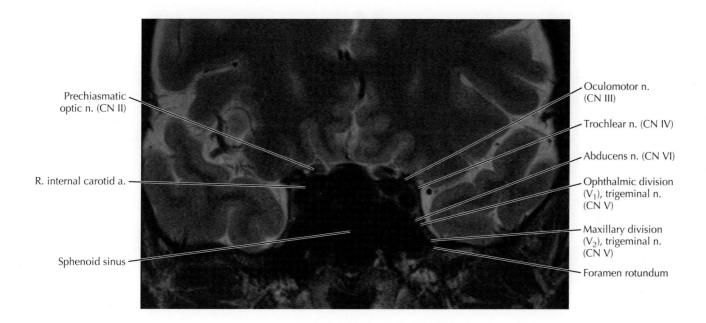

Prechiasmatic optic n. (CN II)

Oculomotor n. (CN III)

Trochlear n. (CN IV)

Abducens n. (CN VI)

R. internal carotid a.

Ophthalmic division (V$_1$), trigeminal n. (CN V)

Maxillary division (V$_2$), trigeminal n. (CN V)

Sphenoid sinus

Foramen rotundum

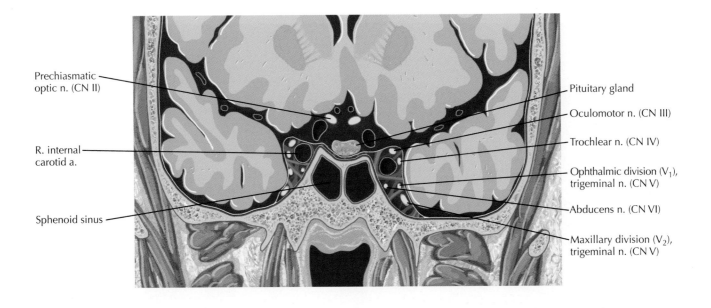

Prechiasmatic optic n. (CN II)

R. internal carotid a.

Sphenoid sinus

Pituitary gland

Oculomotor n. (CN III)

Trochlear n. (CN IV)

Ophthalmic division (V₁), trigeminal n. (CN V)

Abducens n. (CN VI)

Maxillary division (V₂), trigeminal n. (CN V)

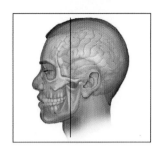

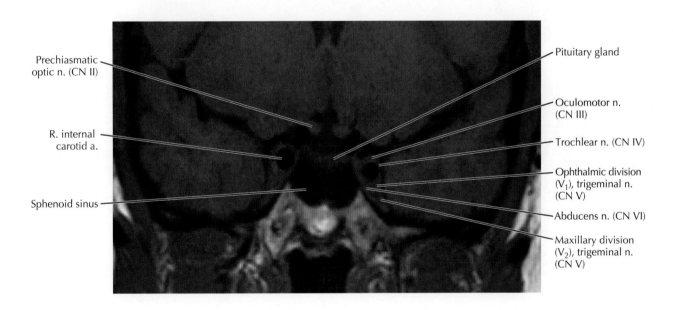

Prechiasmatic optic n. (CN II)

R. internal carotid a.

Sphenoid sinus

Pituitary gland

Oculomotor n. (CN III)

Trochlear n. (CN IV)

Ophthalmic division (V₁), trigeminal n. (CN V)

Abducens n. (CN VI)

Maxillary division (V₂), trigeminal n. (CN V)

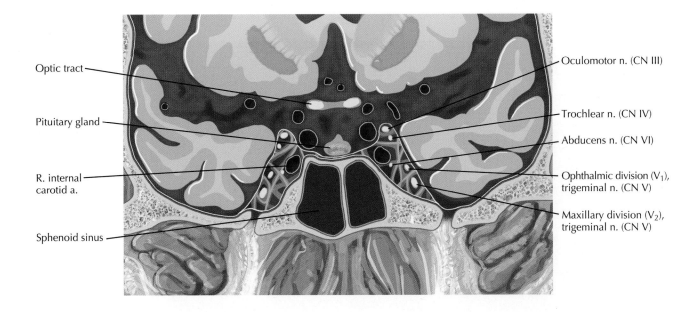

Optic tract

Pituitary gland

R. internal
carotid a.

Sphenoid sinus

Oculomotor n. (CN III)

Trochlear n. (CN IV)

Abducens n. (CN VI)

Ophthalmic division (V_1),
trigeminal n. (CN V)

Maxillary division (V_2),
trigeminal n. (CN V)

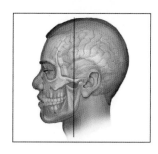

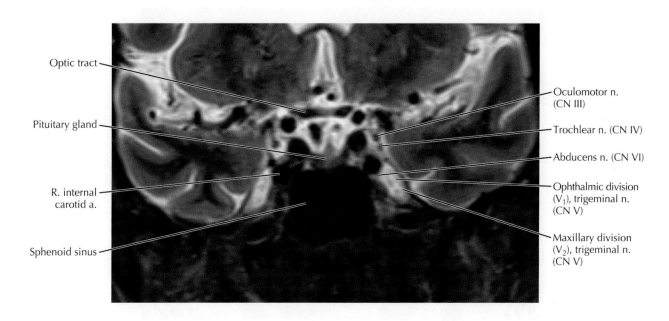

Optic tract

Pituitary gland

R. internal carotid a.

Sphenoid sinus

Oculomotor n. (CN III)

Trochlear n. (CN IV)

Abducens n. (CN VI)

Ophthalmic division (V₁), trigeminal n. (CN V)

Maxillary division (V₂), trigeminal n. (CN V)

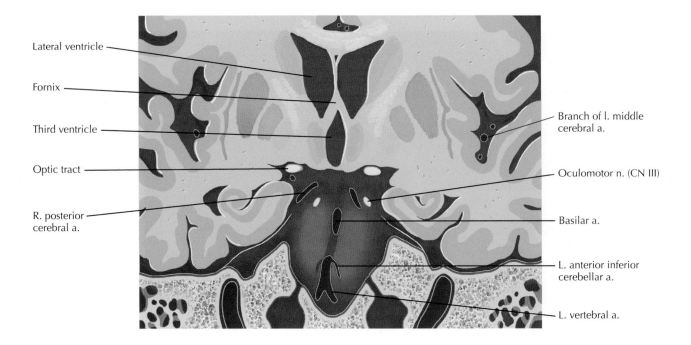

Lateral ventricle

Fornix

Third ventricle

Optic tract

R. posterior
cerebral a.

Branch of l. middle
cerebral a.

Oculomotor n. (CN III)

Basilar a.

L. anterior inferior
cerebellar a.

L. vertebral a.

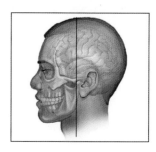

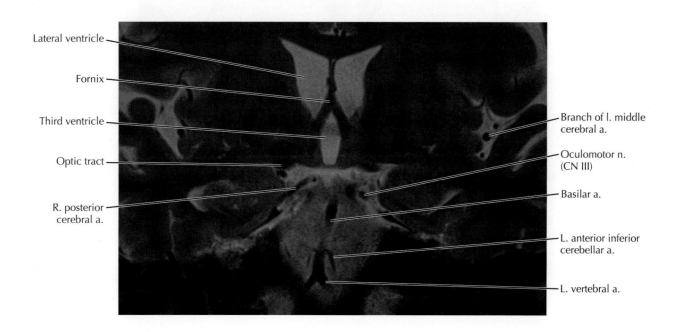

Lateral ventricle

Fornix

Third ventricle

Optic tract

R. posterior
cerebral a.

Branch of l. middle
cerebral a.

Oculomotor n.
(CN III)

Basilar a.

L. anterior inferior
cerebellar a.

L. vertebral a.

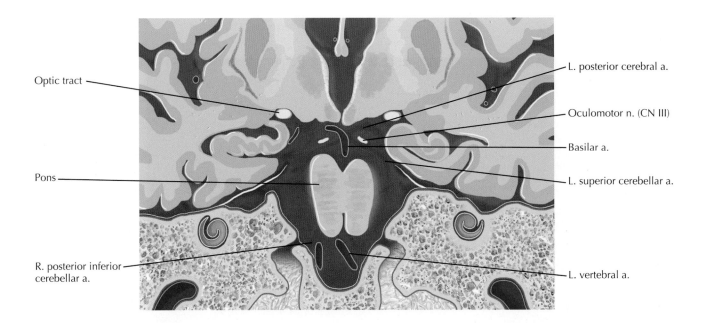

Optic tract

Pons

R. posterior inferior cerebellar a.

L. posterior cerebral a.

Oculomotor n. (CN III)

Basilar a.

L. superior cerebellar a.

L. vertebral a.

NORMAL ANATOMY

Note the oculomotor nerve passing between the posterior cerebral artery and superior cerebellar artery.

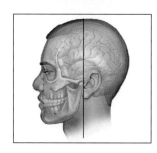

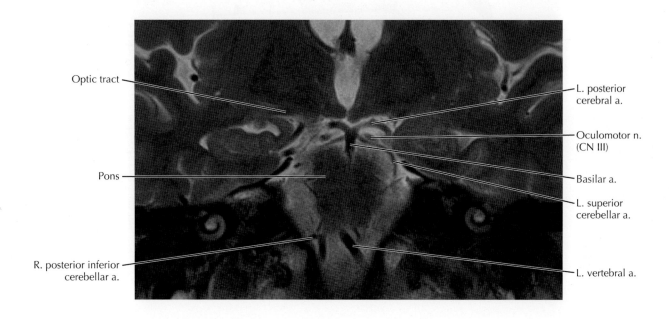

Optic tract

Pons

R. posterior inferior
cerebellar a.

L. posterior
cerebral a.

Oculomotor n.
(CN III)

Basilar a.

L. superior
cerebellar a.

L. vertebral a.

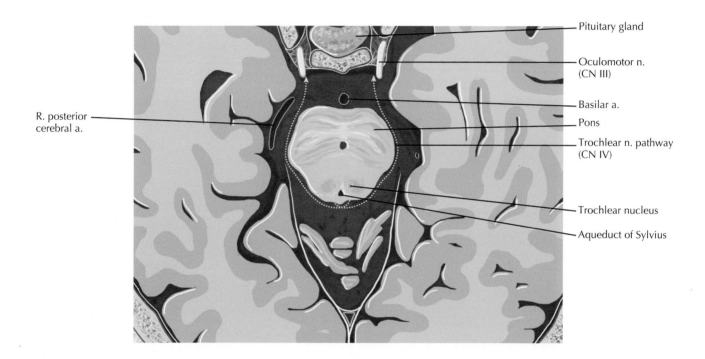

Pituitary gland

Oculomotor n. (CN III)

Basilar a.

Pons

Trochlear n. pathway (CN IV)

Trochlear nucleus

Aqueduct of Sylvius

R. posterior cerebral a.

NORMAL ANATOMY

The trochlear nerve (fourth cranial, CN IV) is a motor nerve innervating the superior oblique muscle of the orbit. Contraction of this muscle will point the eye medially and inferiorly toward the tip of the nose. CN IV is the thinnest cranial nerve but the longest intracranially, the only cranial nerve to exit the brainstem dorsally. The trochlear nerve is also the only cranial nerve to cross the midline posterior to the brainstem, with the medial fibers of the optic nerve the only other cranial nerve to cross the midline.

The tiny incidental cyst in the middle of the pons in this axial MR image is not the aqueduct of Sylvius (cerebral aqueduct), which can be seen between the trochlear nuclei. The dark signal in the middle of the aqueduct is caused by CSF flow.

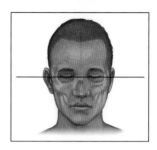

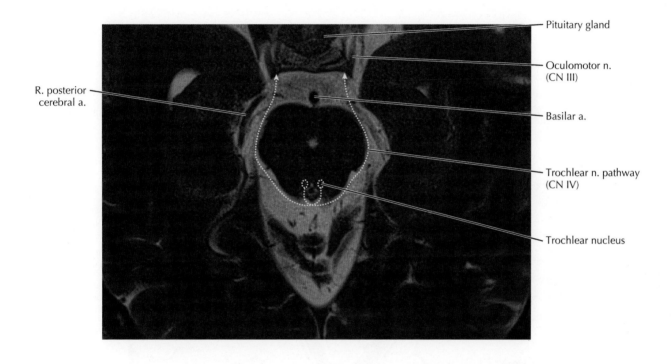

Pituitary gland

Oculomotor n.
(CN III)

R. posterior
cerebral a.

Basilar a.

Trochlear n. pathway
(CN IV)

Trochlear nucleus

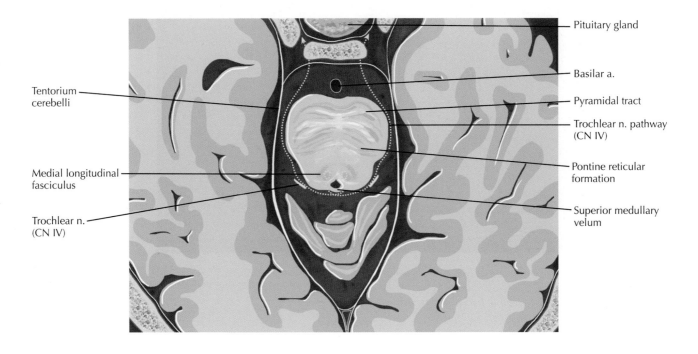

Pituitary gland

Basilar a.

Pyramidal tract

Trochlear n. pathway
(CN IV)

Pontine reticular
formation

Superior medullary
velum

Tentorium
cerebelli

Medial longitudinal
fasciculus

Trochlear n.
(CN IV)

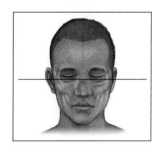

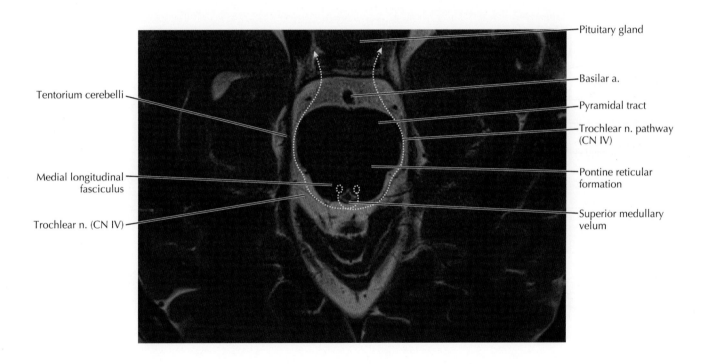

Pituitary gland

Basilar a.

Pyramidal tract

Trochlear n. pathway (CN IV)

Pontine reticular formation

Superior medullary velum

Tentorium cerebelli

Medial longitudinal fasciculus

Trochlear n. (CN IV)

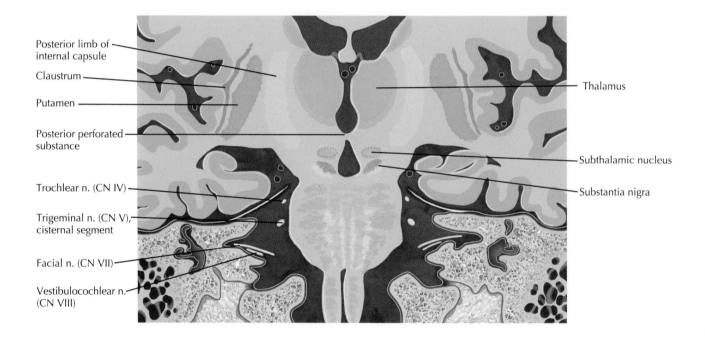

Posterior limb of internal capsule

Claustrum

Putamen

Posterior perforated substance

Trochlear n. (CN IV)

Trigeminal n. (CN V), cisternal segment

Facial n. (CN VII)

Vestibulocochlear n. (CN VIII)

Thalamus

Subthalamic nucleus

Substantia nigra

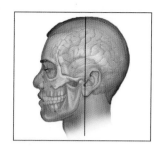

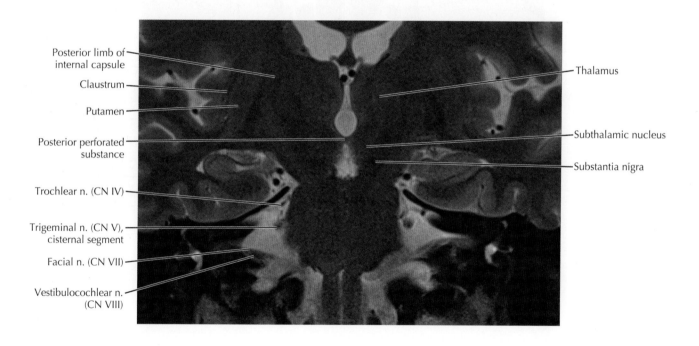

Posterior limb of internal capsule

Claustrum

Putamen

Posterior perforated substance

Trochlear n. (CN IV)

Trigeminal n. (CN V), cisternal segment

Facial n. (CN VII)

Vestibulocochlear n. (CN VIII)

Thalamus

Subthalamic nucleus

Substantia nigra

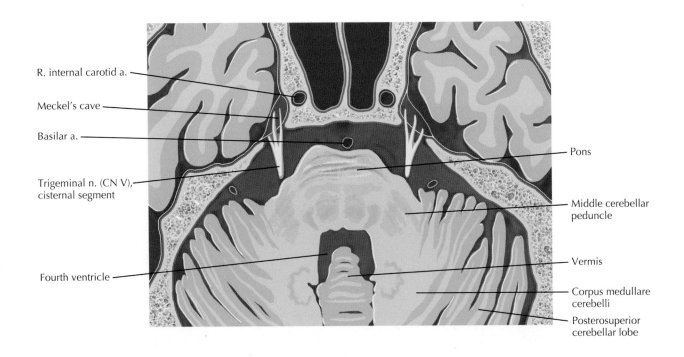

R. internal carotid a.

Meckel's cave

Basilar a.

Trigeminal n. (CN V), cisternal segment

Fourth ventricle

Pons

Middle cerebellar peduncle

Vermis

Corpus medullare cerebelli

Posterosuperior cerebellar lobe

NORMAL ANATOMY

The trigeminal nerve (fifth cranial, CN V) is named for its three major branches: ophthalmic (V_1), maxillary (V_2), and mandibular (V_3). CN V innervates sensation of the face and the muscles of mastication; V_1 and V_2 branches are cutaneous sensory nerves only, whereas V_3 has cutaneous sensory and motor functions.

The trigeminal nerve is the largest of the cranial nerves, and its cisternal segment has a fan-shaped appearance on axial imaging as it courses from the brainstem to Meckel's cave. The ganglion within Meckel's cave is called the *trigeminal*, or Gasserian, *ganglion*. Meckel's ganglion along V_2 is located within the pterygopalatine fossa more anteriorly (see also Trigeminal Axial 9).

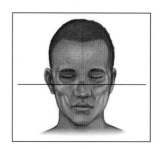

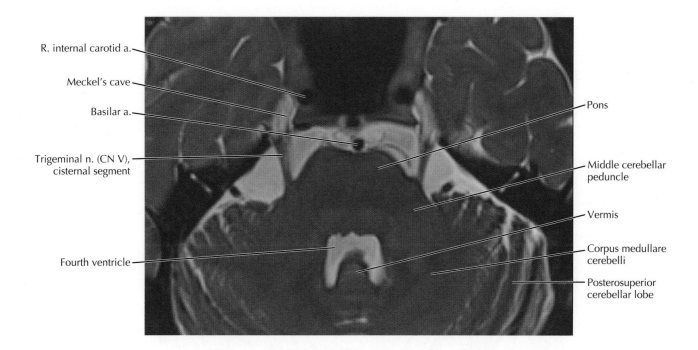

R. internal carotid a.

Meckel's cave

Basilar a.

Trigeminal n. (CN V),
cisternal segment

Fourth ventricle

Pons

Middle cerebellar
peduncle

Vermis

Corpus medullare
cerebelli

Posterosuperior
cerebellar lobe

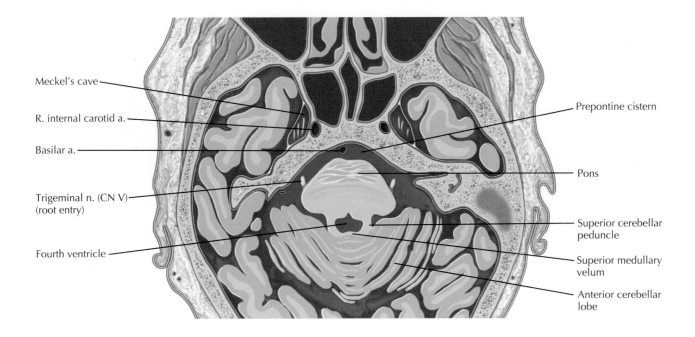

Meckel's cave

R. internal carotid a.

Basilar a.

Trigeminal n. (CN V)
(root entry)

Fourth ventricle

Prepontine cistern

Pons

Superior cerebellar
peduncle

Superior medullary
velum

Anterior cerebellar
lobe

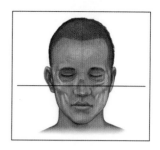

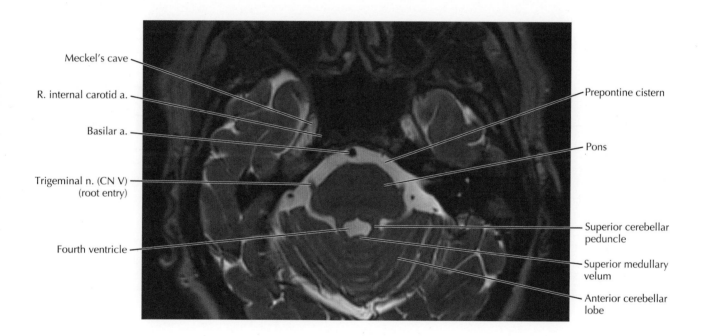

Meckel's cave

R. internal carotid a.

Basilar a.

Trigeminal n. (CN V)
(root entry)

Fourth ventricle

Prepontine cistern

Pons

Superior cerebellar
peduncle

Superior medullary
velum

Anterior cerebellar
lobe

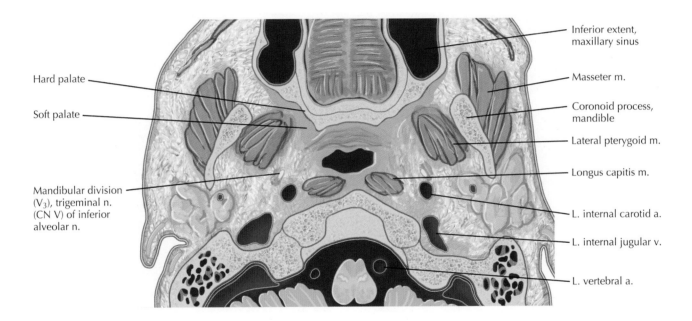

Hard palate

Soft palate

Mandibular division (V₃), trigeminal n. (CN V) of inferior alveolar n.

Inferior extent, maxillary sinus

Masseter m.

Coronoid process, mandible

Lateral pterygoid m.

Longus capitis m.

L. internal carotid a.

L. internal jugular v.

L. vertebral a.

NORMAL ANATOMY

The mandibular branch (V_3) of the trigeminal nerve arises from the trigeminal ganglion and descends vertically out of the skull through the foramen ovale.

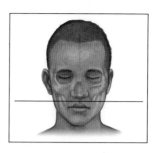

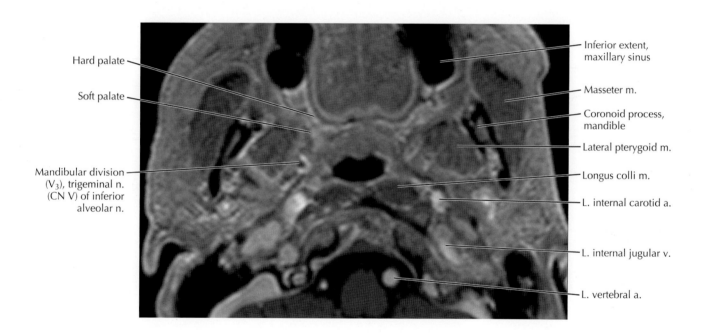

Hard palate

Soft palate

Mandibular division
(V₃), trigeminal n.
(CN V) of inferior
alveolar n.

Inferior extent,
maxillary sinus

Masseter m.

Coronoid process,
mandible

Lateral pterygoid m.

Longus colli m.

L. internal carotid a.

L. internal jugular v.

L. vertebral a.

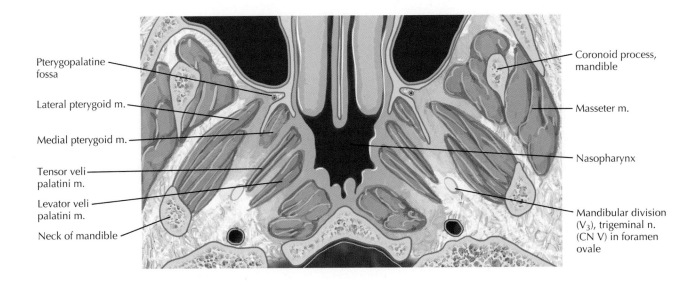

Pterygopalatine fossa

Lateral pterygoid m.

Medial pterygoid m.

Tensor veli palatini m.

Levator veli palatini m.

Neck of mandible

Coronoid process, mandible

Masseter m.

Nasopharynx

Mandibular division (V₃), trigeminal n. (CN V) in foramen ovale

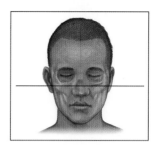

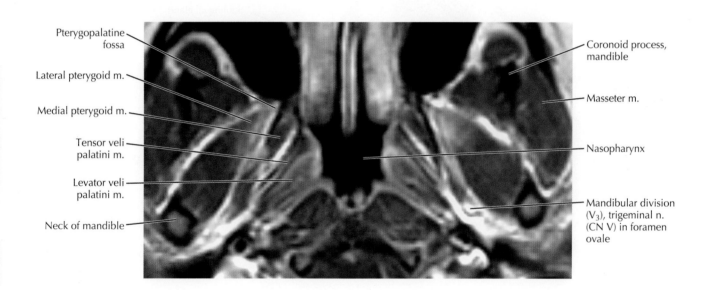

Pterygopalatine fossa

Lateral pterygoid m.

Medial pterygoid m.

Tensor veli palatini m.

Levator veli palatini m.

Neck of mandible

Coronoid process, mandible

Masseter m.

Nasopharynx

Mandibular division (V₃), trigeminal n. (CN V) in foramen ovale

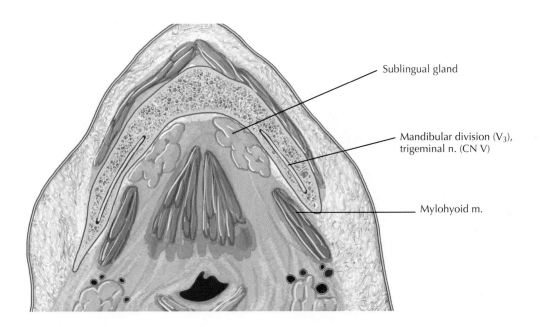

Sublingual gland

Mandibular division (V₃),
trigeminal n. (CN V)

Mylohyoid m.

NORMAL ANATOMY

The mandibular branch (V₃) of the trigeminal nerve gives rise to the alveolar nerve, a sensory branch that courses through the alveolar canal in the mandible and exits the mental foramen into the subcutaneous tissues. A squamous cell carcinoma along the alveolar ridge of the teeth can invade the mandible and infiltrate the mandibular nerve.

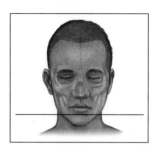

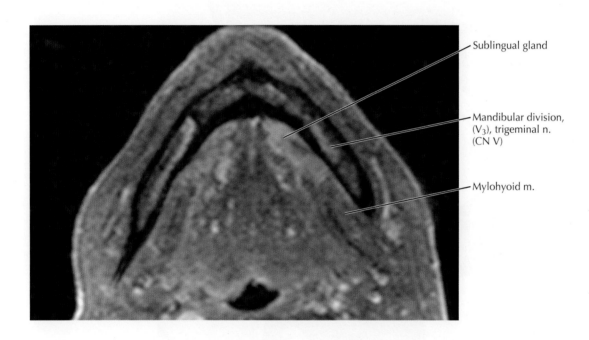

Sublingual gland

Mandibular division, (V₃), trigeminal n. (CN V)

Mylohyoid m.

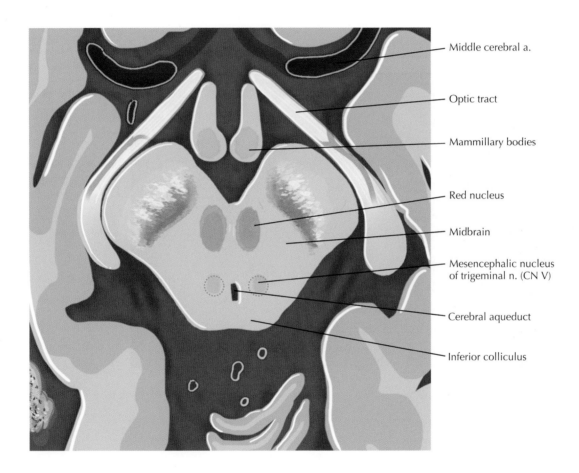

Middle cerebral a.

Optic tract

Mammillary bodies

Red nucleus

Midbrain

Mesencephalic nucleus
of trigeminal n. (CN V)

Cerebral aqueduct

Inferior colliculus

NORMAL ANATOMY

The mesencephalic nucleus of the trigeminal nerve senses the location of the jaw. This nucleus usually is not discernible on MRI.

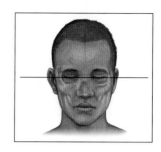

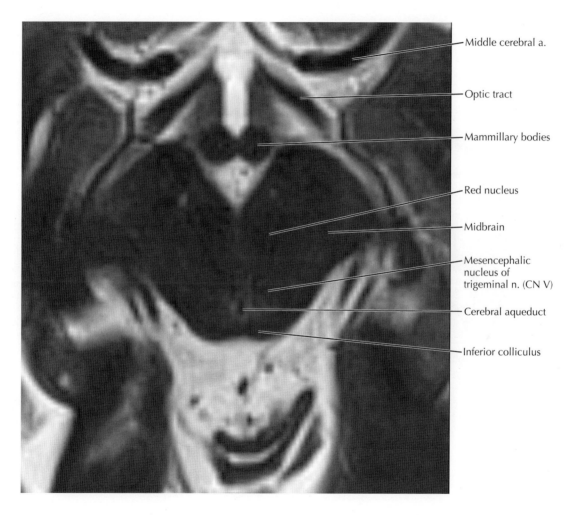

Middle cerebral a.

Optic tract

Mammillary bodies

Red nucleus

Midbrain

Mesencephalic
nucleus of
trigeminal n. (CN V)

Cerebral aqueduct

Inferior colliculus

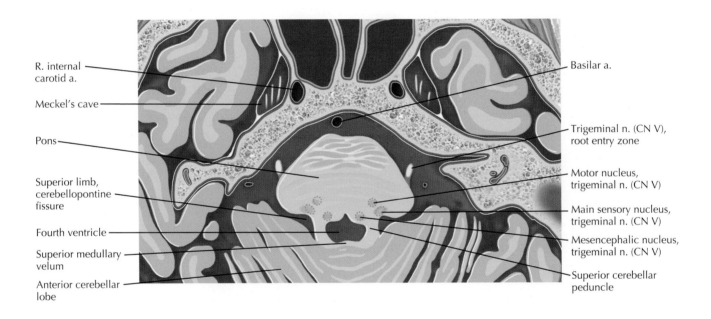

R. internal
carotid a.

Meckel's cave

Pons

Superior limb,
cerebellopontine
fissure

Fourth ventricle

Superior medullary
velum

Anterior cerebellar
lobe

Basilar a.

Trigeminal n. (CN V),
root entry zone

Motor nucleus,
trigeminal n. (CN V)

Main sensory nucleus,
trigeminal n. (CN V)

Mesencephalic nucleus,
trigeminal n. (CN V)

Superior cerebellar
peduncle

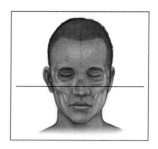

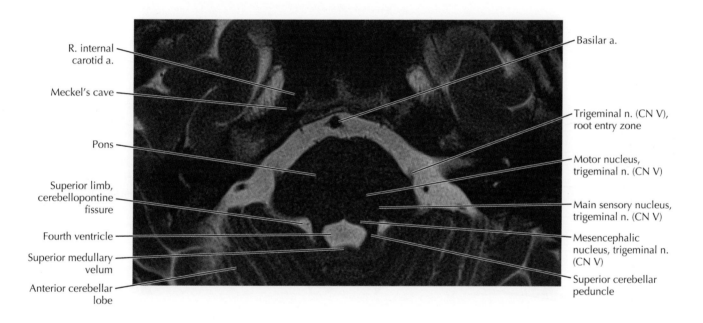

R. internal carotid a.

Meckel's cave

Pons

Superior limb, cerebellopontine fissure

Fourth ventricle

Superior medullary velum

Anterior cerebellar lobe

Basilar a.

Trigeminal n. (CN V), root entry zone

Motor nucleus, trigeminal n. (CN V)

Main sensory nucleus, trigeminal n. (CN V)

Mesencephalic nucleus, trigeminal n. (CN V)

Superior cerebellar peduncle

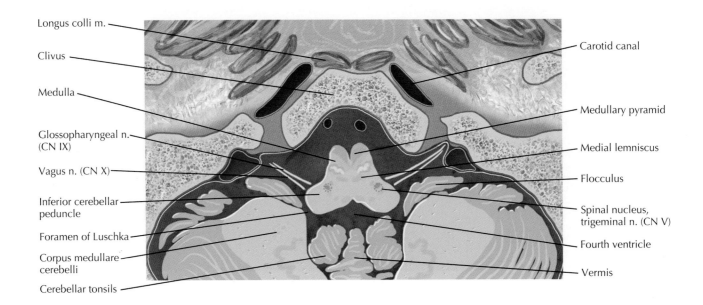

Longus colli m.

Clivus

Medulla

Glossopharyngeal n.
(CN IX)

Vagus n. (CN X)

Inferior cerebellar
peduncle

Foramen of Luschka

Corpus medullare
cerebelli

Cerebellar tonsils

Carotid canal

Medullary pyramid

Medial lemniscus

Flocculus

Spinal nucleus,
trigeminal n. (CN V)

Fourth ventricle

Vermis

NORMAL ANATOMY

The spinal nucleus of the trigeminal nerve receives pain and temperature sensation from the face.

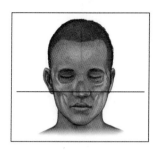

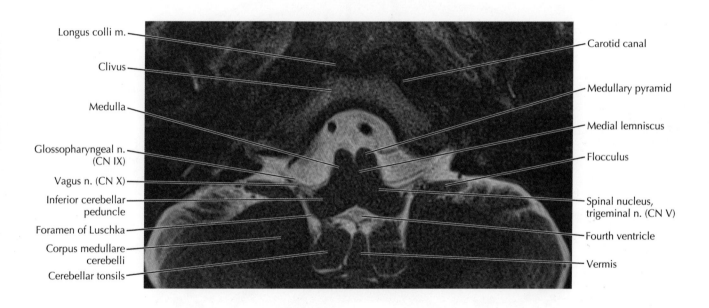

Longus colli m.

Clivus

Medulla

Glossopharyngeal n.
(CN IX)

Vagus n. (CN X)

Inferior cerebellar
peduncle

Foramen of Luschka

Corpus medullare
cerebelli

Cerebellar tonsils

Carotid canal

Medullary pyramid

Medial lemniscus

Flocculus

Spinal nucleus,
trigeminal n. (CN V)

Fourth ventricle

Vermis

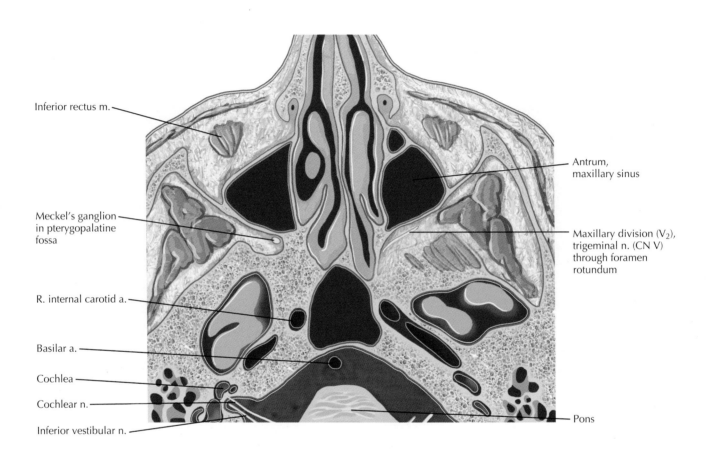

Inferior rectus m.

Meckel's ganglion in pterygopalatine fossa

R. internal carotid a.

Basilar a.

Cochlea

Cochlear n.

Inferior vestibular n.

Antrum, maxillary sinus

Maxillary division (V₂), trigeminal n. (CN V) through foramen rotundum

Pons

DIAGNOSTIC CONSIDERATION

Loss of normally bright T1-weighted fat signal in the pterygopalatine fossa can be a sign of perineural invasion from the face.

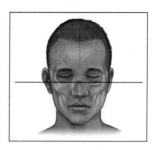

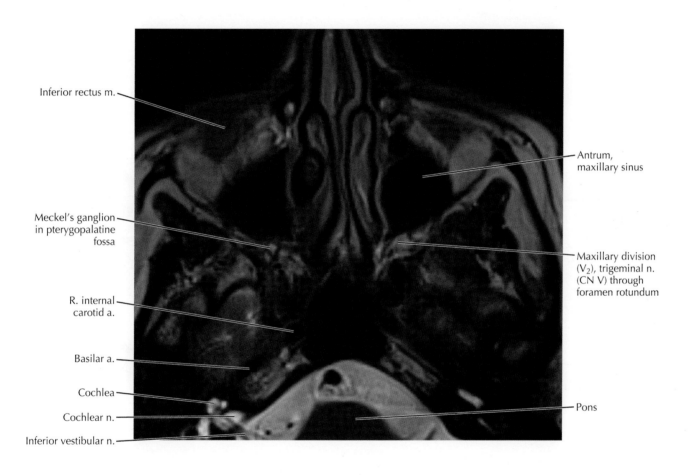

Inferior rectus m.

Antrum, maxillary sinus

Meckel's ganglion in pterygopalatine fossa

Maxillary division (V$_2$), trigeminal n. (CN V) through foramen rotundum

R. internal carotid a.

Basilar a.

Cochlea

Cochlear n.

Pons

Inferior vestibular n.

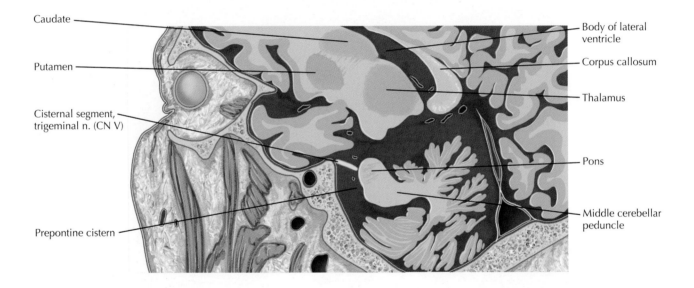

Caudate

Putamen

Cisternal segment,
trigeminal n. (CN V)

Prepontine cistern

Body of lateral
ventricle

Corpus callosum

Thalamus

Pons

Middle cerebellar
peduncle

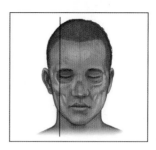

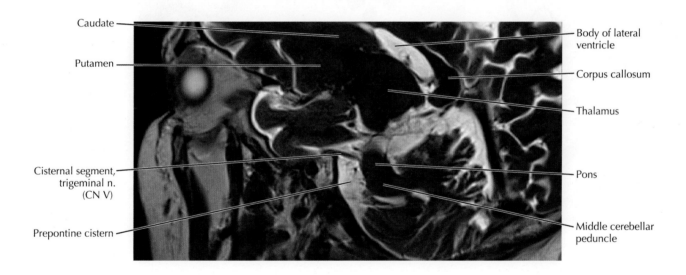

Caudate

Putamen

Cisternal segment, trigeminal n. (CN V)

Prepontine cistern

Body of lateral ventricle

Corpus callosum

Thalamus

Pons

Middle cerebellar peduncle

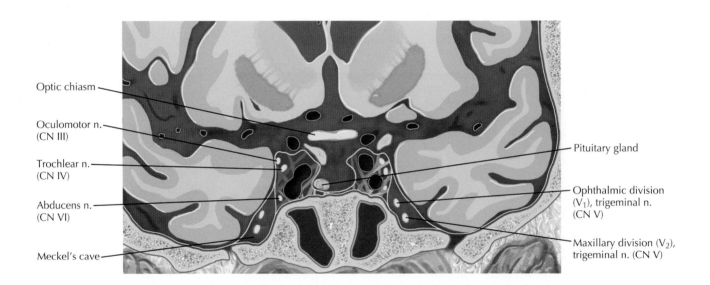

Optic chiasm

Oculomotor n. (CN III)

Trochlear n. (CN IV)

Abducens n. (CN VI)

Meckel's cave

Pituitary gland

Ophthalmic division (V$_1$), trigeminal n. (CN V)

Maxillary division (V$_2$), trigeminal n. (CN V)

DIAGNOSTIC CONSIDERATION

Although the trigeminal ganglion is located within Meckel's cave, on T2-weighted MR images the appearance is that of multiple branches passing through Meckel's cave, bathed in cerebrospinal fluid.

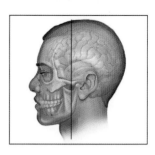

Optic chiasm

Oculomotor n.
(CN III)

Trochlear n.
(CN IV)

Abducens n.
(CN VI)

Meckel's cave

Pituitary gland

Ophthalmic division
(V₁), trigeminal n.
(CN V)

Maxillary division
(V₂), trigeminal n.
(CN V)

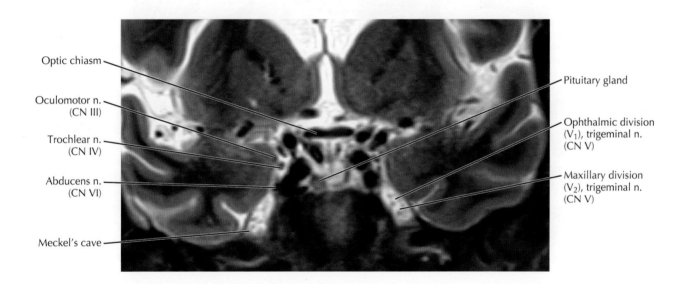

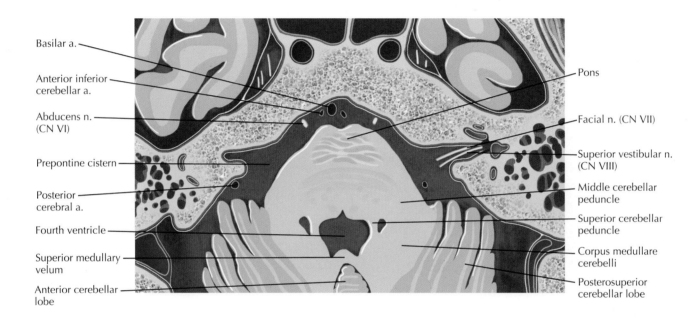

Basilar a.

Anterior inferior cerebellar a.

Abducens n. (CN VI)

Prepontine cistern

Posterior cerebral a.

Fourth ventricle

Superior medullary velum

Anterior cerebellar lobe

Pons

Facial n. (CN VII)

Superior vestibular n. (CN VIII)

Middle cerebellar peduncle

Superior cerebellar peduncle

Corpus medullare cerebelli

Posterosuperior cerebellar lobe

NORMAL ANATOMY

The abducens (or abducent) nerve (sixth cranial, CN VI) is a somatic efferent nerve that controls movement of the lateral rectus muscle of the orbit. Palsy of CN VI leads to a defect in directing the lateral gaze. The cisternal segment of the abducens nerve enters the base of the skull at Dorello's canal.

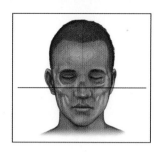

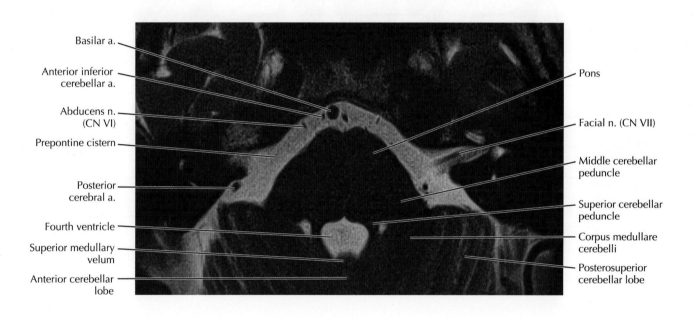

Basilar a.

Anterior inferior
cerebellar a.

Abducens n.
(CN VI)

Prepontine cistern

Posterior
cerebral a.

Fourth ventricle

Superior medullary
velum

Anterior cerebellar
lobe

Pons

Facial n. (CN VII)

Middle cerebellar
peduncle

Superior cerebellar
peduncle

Corpus medullare
cerebelli

Posterosuperior
cerebellar lobe

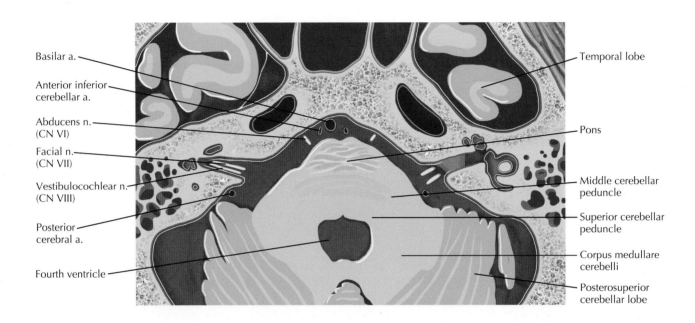

Basilar a.

Anterior inferior cerebellar a.

Abducens n. (CN VI)

Facial n. (CN VII)

Vestibulocochlear n. (CN VIII)

Posterior cerebral a.

Fourth ventricle

Temporal lobe

Pons

Middle cerebellar peduncle

Superior cerebellar peduncle

Corpus medullare cerebelli

Posterosuperior cerebellar lobe

PATHOLOGIC PROCESS

The abducens nerve innervates a single muscle, as does the trochlear nerve, and is only slightly larger than the trochlear. CN VI exits the brainstem between the pons and medulla medial to the facial nerve (CN VII) and passes anteriorly and superiorly to enter the skull base at a slightly acute angle into Dorello's canal. At the tip of the petrous segment of the temporal bone, the abducens nerve makes another acute angle forward to enter the cavernous sinus, coursing alongside the cavernous segment of the internal carotid artery, and enters the orbit through the superior orbital fissure. Because of its long course from brainstem to eye and acute turns at bony structures, the abducens nerve is particularly vulnerable to injury.

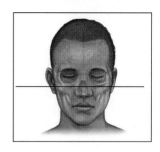

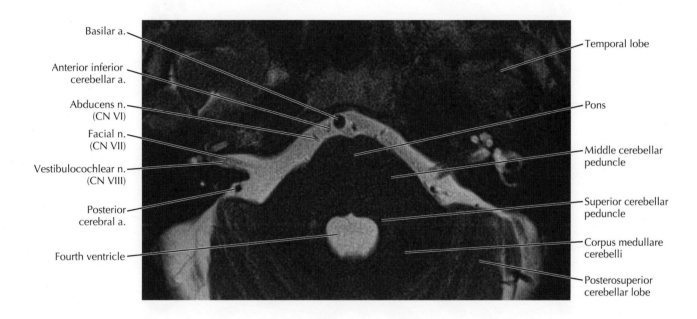

Basilar a.

Anterior inferior
cerebellar a.

Abducens n.
(CN VI)

Facial n.
(CN VII)

Vestibulocochlear n.
(CN VIII)

Posterior
cerebral a.

Fourth ventricle

Temporal lobe

Pons

Middle cerebellar
peduncle

Superior cerebellar
peduncle

Corpus medullare
cerebelli

Posterosuperior
cerebellar lobe

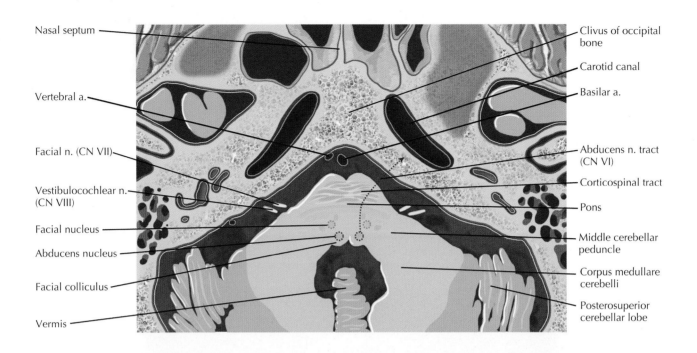

Nasal septum

Vertebral a.

Facial n. (CN VII)

Vestibulocochlear n. (CN VIII)

Facial nucleus

Abducens nucleus

Facial colliculus

Vermis

Clivus of occipital bone

Carotid canal

Basilar a.

Abducens n. tract (CN VI)

Corticospinal tract

Pons

Middle cerebellar peduncle

Corpus medullare cerebelli

Posterosuperior cerebellar lobe

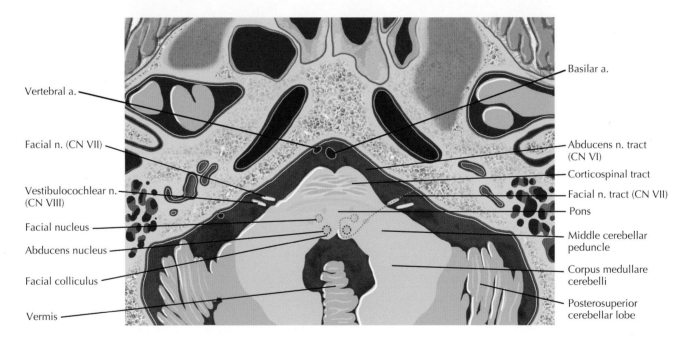

Vertebral a.

Facial n. (CN VII)

Vestibulocochlear n. (CN VIII)

Facial nucleus

Abducens nucleus

Facial colliculus

Vermis

Basilar a.

Abducens n. tract (CN VI)

Corticospinal tract

Facial n. tract (CN VII)

Pons

Middle cerebellar peduncle

Corpus medullare cerebelli

Posterosuperior cerebellar lobe

DIAGNOSTIC CONSIDERATION

The abducens nucleus is located in the pons along the anterior aspect of the fourth ventricle. Nerve fibers from the facial nucleus wrap medially and then posteriorly and laterally to the abducens nucleus, forming a bump on the anterior wall of the fourth ventricle called the *facial colliculus*. The abducens nuclei are close to the midline, as with the other nuclei that control ocular movement. The abducens axons pass from the nucleus anteriorly through the pons lateral to the corticospinal tract before exiting the brainstem and the pontomedullary junction.

Infarcts of the dorsal pons can injure both the abducens nucleus, causing lateral rectus palsy, and the facial nerve fibers, resulting in an ipsilateral facial palsy. Infarcts of the ventral pons can affect the abducens nerve and the corticospinal tract, producing lateral rectus muscle palsy and contralateral hemiparesis.

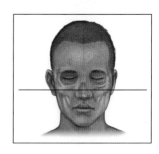

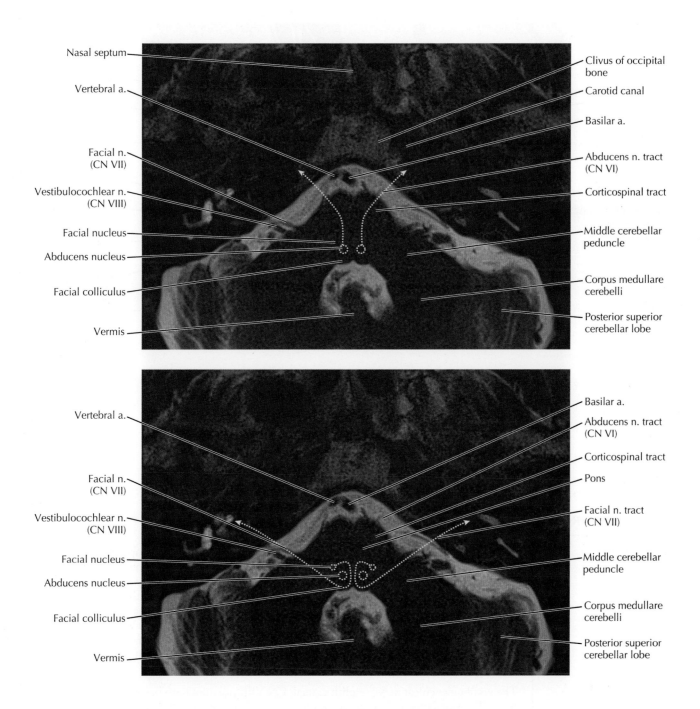

Nasal septum

Vertebral a.

Facial n.
(CN VII)

Vestibulocochlear n.
(CN VIII)

Facial nucleus

Abducens nucleus

Facial colliculus

Vermis

Clivus of occipital bone

Carotid canal

Basilar a.

Abducens n. tract
(CN VI)

Corticospinal tract

Middle cerebellar peduncle

Corpus medullare cerebelli

Posterior superior cerebellar lobe

Vertebral a.

Facial n.
(CN VII)

Vestibulocochlear n.
(CN VIII)

Facial nucleus

Abducens nucleus

Facial colliculus

Vermis

Basilar a.

Abducens n. tract
(CN VI)

Corticospinal tract

Pons

Facial n. tract
(CN VII)

Middle cerebellar peduncle

Corpus medullare cerebelli

Posterior superior cerebellar lobe

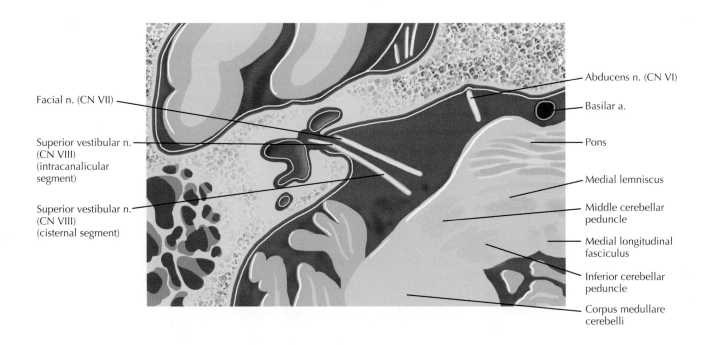

Facial n. (CN VII)

Superior vestibular n.
(CN VIII)
(intracanalicular
segment)

Superior vestibular n.
(CN VIII)
(cisternal segment)

Abducens n. (CN VI)

Basilar a.

Pons

Medial lemniscus

Middle cerebellar
peduncle

Medial longitudinal
fasciculus

Inferior cerebellar
peduncle

Corpus medullare
cerebelli

NORMAL ANATOMY

The facial nerve (seventh cranial, CN VII) exits the facial nucleus and wraps medial and posterior to the abducens nucleus to form a bump in the anterior wall of the fourth ventricle, called the *facial colliculus*. CN VII exits the brainstem at the lateral pontomedullary junction and courses through the CSF in the cerebellopontine angle anterior and parallel to the vestibulocochlear nerve (CN VIII) into the internal auditory canal. (For the segments of the facial nerve passing through bony canals as well as the semicircular canals, see Chapter 12.) The facial nerve is a motor nerve that supplies the muscles of the face. Injury to CN VII is of great clinical significance because of the stigma of ipsilateral facial palsy mimicking stroke and the impact on social interaction.

The vestibulocochlear nerve (eighth cranial, CN VIII) provides both balance and hearing functions. The vestibulocochlear nerve was formerly called the "acoustic" or "auditory" nerve, but these terms did not recognize the nerve's role in the vestibular system.

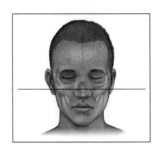

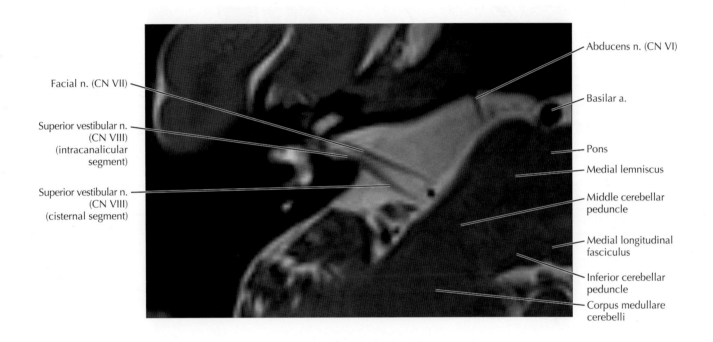

Facial n. (CN VII)

Superior vestibular n.
(CN VIII)
(intracanalicular
segment)

Superior vestibular n.
(CN VIII)
(cisternal segment)

Abducens n. (CN VI)

Basilar a.

Pons

Medial lemniscus

Middle cerebellar
peduncle

Medial longitudinal
fasciculus

Inferior cerebellar
peduncle

Corpus medullare
cerebelli

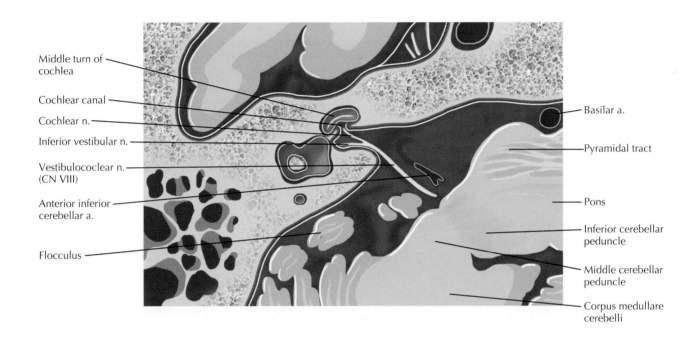

Middle turn of cochlea

Cochlear canal

Cochlear n.

Inferior vestibular n.

Vestibulococlear n. (CN VIII)

Anterior inferior cerebellar a.

Flocculus

Basilar a.

Pyramidal tract

Pons

Inferior cerebellar peduncle

Middle cerebellar peduncle

Corpus medullare cerebelli

NORMAL ANATOMY

The cochlear branch of the vestibulocochlear nerve (CN VIII) courses in the anteroinferior quadrant of the internal auditory canal. The cochlear nerve passes laterally into the small cochlear canal and winds within the cochlea.

The inferior and posterior divisions of the vestibular branch of the vestibulocochlear nerve pass in the posterior quadrants of the internal auditory canal and provide innervation for equilibrium to the three semicircular canals.

DIAGNOSTIC CONSIDERATION

The anterior inferior cerebellary artery passes close to the porous acoustic meatus (auditory canal). In some people the anterior inferior cerebellar artery can pass into the internal auditory canal. Looping of this artery into the canal, particularly deeper than halfway, may be associated with pressure symptoms on the facial or vestibulocochlear nerves, including potentially debilitating pulsatile tinnitus.

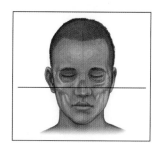

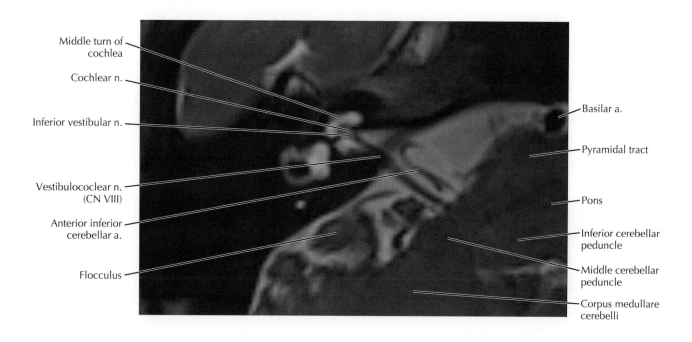

Middle turn of cochlea

Cochlear n.

Inferior vestibular n.

Vestibulococlear n. (CN VIII)

Anterior inferior cerebellar a.

Flocculus

Basilar a.

Pyramidal tract

Pons

Inferior cerebellar peduncle

Middle cerebellar peduncle

Corpus medullare cerebelli

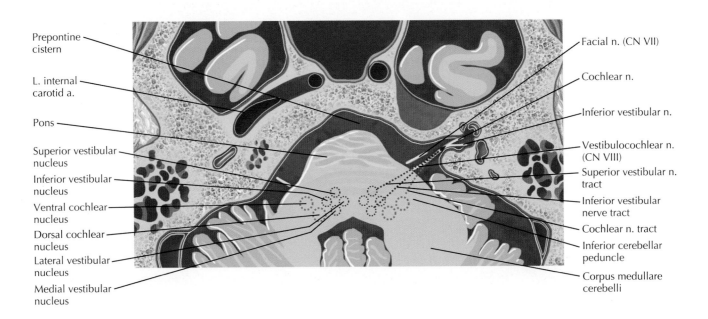

Prepontine cistern

L. internal carotid a.

Pons

Superior vestibular nucleus

Inferior vestibular nucleus

Ventral cochlear nucleus

Dorsal cochlear nucleus

Lateral vestibular nucleus

Medial vestibular nucleus

Facial n. (CN VII)

Cochlear n.

Inferior vestibular n.

Vestibulocochlear n. (CN VIII)

Superior vestibular n. tract

Inferior vestibular nerve tract

Cochlear n. tract

Inferior cerebellar peduncle

Corpus medullare cerebelli

NORMAL ANATOMY

The four vestibular nuclei include the medial, lateral, and inferior nuclei, located within the medulla, and the superior nucleus within the pons. The vestibular nuclei are medial to the ventral and dorsal cochlear nuclei.

PATHOLOGIC PROCESS

Note that this axial image is slightly tilted, showing a slightly lower aspect of the right side of the patient's head. The basal turn of the right cochlea is seen, as well as the middle and apical turns of the left cochlea. Note also the proximity of the petrous segment of the internal auditory canal to the basal turn. When the bony wall between this petrous segment and the basal turn is dehiscent, the patient may experience pulsatile tinnitus.

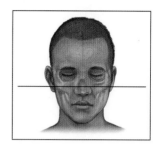

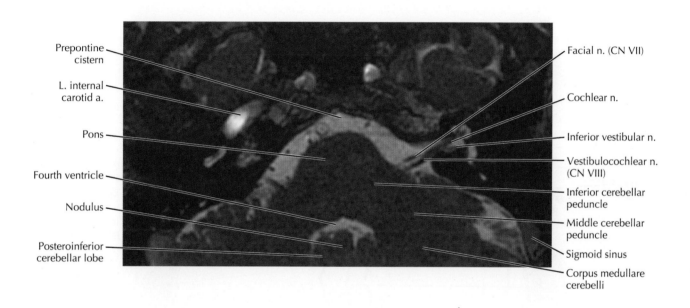

Prepontine cistern

L. internal carotid a.

Pons

Fourth ventricle

Nodulus

Posteroinferior cerebellar lobe

Facial n. (CN VII)

Cochlear n.

Inferior vestibular n.

Vestibulocochlear n. (CN VIII)

Inferior cerebellar peduncle

Middle cerebellar peduncle

Sigmoid sinus

Corpus medullare cerebelli

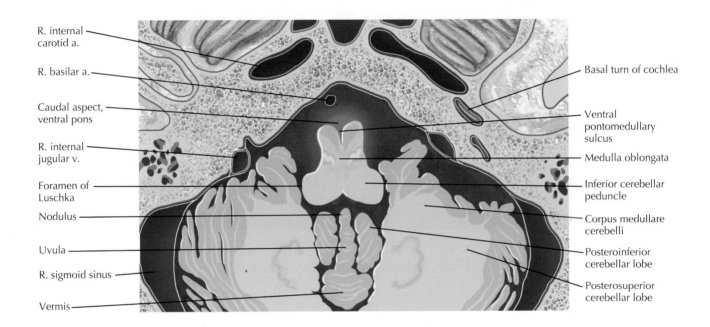

R. internal carotid a.

R. basilar a.

Caudal aspect, ventral pons

R. internal jugular v.

Foramen of Luschka

Nodulus

Uvula

R. sigmoid sinus

Vermis

Basal turn of cochlea

Ventral pontomedullary sulcus

Medulla oblongata

Inferior cerebellar peduncle

Corpus medullare cerebelli

Posteroinferior cerebellar lobe

Posterosuperior cerebellar lobe

NORMAL ANATOMY

This image is slightly more caudal than the Axial 6 image, and the basal turn of the left cochlear has now come into view. The part of the cochlear nerve in this basal turn registers higher frequencies, up to 20,000 Hz. As the cochlear nerve winds deeper into the middle and apical turns, it registers lower frequencies, down to 20 Hz.

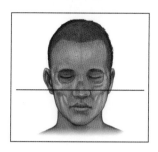

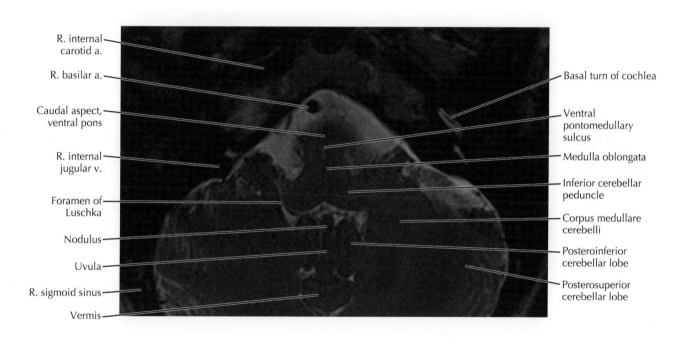

R. internal carotid a.

R. basilar a.

Caudal aspect, ventral pons

R. internal jugular v.

Foramen of Luschka

Nodulus

Uvula

R. sigmoid sinus

Vermis

Basal turn of cochlea

Ventral pontomedullary sulcus

Medulla oblongata

Inferior cerebellar peduncle

Corpus medullare cerebelli

Posteroinferior cerebellar lobe

Posterosuperior cerebellar lobe

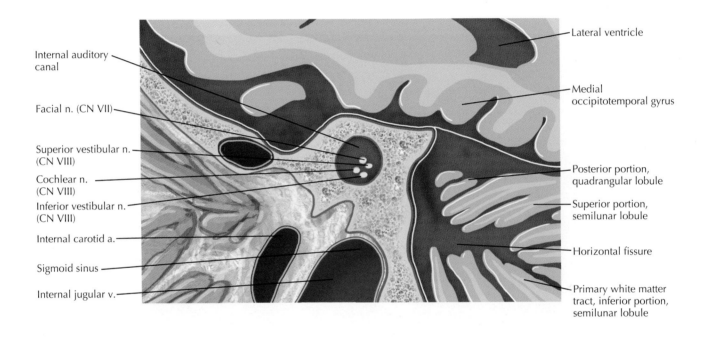

Internal auditory canal

Facial n. (CN VII)

Superior vestibular n. (CN VIII)

Cochlear n. (CN VIII)

Inferior vestibular n. (CN VIII)

Internal carotid a.

Sigmoid sinus

Internal jugular v.

Lateral ventricle

Medial occipitotemporal gyrus

Posterior portion, quadrangular lobule

Superior portion, semilunar lobule

Horizontal fissure

Primary white matter tract, inferior portion, semilunar lobule

NORMAL ANATOMY

The sagittal MR projection is the best imaging plane for distinguishing the facial nerve and the cochlear and vestibular branches of the vestibulocochlear nerve. In this sagittal image the nerves are seen in cross section to their long axis, with the facial nerve in the anterosuperior quadrant, the cochlear nerve in the anteroinferior quadrant, the superior vestibular branch in the posterosuperior quadrant, and the inferior vestibular branch in the posteroinferior quadrant. The patient's neck is slightly extended, tilting the facial nerve into the most superior position.

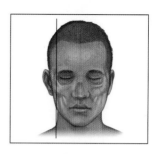

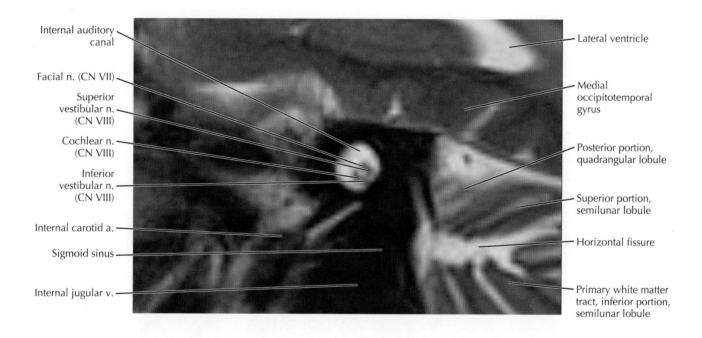

Internal auditory canal

Facial n. (CN VII)

Superior vestibular n. (CN VIII)

Cochlear n. (CN VIII)

Inferior vestibular n. (CN VIII)

Internal carotid a.

Sigmoid sinus

Internal jugular v.

Lateral ventricle

Medial occipitotemporal gyrus

Posterior portion, quadrangular lobule

Superior portion, semilunar lobule

Horizontal fissure

Primary white matter tract, inferior portion, semilunar lobule

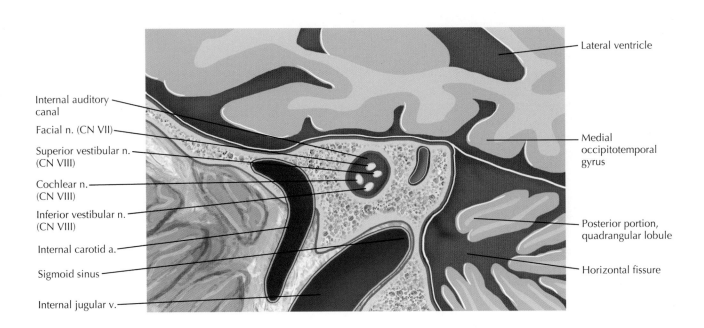

Lateral ventricle

Internal auditory canal

Facial n. (CN VII)

Superior vestibular n. (CN VIII)

Cochlear n. (CN VIII)

Inferior vestibular n. (CN VIII)

Internal carotid a.

Sigmoid sinus

Internal jugular v.

Medial occipitotemporal gyrus

Posterior portion, quadrangular lobule

Horizontal fissure

PATHOLOGIC PROCESS

Acoustic neuroma (schwannoma) may be seen in the patient with neurofibromatosis 2 and typically arises from the vestibular branches of CN VIII.

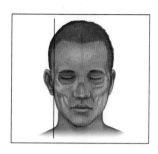

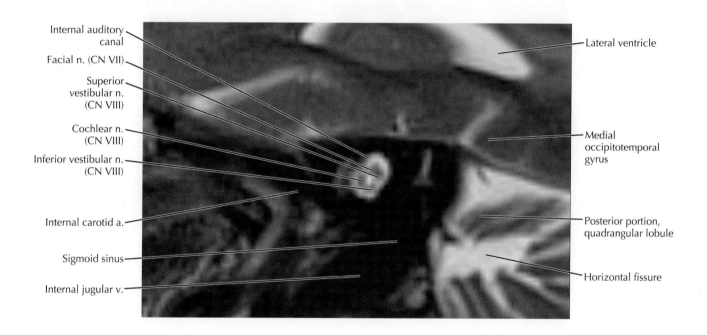

Internal auditory canal

Facial n. (CN VII)

Superior vestibular n. (CN VIII)

Cochlear n. (CN VIII)

Inferior vestibular n. (CN VIII)

Internal carotid a.

Sigmoid sinus

Internal jugular v.

Lateral ventricle

Medial occipitotemporal gyrus

Posterior portion, quadrangular lobule

Horizontal fissure

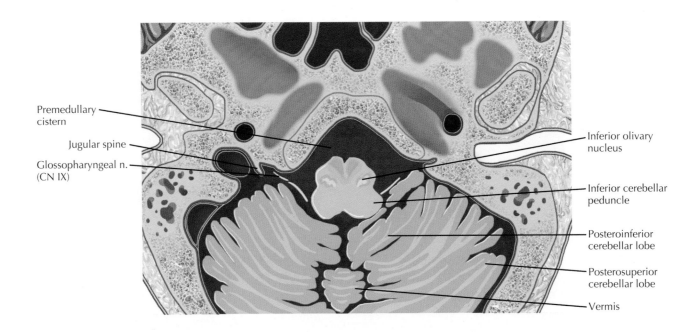

Premedullary cistern

Jugular spine

Glossopharyngeal n. (CN IX)

Inferior olivary nucleus

Inferior cerebellar peduncle

Posteroinferior cerebellar lobe

Posterosuperior cerebellar lobe

Vermis

NORMAL ANATOMY

The glossopharyngeal nerve (ninth cranial, CN IX) exits the brainstem from the lateral aspect of the upper medulla just anterior to the vagus nerve. The glossopharyngeal nerve exits the skull base through the *pars nervosa,* a small anteromedial compartment of the jugular foramen separated from the larger posterolateral compartment by a small bony ridge called the "jugular spine."

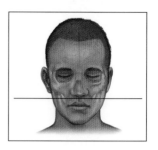

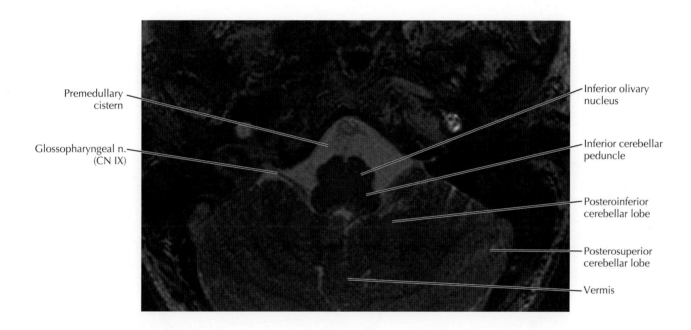

Premedullary cistern

Glossopharyngeal n. (CN IX)

Inferior olivary nucleus

Inferior cerebellar peduncle

Posteroinferior cerebellar lobe

Posterosuperior cerebellar lobe

Vermis

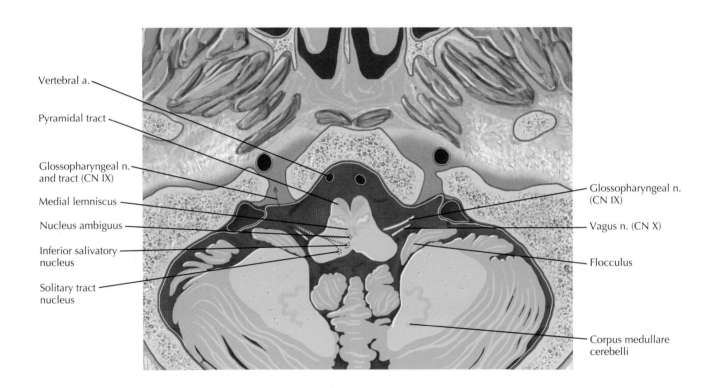

Vertebral a.

Pyramidal tract

Glossopharyngeal n.
and tract (CN IX)

Medial lemniscus

Nucleus ambiguus

Inferior salivatory
nucleus

Solitary tract
nucleus

Glossopharyngeal n.
(CN IX)

Vagus n. (CN X)

Flocculus

Corpus medullare
cerebelli

NORMAL ANATOMY

The nucleus ambiguus gives rise to motor fibers of the glossopharyngeal nerve and motor fibers of the vagus nerve. The inferior salivatory nucleus controls the parasympathetic input to the parotid gland and gives rise to axons traveling in the glossopharyngeal nerve. The solitary tract nucleus gives rise to fibers supplying the facial, glossopharyngeal, and vagus nerves and forms a circuit that contributes to autonomic regulation.

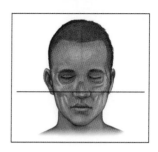

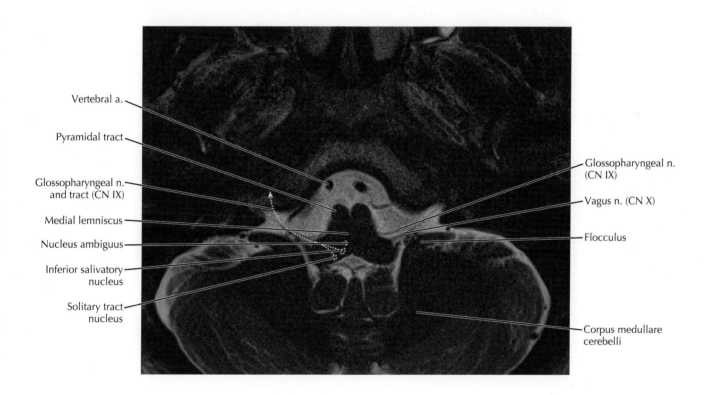

Vertebral a.

Pyramidal tract

Glossopharyngeal n. and tract (CN IX)

Medial lemniscus

Nucleus ambiguus

Inferior salivatory nucleus

Solitary tract nucleus

Glossopharyngeal n. (CN IX)

Vagus n. (CN X)

Flocculus

Corpus medullare cerebelli

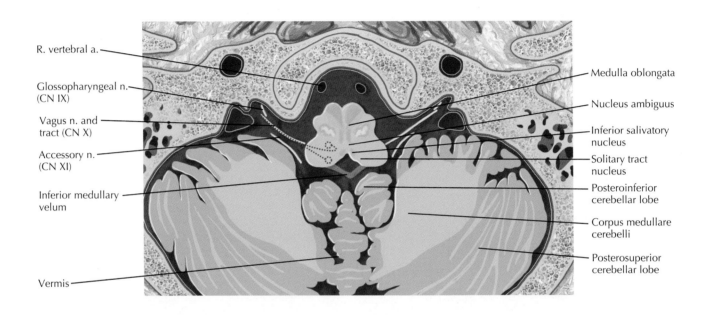

R. vertebral a.

Glossopharyngeal n.
(CN IX)

Vagus n. and
tract (CN X)

Accessory n.
(CN XI)

Inferior medullary
velum

Vermis

Medulla oblongata

Nucleus ambiguus

Inferior salivatory
nucleus

Solitary tract
nucleus

Posteroinferior
cerebellar lobe

Corpus medullare
cerebelli

Posterosuperior
cerebellar lobe

NORMAL ANATOMY

The vagus nerve (tenth cranial, CN X) is the longest cranial nerve. CN X exits the medulla between the medullary pyramid and inferior cerebellar peduncle, passes through the pars vascularis of the jugular foramen, courses inferior into the carotid sheath between the internal carotid artery the internal jugular vein, and then passes down into the neck, chest, and abdomen to innervate the viscera (Latin *vagus*, "wandering"). Most vagus nerve fibers provide sensory information about the state of organs to the brain, although some output also occurs.

The accessory nerve (CN XI) innervates the sternocleidomastoid and trapezius muscles of the neck and shoulder. Originally thought to be part of the brain, this nerve was designated the "eleventh cranial nerve" based on its location relative to other cranial nerves. However, the cranial component soon joins the vagus nerve, so more recently the accessory nerve is deemed to be synonymous with its spinal component and simply labeled *spinal accessory nerve.*

The spinal accessory nerve is the only cranial nerve that forms outside the skull. Nerve outlets originate from the upper spinal cord and coalesce to form the spinal accessory nerve, which then enters the skull through the foramen magnum, joining the vagus nerve to exit the skull through the pars vascularis compartment of the jugular foramen.

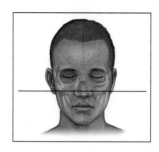

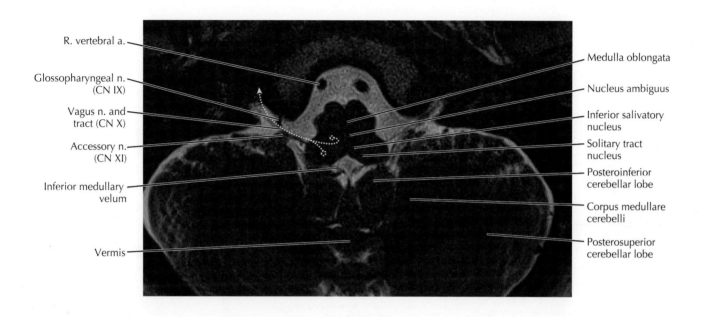

R. vertebral a.

Glossopharyngeal n. (CN IX)

Vagus n. and tract (CN X)

Accessory n. (CN XI)

Inferior medullary velum

Vermis

Medulla oblongata

Nucleus ambiguus

Inferior salivatory nucleus

Solitary tract nucleus

Posteroinferior cerebellar lobe

Corpus medullare cerebelli

Posterosuperior cerebellar lobe

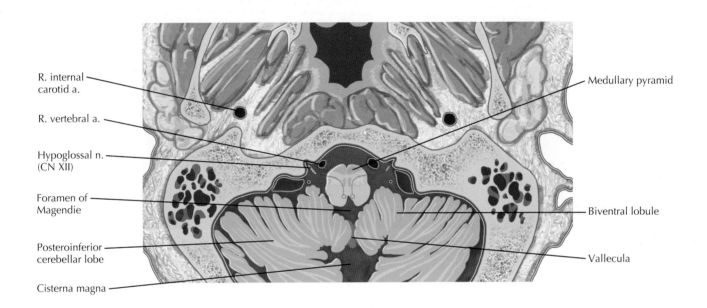

R. internal carotid a.

R. vertebral a.

Hypoglossal n. (CN XII)

Foramen of Magendie

Posteroinferior cerebellar lobe

Cisterna magna

Medullary pyramid

Biventral lobule

Vallecula

DIAGNOSTIC CONSIDERATION

The hypoglossal nerve (twelfth cranial, CN XII) innervates the muscles of the tongue. After exiting the medulla, CN XII exits the skull through its own canal, the hypoglossal canal, and courses anteriorly to innervate the tongue from inferiorly. This axial image shows its cisternal course immediately posterior to the intracranial segment of the vertebral artery.

Damage to the hypoglossal nerve can lead to atrophy of the ipsilateral muscles of the tongue and on protrusion of the tongue, deviation toward the affected side.

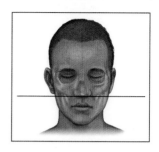

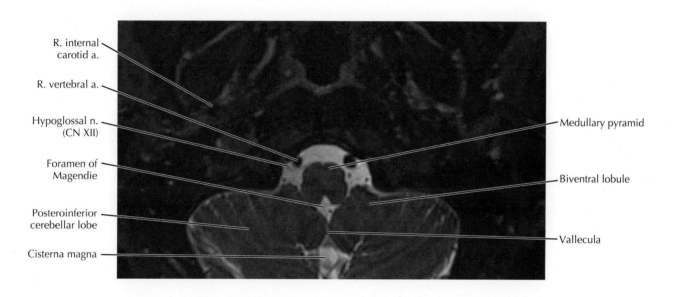

R. internal
carotid a.

R. vertebral a.

Hypoglossal n.
(CN XII)

Foramen of
Magendie

Posteroinferior
cerebellar lobe

Cisterna magna

Medullary pyramid

Biventral lobule

Vallecula

Chapter 6 VENTRICLES AND CEREBROSPINAL FLUID CISTERNS

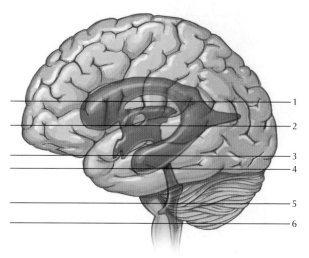

AXIAL   274

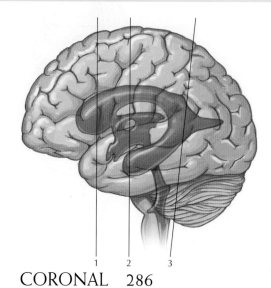

CORONAL   286

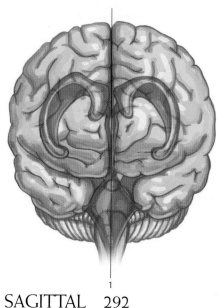

SAGITTAL   292

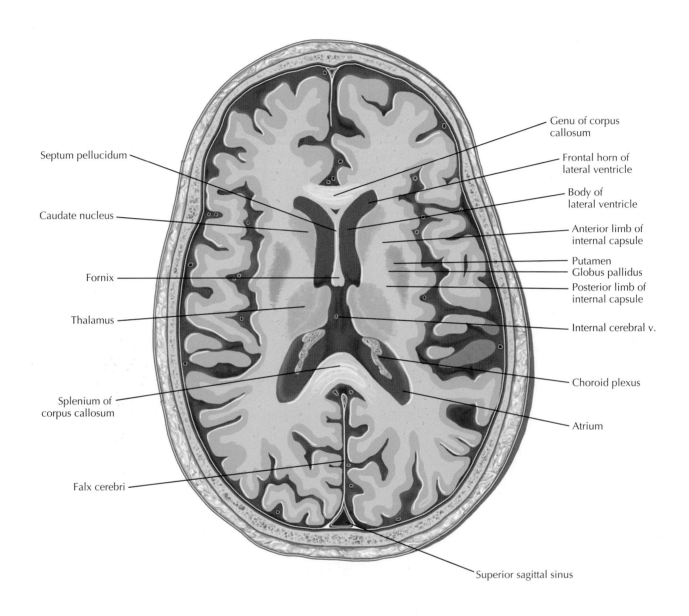

Septum pellucidum

Caudate nucleus

Fornix

Thalamus

Splenium of
corpus callosum

Falx cerebri

Genu of corpus
callosum

Frontal horn of
lateral ventricle

Body of
lateral ventricle

Anterior limb of
internal capsule

Putamen
Globus pallidus
Posterior limb of
internal capsule

Internal cerebral v.

Choroid plexus

Atrium

Superior sagittal sinus

NORMAL ANATOMY

The ventricular system is located deep within the brain and is filled with cerebrospinal fluid (CSF). The normal appearance of CSF on magnetic resonance images is that of water. This axial MR image shows the *choroid plexus* within the ventricles, where CSF is produced. CSF is also seen outside the brain and within the sulci (subarachnoid space).

PATHOLOGIC PROCESS

A *colloid cyst* is a benign lesion located near the foramen of Munro that may lead to sudden CSF obstruction, brain edema, and death if not treated with drainage and resection. CSF is produced at a rate of 500 mL daily; the intracranial vault and spinal canal contain only 150 mL, so the CSF turns over about three times each day.

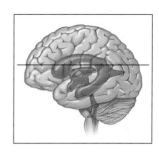

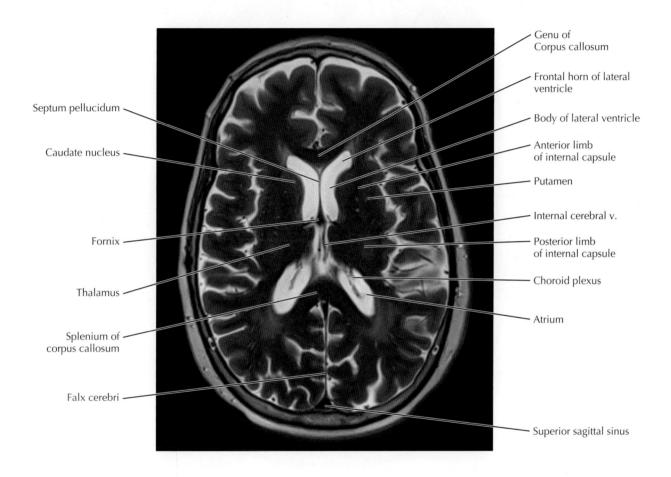

Genu of
Corpus callosum

Frontal horn of lateral
ventricle

Body of lateral ventricle

Anterior limb
of internal capsule

Putamen

Internal cerebral v.

Posterior limb
of internal capsule

Choroid plexus

Atrium

Superior sagittal sinus

Septum pellucidum

Caudate nucleus

Fornix

Thalamus

Splenium of
corpus callosum

Falx cerebri

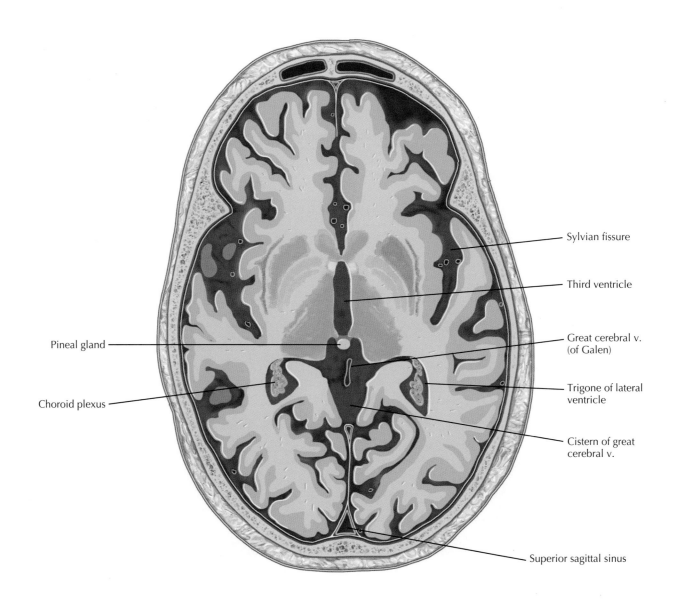

Sylvian fissure

Third ventricle

Pineal gland

Great cerebral v. (of Galen)

Trigone of lateral ventricle

Choroid plexus

Cistern of great cerebral v.

Superior sagittal sinus

NORMAL ANATOMY

At this axial level, the atrium has a triangular appearance and thus is often referred to as the *trigone*.

IMAGING TECHNIQUE CONSIDERATION

Note that fluid is bright on T2-weighted MRI. The subcutaneous fat shows some brightness on T2-weighted images when multiple spin-echo pulses are applied (fast, or "turbo," spin echo), as opposed to conventional spin echo T2-weighted imaging, where fat appears dark.

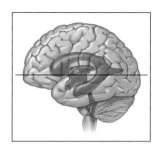

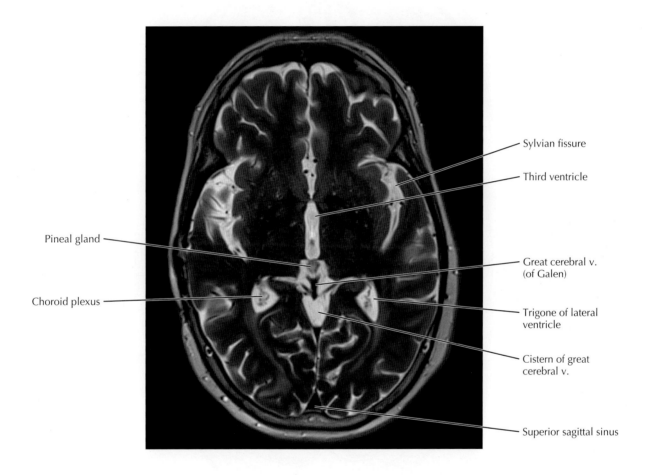

Sylvian fissure

Third ventricle

Pineal gland

Great cerebral v. (of Galen)

Choroid plexus

Trigone of lateral ventricle

Cistern of great cerebral v.

Superior sagittal sinus

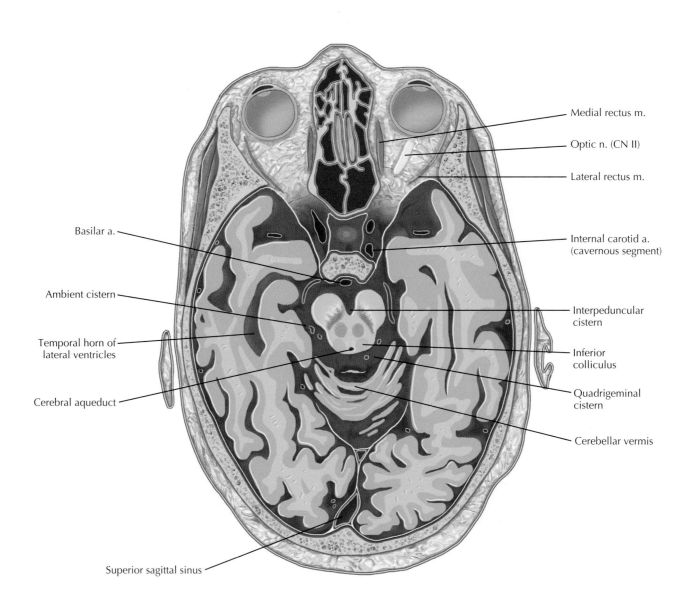

Medial rectus m.

Optic n. (CN II)

Lateral rectus m.

Basilar a.

Internal carotid a.
(cavernous segment)

Ambient cistern

Interpeduncular
cistern

Temporal horn of
lateral ventricles

Inferior
colliculus

Cerebral aqueduct

Quadrigeminal
cistern

Cerebellar vermis

Superior sagittal sinus

PATHOLOGIC PROCESS

Note that the temporal horn is a contiguous part of the lateral ventricles. Dilatation of the temporal horns is frequently a sign of hydrocephalus.

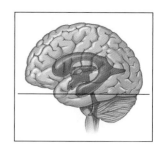

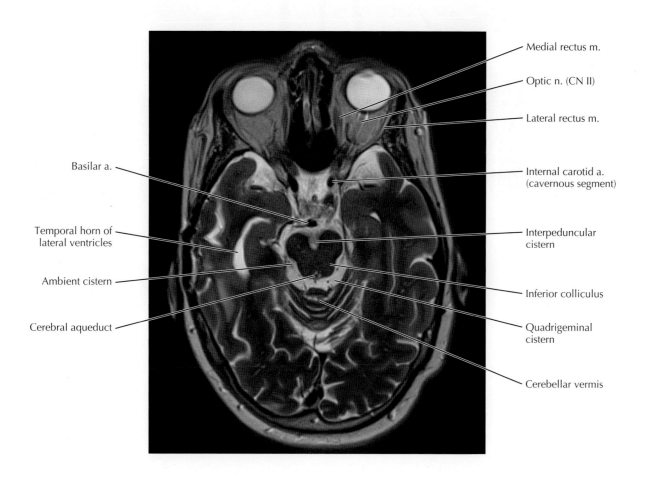

Medial rectus m.

Optic n. (CN II)

Lateral rectus m.

Internal carotid a.
(cavernous segment)

Interpeduncular
cistern

Inferior colliculus

Quadrigeminal
cistern

Cerebellar vermis

Basilar a.

Temporal horn of
lateral ventricles

Ambient cistern

Cerebral aqueduct

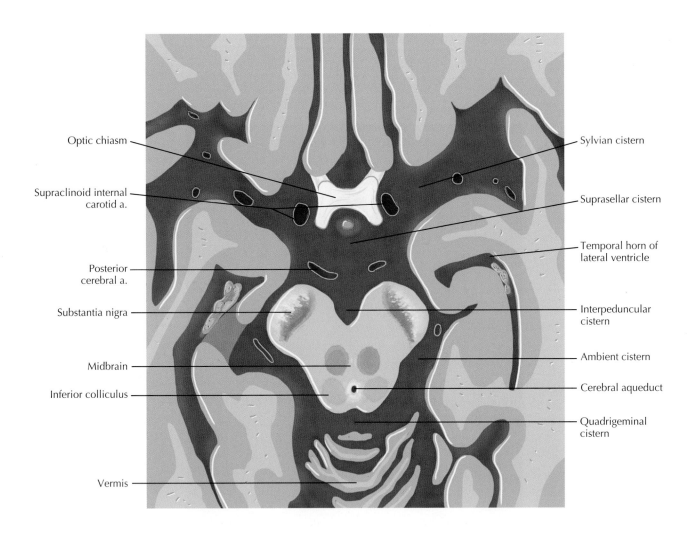

Optic chiasm

Supraclinoid internal
carotid a.

Posterior
cerebral a.

Substantia nigra

Midbrain

Inferior colliculus

Vermis

Sylvian cistern

Suprasellar cistern

Temporal horn of
lateral ventricle

Interpeduncular
cistern

Ambient cistern

Cerebral aqueduct

Quadrigeminal
cistern

PATHOLOGIC PROCESS

The suprasellar cistern has the shape of a six-pointed star. The interpeduncular cistern forms the posterior point of the star and is often the first location where a small amount of subarachnoid hemorrhage will layer when an aneurysm of the circle of Willis ruptures.

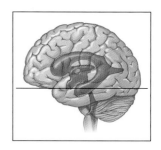

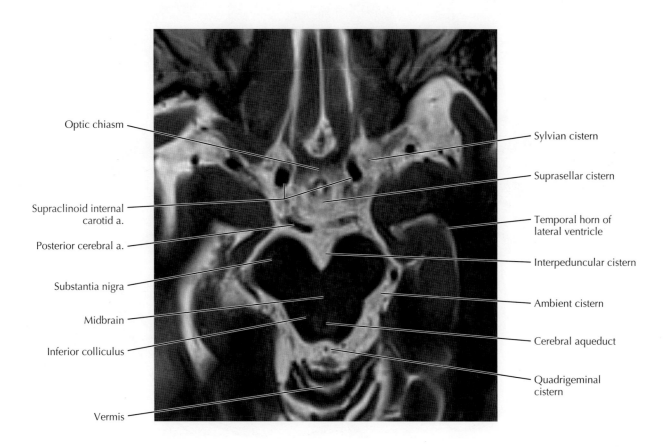

Optic chiasm

Supraclinoid internal carotid a.

Posterior cerebral a.

Substantia nigra

Midbrain

Inferior colliculus

Vermis

Sylvian cistern

Suprasellar cistern

Temporal horn of lateral ventricle

Interpeduncular cistern

Ambient cistern

Cerebral aqueduct

Quadrigeminal cistern

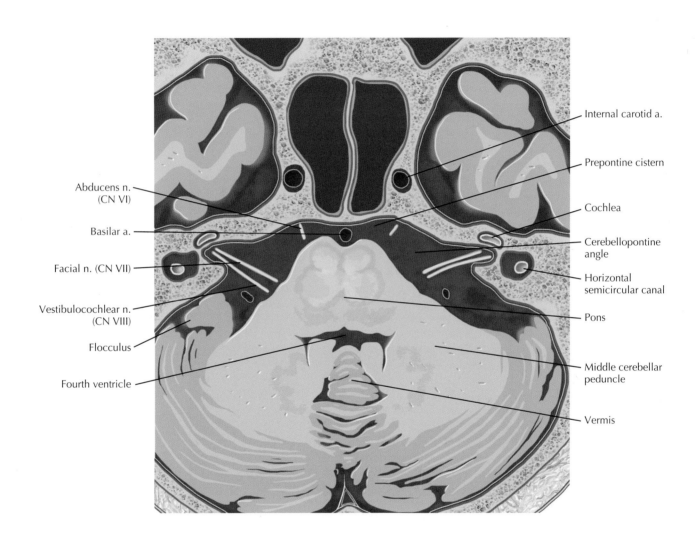

Abducens n.
(CN VI)

Basilar a.

Facial n. (CN VII)

Vestibulocochlear n.
(CN VIII)

Flocculus

Fourth ventricle

Internal carotid a.

Prepontine cistern

Cochlea

Cerebellopontine
angle

Horizontal
semicircular canal

Pons

Middle cerebellar
peduncle

Vermis

NORMAL ANATOMY

The fluid in the semicircular canal is called *endolymph.*

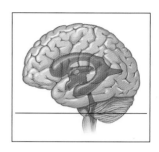

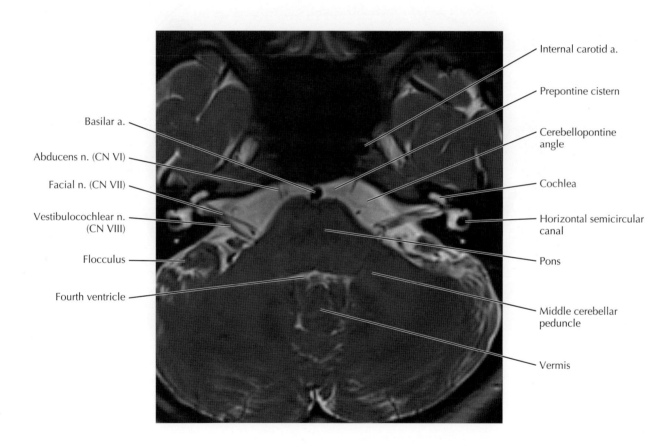

Basilar a.

Abducens n. (CN VI)

Facial n. (CN VII)

Vestibulocochlear n.
(CN VIII)

Flocculus

Fourth ventricle

Internal carotid a.

Prepontine cistern

Cerebellopontine
angle

Cochlea

Horizontal semicircular
canal

Pons

Middle cerebellar
peduncle

Vermis

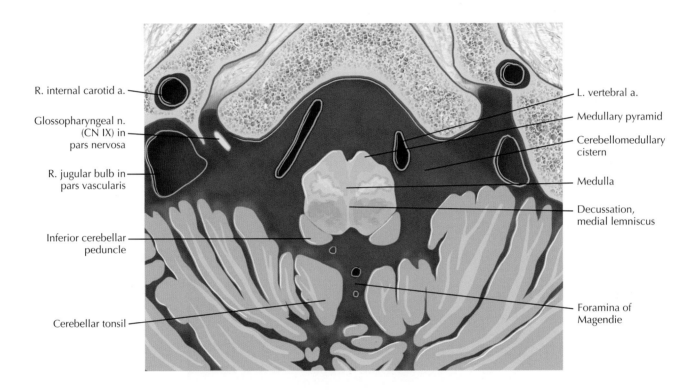

R. internal carotid a.

Glossopharyngeal n. (CN IX) in pars nervosa

R. jugular bulb in pars vascularis

Inferior cerebellar peduncle

Cerebellar tonsil

L. vertebral a.

Medullary pyramid

Cerebellomedullary cistern

Medulla

Decussation, medial lemniscus

Foramina of Magendie

NORMAL ANATOMY

Cerebrospinal fluid produced by the choroid plexus flows downward from the lateral ventricles, third ventricle, aqueduct of Sylvius (cerebral aqueduct), and fourth ventricle. CSF then flows out laterally through the foramina of Luschka or the midline through the foramen of Magendie. From here the CSF flows caudally around the spinal cord or cranially around the brain to the convexity, where it is absorbed by arachnoid granulations.

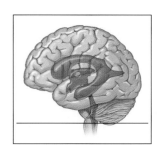

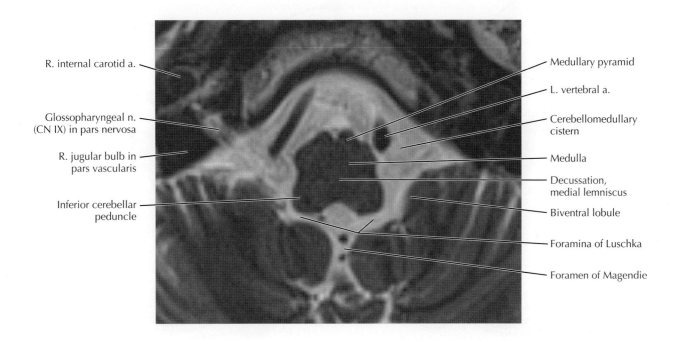

R. internal carotid a.

Glossopharyngeal n. (CN IX) in pars nervosa

R. jugular bulb in pars vascularis

Inferior cerebellar peduncle

Medullary pyramid

L. vertebral a.

Cerebellomedullary cistern

Medulla

Decussation, medial lemniscus

Biventral lobule

Foramina of Luschka

Foramen of Magendie

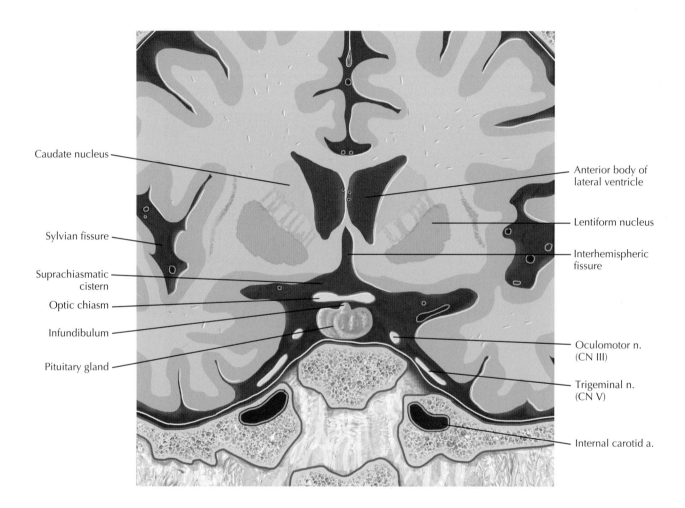

Caudate nucleus

Sylvian fissure

Suprachiasmatic cistern

Optic chiasm

Infundibulum

Pituitary gland

Anterior body of lateral ventricle

Lentiform nucleus

Interhemispheric fissure

Oculomotor n. (CN III)

Trigeminal n. (CN V)

Internal carotid a.

DIAGNOSTIC CONSIDERATION

Coronal imaging is not used as often as axial MRI for assessment of the ventricles and cisterns, although the cerebrospinal fluid does provide good contrast in assessment of midline structures such as the optic chiasm, infundibulum, and pituitary gland (hypophysis).

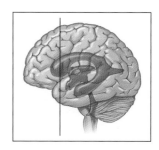

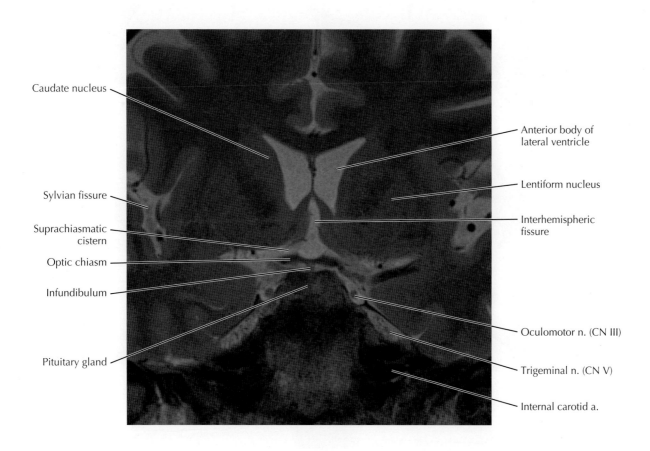

Caudate nucleus

Sylvian fissure

Suprachiasmatic cistern

Optic chiasm

Infundibulum

Pituitary gland

Anterior body of lateral ventricle

Lentiform nucleus

Interhemispheric fissure

Oculomotor n. (CN III)

Trigeminal n. (CN V)

Internal carotid a.

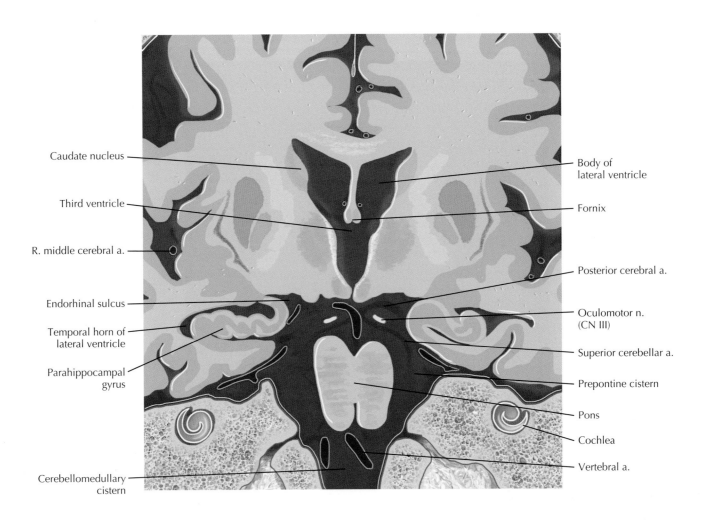

Caudate nucleus

Third ventricle

R. middle cerebral a.

Endorhinal sulcus

Temporal horn of
lateral ventricle

Parahippocampal
gyrus

Cerebellomedullary
cistern

Body of
lateral ventricle

Fornix

Posterior cerebral a.

Oculomotor n.
(CN III)

Superior cerebellar a.

Prepontine cistern

Pons

Cochlea

Vertebral a.

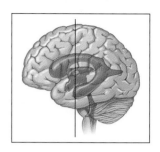

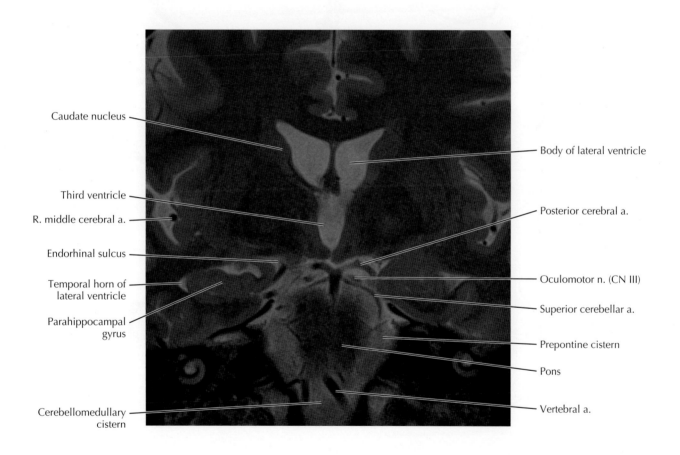

Caudate nucleus

Third ventricle

R. middle cerebral a.

Endorhinal sulcus

Temporal horn of
lateral ventricle

Parahippocampal
gyrus

Cerebellomedullary
cistern

Body of lateral ventricle

Posterior cerebral a.

Oculomotor n. (CN III)

Superior cerebellar a.

Prepontine cistern

Pons

Vertebral a.

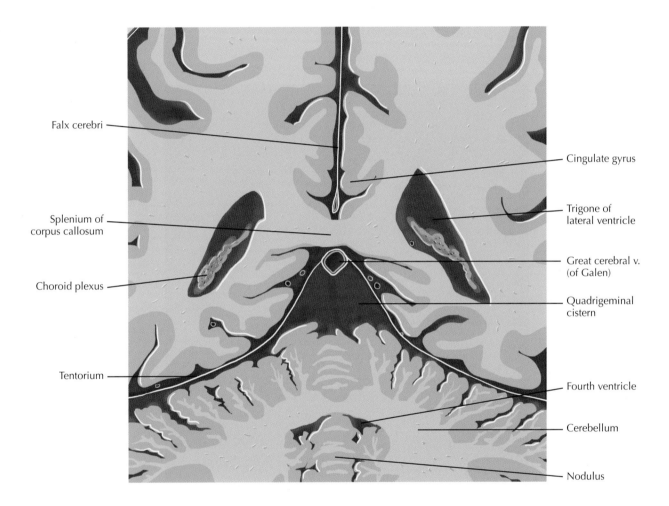

Falx cerebri

Splenium of corpus callosum

Choroid plexus

Tentorium

Cingulate gyrus

Trigone of lateral ventricle

Great cerebral v. (of Galen)

Quadrigeminal cistern

Fourth ventricle

Cerebellum

Nodulus

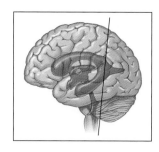

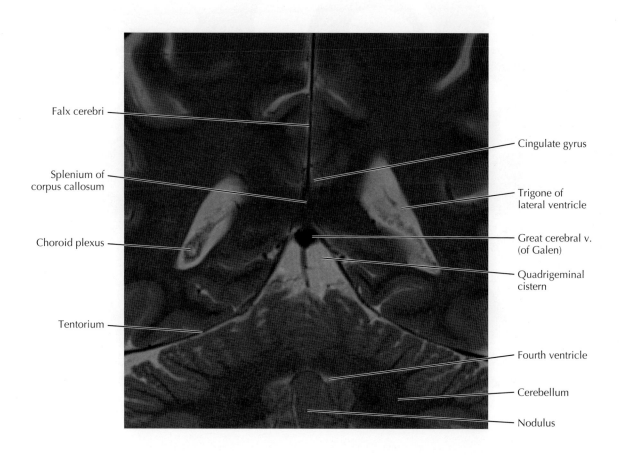

Falx cerebri

Splenium of corpus callosum

Choroid plexus

Tentorium

Cingulate gyrus

Trigone of lateral ventricle

Great cerebral v. (of Galen)

Quadrigeminal cistern

Fourth ventricle

Cerebellum

Nodulus

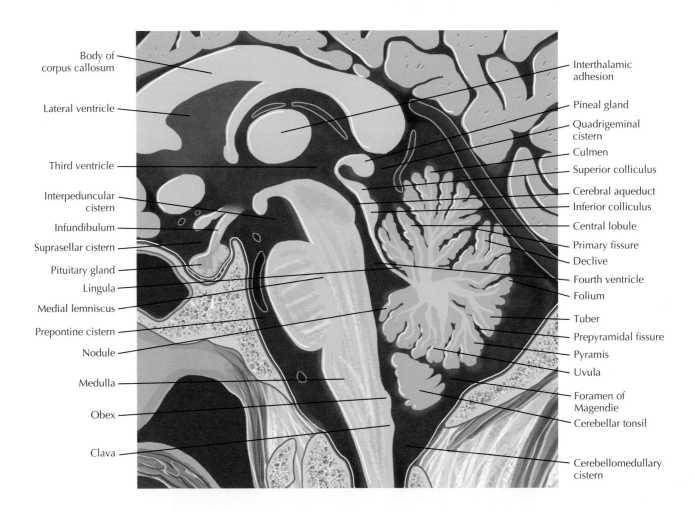

Body of corpus callosum

Lateral ventricle

Third ventricle

Interpeduncular cistern

Infundibulum

Suprasellar cistern

Pituitary gland

Lingula

Medial lemniscus

Prepontine cistern

Nodule

Medulla

Obex

Clava

Interthalamic adhesion

Pineal gland

Quadrigeminal cistern

Culmen

Superior colliculus

Cerebral aqueduct

Inferior colliculus

Central lobule

Primary fissure

Declive

Fourth ventricle

Folium

Tuber

Prepyramidal fissure

Pyramis

Uvula

Foramen of Magendie

Cerebellar tonsil

Cerebellomedullary cistern

DIAGNOSTIC CONSIDERATION

The midline sagittal plane on MR images provides a good view of the aqueduct of Sylvius (cerebral aqueduct). This long, thin, narrow channel is a relatively easy point for obstruction of CSF flow from a mass or adhesions. Dynamic MRI can be obtained in this sagittal plane to assess whether there is movement of CSF through the cerebral aqueduct.

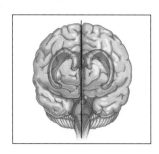

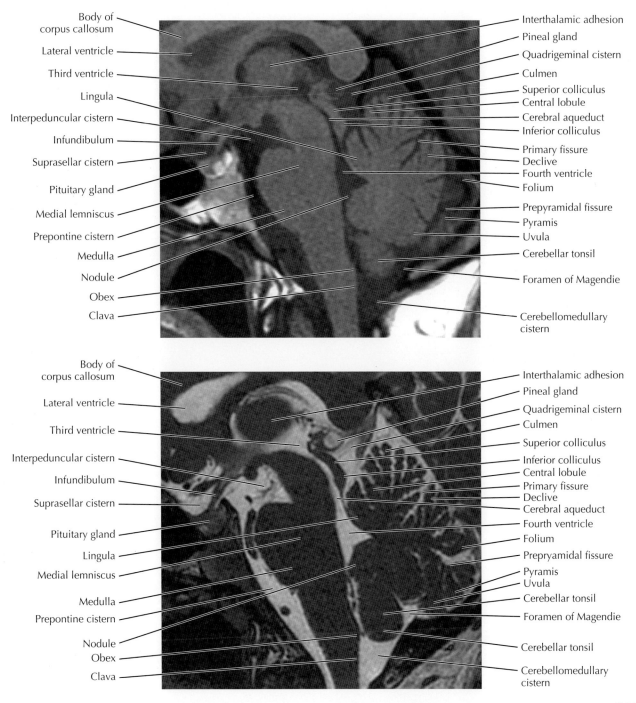

Body of corpus callosum

Lateral ventricle

Third ventricle

Lingula

Interpeduncular cistern

Infundibulum

Suprasellar cistern

Pituitary gland

Medial lemniscus

Prepontine cistern

Medulla

Nodule

Obex

Clava

Interthalamic adhesion

Pineal gland

Quadrigeminal cistern

Culmen

Superior colliculus

Central lobule

Cerebral aqueduct

Inferior colliculus

Primary fissure

Declive

Fourth ventricle

Folium

Prepyramidal fissure

Pyramis

Uvula

Cerebellar tonsil

Foramen of Magendie

Cerebellomedullary cistern

Body of corpus callosum

Lateral ventricle

Third ventricle

Interpeduncular cistern

Infundibulum

Suprasellar cistern

Pituitary gland

Lingula

Medial lemniscus

Medulla

Prepontine cistern

Nodule

Obex

Clava

Interthalamic adhesion

Pineal gland

Quadrigeminal cistern

Culmen

Superior colliculus

Inferior colliculus

Central lobule

Primary fissure

Declive

Cerebral aqueduct

Fourth ventricle

Folium

Prepryamidal fissure

Pyramis

Uvula

Cerebellar tonsil

Foramen of Magendie

Cerebellar tonsil

Cerebellomedullary cistern

Chapter 7 SELLA TURCICA

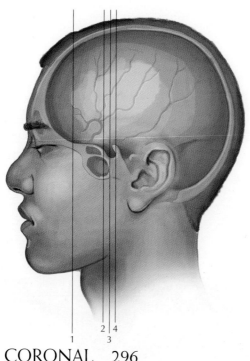

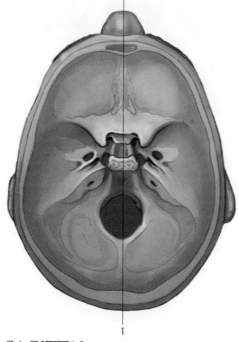

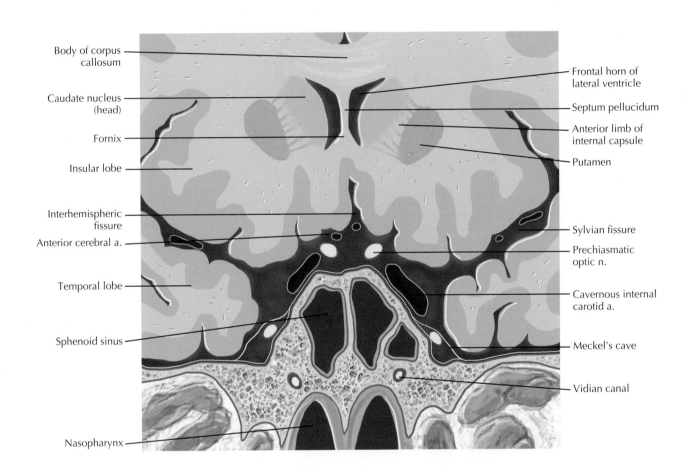

Body of corpus callosum

Caudate nucleus (head)

Fornix

Insular lobe

Interhemispheric fissure

Anterior cerebral a.

Temporal lobe

Sphenoid sinus

Nasopharynx

Frontal horn of lateral ventricle

Septum pellucidum

Anterior limb of internal capsule

Putamen

Sylvian fissure

Prechiasmatic optic n.

Cavernous internal carotid a.

Meckel's cave

Vidian canal

TECHNICAL NOTE

The upper MR image is a coronal T1-weighted pre-contrast sequence and the lower is a coronal T1-weighted post-contrast sequence.

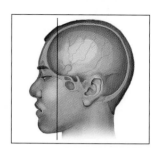

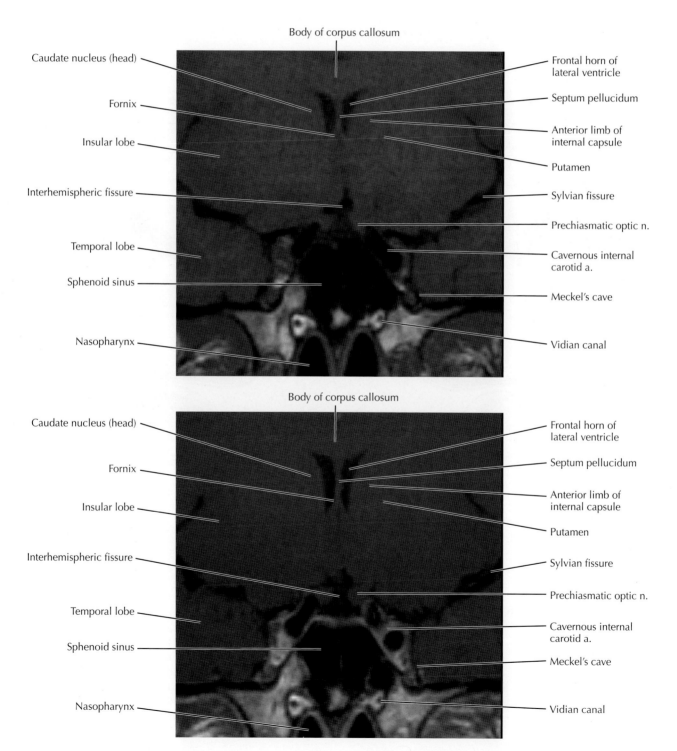

Body of corpus callosum

Caudate nucleus (head)

Fornix

Insular lobe

Interhemispheric fissure

Temporal lobe

Sphenoid sinus

Nasopharynx

Frontal horn of
lateral ventricle

Septum pellucidum

Anterior limb of
internal capsule

Putamen

Sylvian fissure

Prechiasmatic optic n.

Cavernous internal
carotid a.

Meckel's cave

Vidian canal

Body of corpus callosum

Caudate nucleus (head)

Fornix

Insular lobe

Interhemispheric fissure

Temporal lobe

Sphenoid sinus

Nasopharynx

Frontal horn of
lateral ventricle

Septum pellucidum

Anterior limb of
internal capsule

Putamen

Sylvian fissure

Prechiasmatic optic n.

Cavernous internal
carotid a.

Meckel's cave

Vidian canal

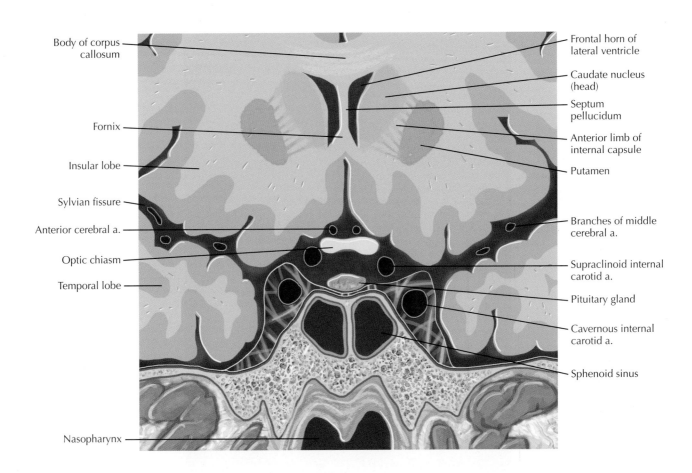

Body of corpus callosum

Fornix

Insular lobe

Sylvian fissure

Anterior cerebral a.

Optic chiasm

Temporal lobe

Nasopharynx

Frontal horn of lateral ventricle

Caudate nucleus (head)

Septum pellucidum

Anterior limb of internal capsule

Putamen

Branches of middle cerebral a.

Supraclinoid internal carotid a.

Pituitary gland

Cavernous internal carotid a.

Sphenoid sinus

DIAGNOSTIC CONSIDERATIONS

The best magnetic resonance sequence to identify a pituitary lesion is coronal, thin, 3-mm magnified postcontrast images of the sella turcica. The sella is a transverse depression crossing the midline at the superior surface of the sphenoid bone that contains the pituitary gland, or *hypophysis*. Pituitary adenomas are typically less enhancing than the normal gland. Precontrast imaging is used to determine that the apparent enhancement is not intrinsic high T1-weighted signal. Intrinsically high T1 signal is most frequently seen with fat, some forms of protein, acute hemorrhage (methemoglobin), and microcalcifications.

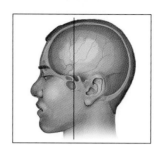

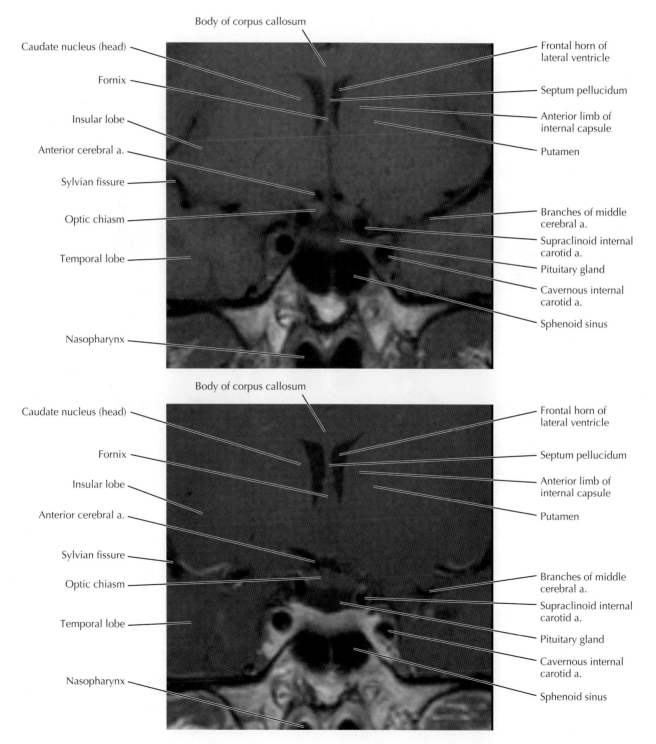

Body of corpus callosum

Caudate nucleus (head)

Fornix

Insular lobe

Anterior cerebral a.

Sylvian fissure

Optic chiasm

Temporal lobe

Nasopharynx

Frontal horn of lateral ventricle

Septum pellucidum

Anterior limb of internal capsule

Putamen

Branches of middle cerebral a.

Supraclinoid internal carotid a.

Pituitary gland

Cavernous internal carotid a.

Sphenoid sinus

Body of corpus callosum

Caudate nucleus (head)

Fornix

Insular lobe

Anterior cerebral a.

Sylvian fissure

Optic chiasm

Temporal lobe

Nasopharynx

Frontal horn of lateral ventricle

Septum pellucidum

Anterior limb of internal capsule

Putamen

Branches of middle cerebral a.

Supraclinoid internal carotid a.

Pituitary gland

Cavernous internal carotid a.

Sphenoid sinus

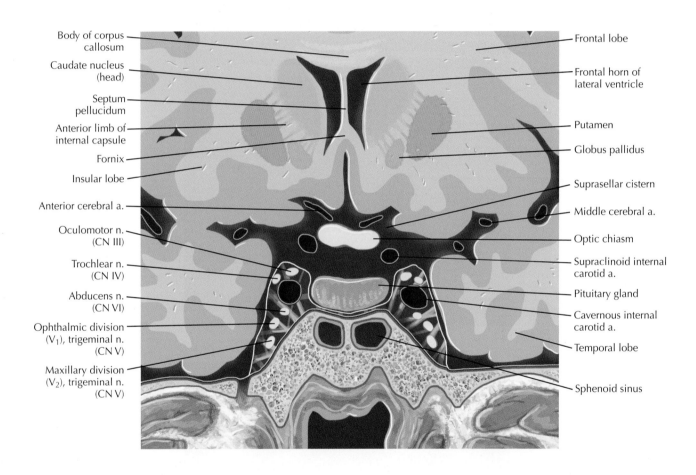

Body of corpus callosum

Caudate nucleus (head)

Septum pellucidum

Anterior limb of internal capsule

Fornix

Insular lobe

Anterior cerebral a.

Oculomotor n. (CN III)

Trochlear n. (CN IV)

Abducens n. (CN VI)

Ophthalmic division (V₁), trigeminal n. (CN V)

Maxillary division (V₂), trigeminal n. (CN V)

Frontal lobe

Frontal horn of lateral ventricle

Putamen

Globus pallidus

Suprasellar cistern

Middle cerebral a.

Optic chiasm

Supraclinoid internal carotid a.

Pituitary gland

Cavernous internal carotid a.

Temporal lobe

Sphenoid sinus

PATHOLOGIC PROCESS

On this coronal MR image, note the 4-mm, ovoid, hypoenhancing lesion within the inferior aspect of the pituitary gland, slightly larger toward the right. The lesion does not cause obvious displacement of the infundibulum or extend into the cavernous sinuses or sphenoid sinuses. This is consistent with a pituitary "microadenoma." This term is a misnomer in that the lesion is not micrometers in size, but rather defined as a lesion less than a centimeter in size, versus a "macroadenoma," which is larger than 1 cm.

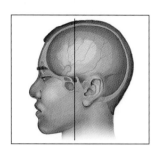

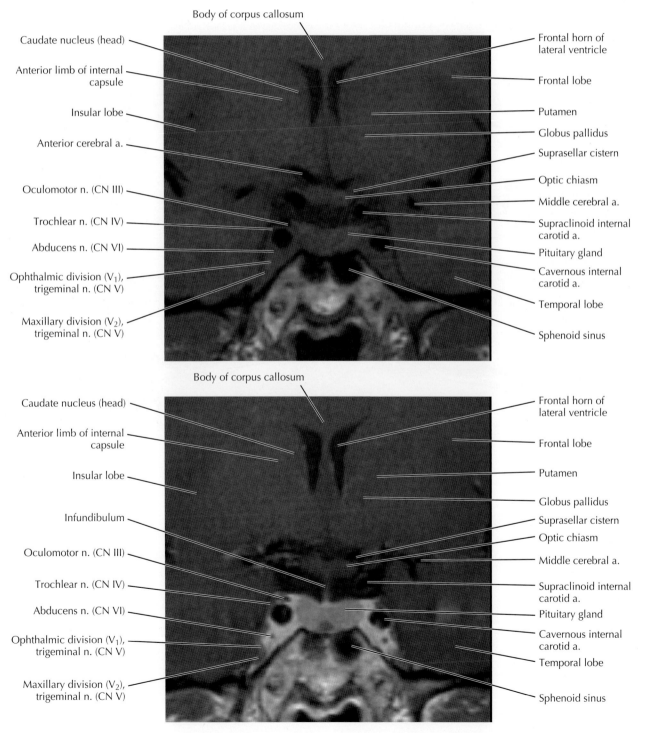

Body of corpus callosum

Caudate nucleus (head)

Anterior limb of internal capsule

Insular lobe

Anterior cerebral a.

Oculomotor n. (CN III)

Trochlear n. (CN IV)

Abducens n. (CN VI)

Ophthalmic division (V₁), trigeminal n. (CN V)

Maxillary division (V₂), trigeminal n. (CN V)

Frontal horn of lateral ventricle

Frontal lobe

Putamen

Globus pallidus

Suprasellar cistern

Optic chiasm

Middle cerebral a.

Supraclinoid internal carotid a.

Pituitary gland

Cavernous internal carotid a.

Temporal lobe

Sphenoid sinus

Body of corpus callosum

Caudate nucleus (head)

Anterior limb of internal capsule

Insular lobe

Infundibulum

Oculomotor n. (CN III)

Trochlear n. (CN IV)

Abducens n. (CN VI)

Ophthalmic division (V₁), trigeminal n. (CN V)

Maxillary division (V₂), trigeminal n. (CN V)

Frontal horn of lateral ventricle

Frontal lobe

Putamen

Globus pallidus

Suprasellar cistern

Optic chiasm

Middle cerebral a.

Supraclinoid internal carotid a.

Pituitary gland

Cavernous internal carotid a.

Temporal lobe

Sphenoid sinus

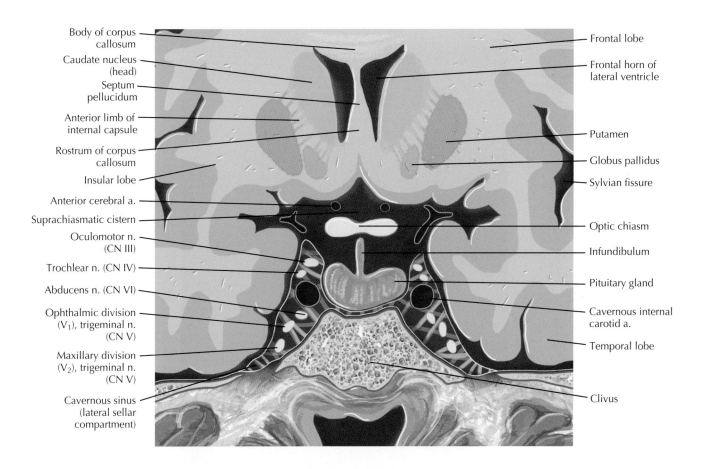

Body of corpus callosum

Caudate nucleus (head)

Septum pellucidum

Anterior limb of internal capsule

Rostrum of corpus callosum

Insular lobe

Anterior cerebral a.

Suprachiasmatic cistern

Oculomotor n. (CN III)

Trochlear n. (CN IV)

Abducens n. (CN VI)

Ophthalmic division (V₁), trigeminal n. (CN V)

Maxillary division (V₂), trigeminal n. (CN V)

Cavernous sinus (lateral sellar compartment)

Frontal lobe

Frontal horn of lateral ventricle

Putamen

Globus pallidus

Sylvian fissure

Optic chiasm

Infundibulum

Pituitary gland

Cavernous internal carotid a.

Temporal lobe

Clivus

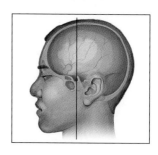

Body of corpus callosum

Caudate nucleus (head)

Anterior limb of internal capsule

Septum pellucidum

Rostrum of corpus callosum

Anterior cerebral a.

Suprachiasmatic cistern

Oculomotor n. (CN III)

Trochlear n. (CN IV)

Abducens n. (CN VI)

Ophthalmic division (V₁), trigeminal n. (CN V)

Maxillary division (V₂) trigeminal n. (CN V)

Cavernous sinus (lateral sellar compartment)

Frontal horn of lateral ventricle

Frontal lobe

Putamen

Globus pallidus

Sylvian fissure

Optic chiasm

Infundibulum

Pituitary gland

Cavernous internal carotid a.

Temporal lobe

Clivus

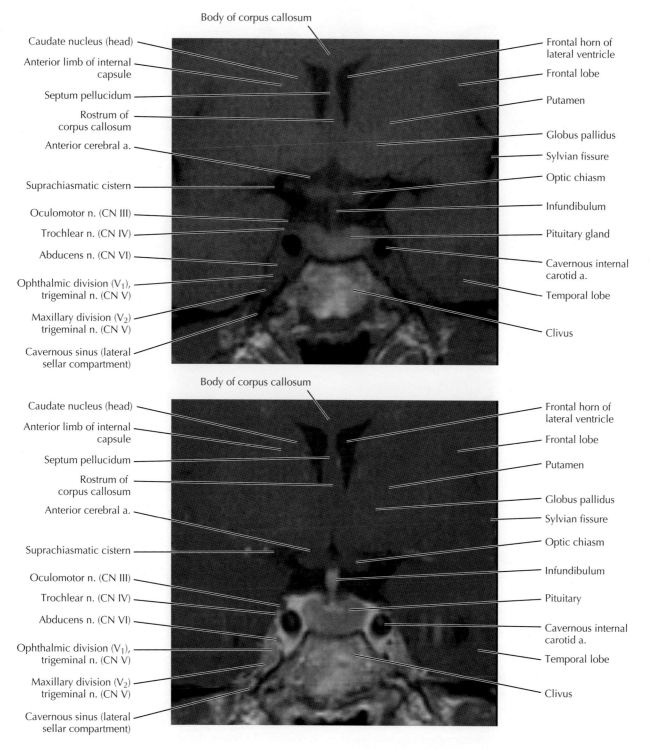

Body of corpus callosum

Caudate nucleus (head)

Anterior limb of internal capsule

Septum pellucidum

Rostrum of corpus callosum

Anterior cerebral a.

Suprachiasmatic cistern

Oculomotor n. (CN III)

Trochlear n. (CN IV)

Abducens n. (CN VI)

Ophthalmic division (V₁), trigeminal n. (CN V)

Maxillary division (V₂) trigeminal n. (CN V)

Cavernous sinus (lateral sellar compartment)

Frontal horn of lateral ventricle

Frontal lobe

Putamen

Globus pallidus

Sylvian fissure

Optic chiasm

Infundibulum

Pituitary

Cavernous internal carotid a.

Temporal lobe

Clivus

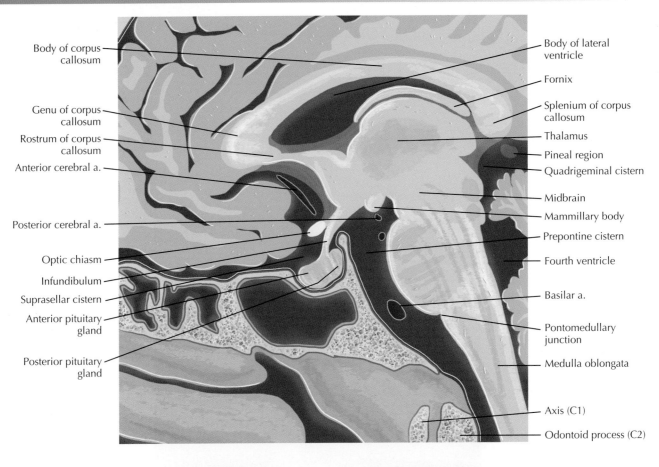

Body of corpus callosum

Genu of corpus callosum

Rostrum of corpus callosum

Anterior cerebral a.

Posterior cerebral a.

Optic chiasm

Infundibulum

Suprasellar cistern

Anterior pituitary gland

Posterior pituitary gland

Body of lateral ventricle

Fornix

Splenium of corpus callosum

Thalamus

Pineal region

Quadrigeminal cistern

Midbrain

Mammillary body

Prepontine cistern

Fourth ventricle

Basilar a.

Pontomedullary junction

Medulla oblongata

Axis (C1)

Odontoid process (C2)

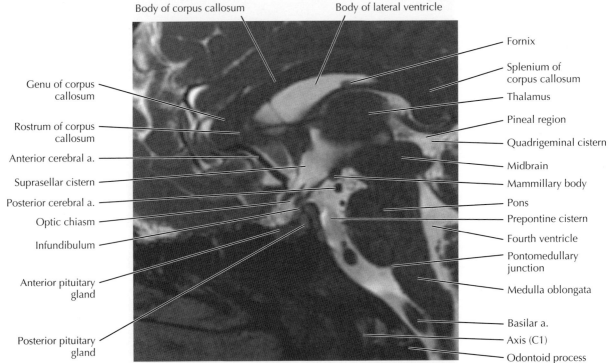

Body of corpus callosum

Body of lateral ventricle

Genu of corpus callosum

Rostrum of corpus callosum

Anterior cerebral a.

Suprasellar cistern

Posterior cerebral a.

Optic chiasm

Infundibulum

Anterior pituitary gland

Posterior pituitary gland

Fornix

Splenium of corpus callosum

Thalamus

Pineal region

Quadrigeminal cistern

Midbrain

Mammillary body

Pons

Prepontine cistern

Fourth ventricle

Pontomedullary junction

Medulla oblongata

Basilar a.

Axis (C1)

Odontoid process

PATHOLOGIC PROCESS

Acute hemorrhage may be seen with *pituitary apoplexy*. In these patients, attention should focus on the posterior aspect of the clivus for signs of hemorrhage extension. Note that the posterior aspect of the pituitary gland, the *neurohypophysis*, is normally T1 bright, the absence of which may be pathologic.

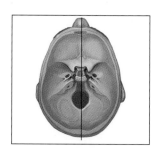

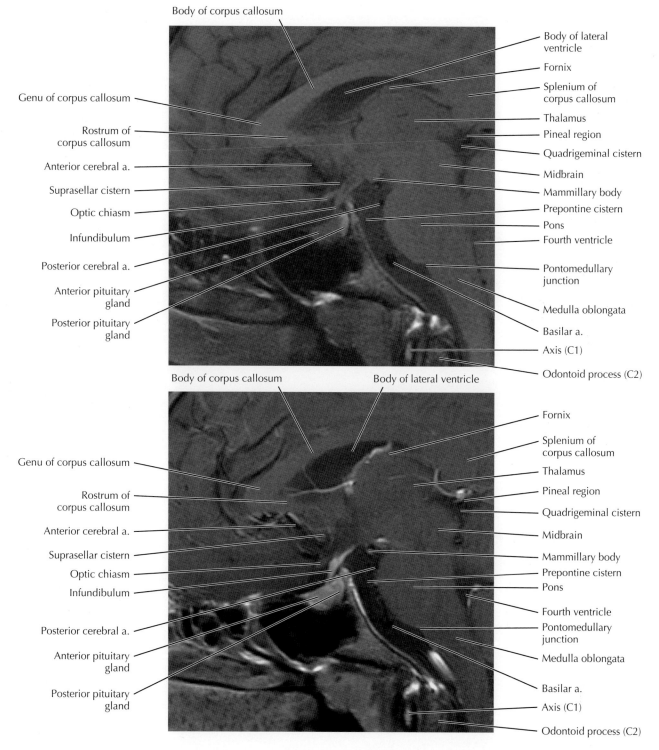

Body of corpus callosum

Genu of corpus callosum

Rostrum of
corpus callosum

Anterior cerebral a.

Suprasellar cistern

Optic chiasm

Infundibulum

Posterior cerebral a.

Anterior pituitary
gland

Posterior pituitary
gland

Body of lateral
ventricle

Fornix

Splenium of
corpus callosum

Thalamus

Pineal region

Quadrigeminal cistern

Midbrain

Mammillary body

Prepontine cistern

Pons

Fourth ventricle

Pontomedullary
junction

Medulla oblongata

Basilar a.

Axis (C1)

Odontoid process (C2)

Body of corpus callosum

Body of lateral ventricle

Genu of corpus callosum

Rostrum of
corpus callosum

Anterior cerebral a.

Suprasellar cistern

Optic chiasm

Infundibulum

Posterior cerebral a.

Anterior pituitary
gland

Posterior pituitary
gland

Fornix

Splenium of
corpus callosum

Thalamus

Pineal region

Quadrigeminal cistern

Midbrain

Mammillary body

Prepontine cistern

Pons

Fourth ventricle

Pontomedullary
junction

Medulla oblongata

Basilar a.

Axis (C1)

Odontoid process (C2)

PART HEAD AND NECK

Chapter 8 OVERVIEW OF HEAD AND NECK

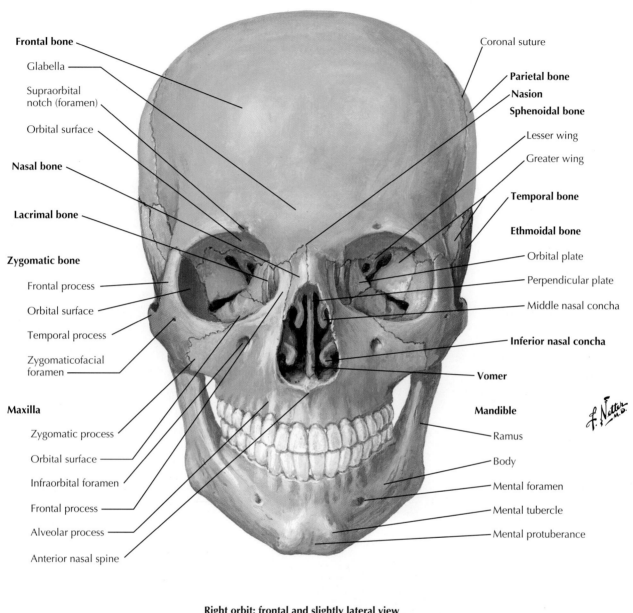

Frontal bone
Glabella
Supraorbital notch (foramen)
Orbital surface

Nasal bone

Lacrimal bone

Zygomatic bone
Frontal process
Orbital surface
Temporal process
Zygomaticofacial foramen

Maxilla
Zygomatic process
Orbital surface
Infraorbital foramen
Frontal process
Alveolar process
Anterior nasal spine

Coronal suture
Parietal bone
Nasion
Sphenoidal bone
Lesser wing
Greater wing
Temporal bone
Ethmoidal bone
Orbital plate
Perpendicular plate
Middle nasal concha
Inferior nasal concha
Vomer
Mandible
Ramus
Body
Mental foramen
Mental tubercle
Mental protuberance

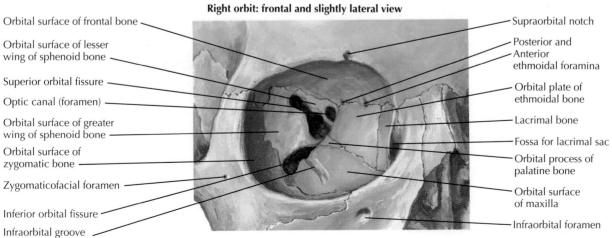

Right orbit: frontal and slightly lateral view

Orbital surface of frontal bone
Orbital surface of lesser wing of sphenoid bone
Superior orbital fissure
Optic canal (foramen)
Orbital surface of greater wing of sphenoid bone
Orbital surface of zygomatic bone
Zygomaticofacial foramen
Inferior orbital fissure
Infraorbital groove

Supraorbital notch
Posterior and Anterior ethmoidal foramina
Orbital plate of ethmoidal bone
Lacrimal bone
Fossa for lacrimal sac
Orbital process of palatine bone
Orbital surface of maxilla
Infraorbital foramen

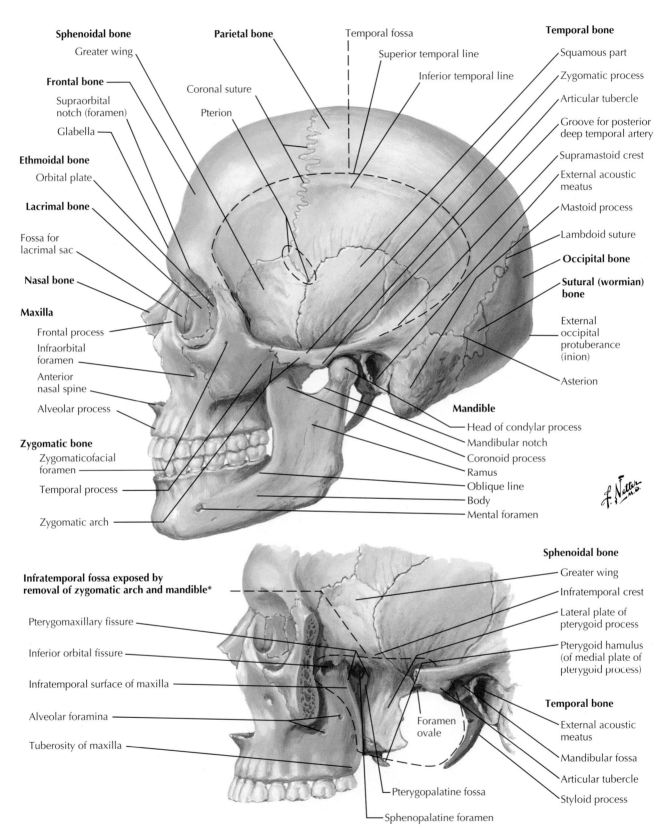

Sphenoidal bone
Greater wing

Frontal bone
Supraorbital notch (foramen)
Glabella

Ethmoidal bone
Orbital plate

Lacrimal bone
Fossa for lacrimal sac

Nasal bone

Maxilla
Frontal process
Infraorbital foramen
Anterior nasal spine
Alveolar process

Zygomatic bone
Zygomaticofacial foramen
Temporal process
Zygomatic arch

Parietal bone
Coronal suture
Pterion

Temporal fossa
Superior temporal line
Inferior temporal line

Temporal bone
Squamous part
Zygomatic process
Articular tubercle
Groove for posterior deep temporal artery
Supramastoid crest
External acoustic meatus
Mastoid process
Lambdoid suture

Occipital bone

Sutural (wormian) bone
External occipital protuberance (inion)
Asterion

Mandible
Head of condylar process
Mandibular notch
Coronoid process
Ramus
Oblique line
Body
Mental foramen

Infratemporal fossa exposed by removal of zygomatic arch and mandible*

Pterygomaxillary fissure
Inferior orbital fissure
Infratemporal surface of maxilla
Alveolar foramina
Tuberosity of maxilla

Foramen ovale

Pterygopalatine fossa
Sphenopalatine foramen

Sphenoidal bone
Greater wing
Infratemporal crest
Lateral plate of pterygoid process
Pterygoid hamulus (of medial plate of pterygoid process)

Temporal bone
External acoustic meatus
Mandibular fossa
Articular tubercle
Styloid process

*Superficially, mastoid process forms posterior boundary.

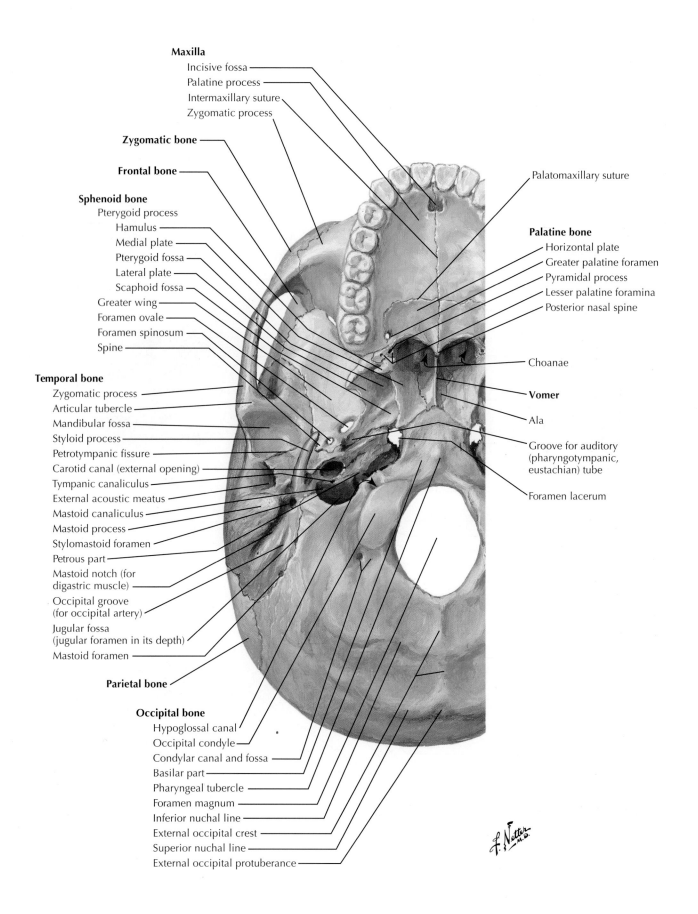

Maxilla
Incisive fossa
Palatine process
Intermaxillary suture
Zygomatic process

Zygomatic bone

Frontal bone

Sphenoid bone
Pterygoid process
Hamulus
Medial plate
Pterygoid fossa
Lateral plate
Scaphoid fossa
Greater wing
Foramen ovale
Foramen spinosum
Spine

Temporal bone
Zygomatic process
Articular tubercle
Mandibular fossa
Styloid process
Petrotympanic fissure
Carotid canal (external opening)
Tympanic canaliculus
External acoustic meatus
Mastoid canaliculus
Mastoid process
Stylomastoid foramen
Petrous part
Mastoid notch (for digastric muscle)
Occipital groove (for occipital artery)
Jugular fossa (jugular foramen in its depth)
Mastoid foramen

Parietal bone

Occipital bone
Hypoglossal canal
Occipital condyle
Condylar canal and fossa
Basilar part
Pharyngeal tubercle
Foramen magnum
Inferior nuchal line
External occipital crest
Superior nuchal line
External occipital protuberance

Palatomaxillary suture

Palatine bone
Horizontal plate
Greater palatine foramen
Pyramidal process
Lesser palatine foramina
Posterior nasal spine

Choanae

Vomer

Ala

Groove for auditory (pharyngotympanic, eustachian) tube

Foramen lacerum

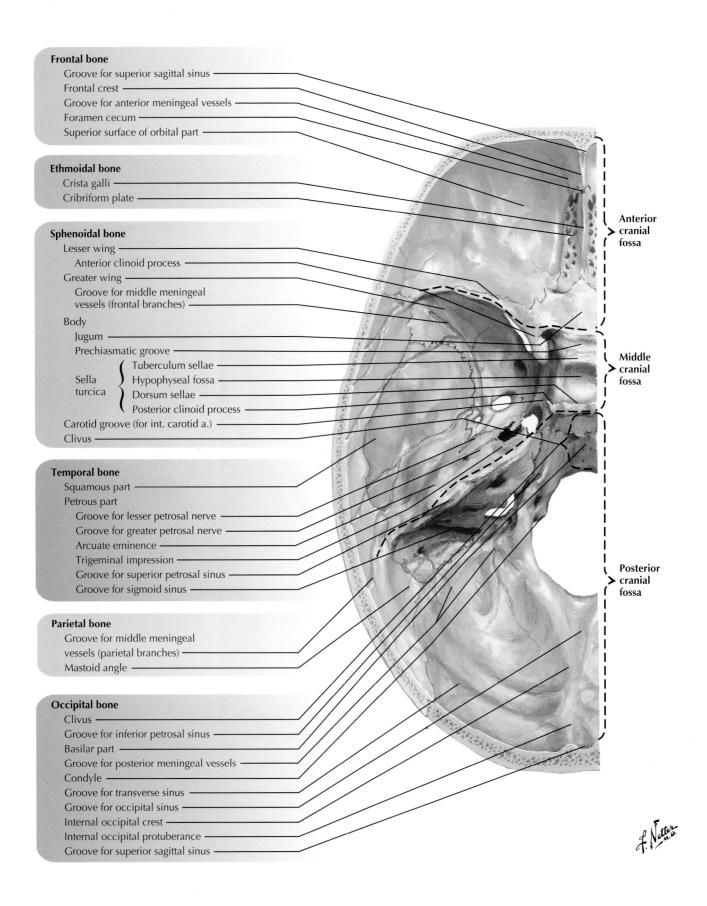

Frontal bone
- Groove for superior sagittal sinus
- Frontal crest
- Groove for anterior meningeal vessels
- Foramen cecum
- Superior surface of orbital part

Ethmoidal bone
- Crista galli
- Cribriform plate

Sphenoidal bone
- Lesser wing
  - Anterior clinoid process
- Greater wing
  - Groove for middle meningeal vessels (frontal branches)
- Body
  - Jugum
  - Prechiasmatic groove
  - Sella turcica
    - Tuberculum sellae
    - Hypophyseal fossa
    - Dorsum sellae
    - Posterior clinoid process
- Carotid groove (for int. carotid a.)
- Clivus

Temporal bone
- Squamous part
- Petrous part
  - Groove for lesser petrosal nerve
  - Groove for greater petrosal nerve
  - Arcuate eminence
  - Trigeminal impression
  - Groove for superior petrosal sinus
  - Groove for sigmoid sinus

Parietal bone
- Groove for middle meningeal vessels (parietal branches)
- Mastoid angle

Occipital bone
- Clivus
- Groove for inferior petrosal sinus
- Basilar part
- Groove for posterior meningeal vessels
- Condyle
- Groove for transverse sinus
- Groove for occipital sinus
- Internal occipital crest
- Internal occipital protuberance
- Groove for superior sagittal sinus

Anterior cranial fossa

Middle cranial fossa

Posterior cranial fossa

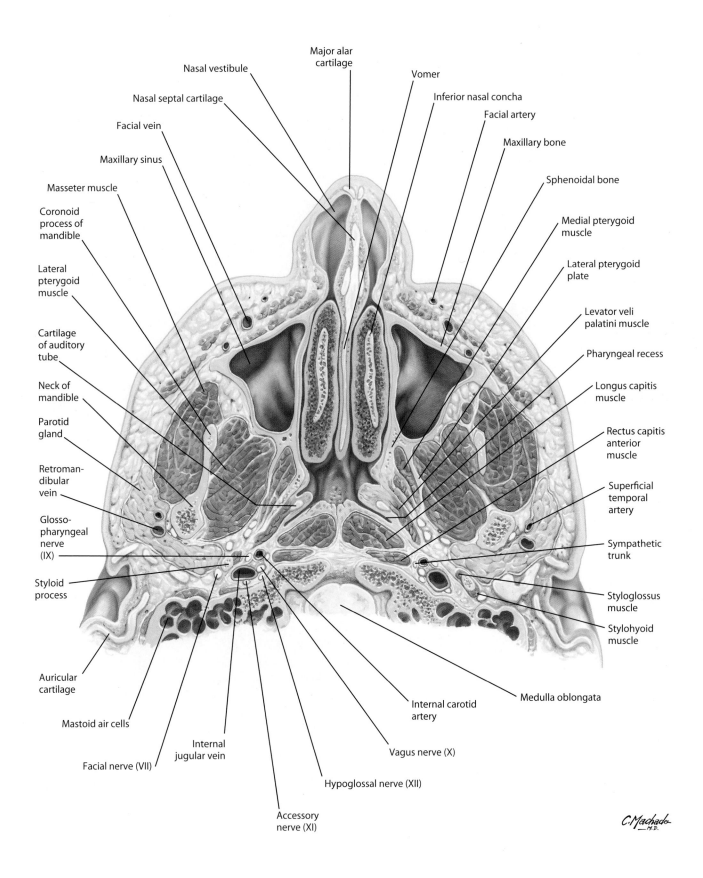

Major alar cartilage

Nasal vestibule

Vomer

Nasal septal cartilage

Inferior nasal concha

Facial vein

Facial artery

Maxillary sinus

Maxillary bone

Masseter muscle

Sphenoidal bone

Coronoid process of mandible

Medial pterygoid muscle

Lateral pterygoid muscle

Lateral pterygoid plate

Cartilage of auditory tube

Levator veli palatini muscle

Pharyngeal recess

Neck of mandible

Longus capitis muscle

Parotid gland

Rectus capitis anterior muscle

Retromandibular vein

Superficial temporal artery

Glossopharyngeal nerve (IX)

Sympathetic trunk

Styloid process

Styloglossus muscle

Stylohyoid muscle

Auricular cartilage

Medulla oblongata

Mastoid air cells

Internal carotid artery

Facial nerve (VII)

Internal jugular vein

Vagus nerve (X)

Accessory nerve (XI)

Hypoglossal nerve (XII)

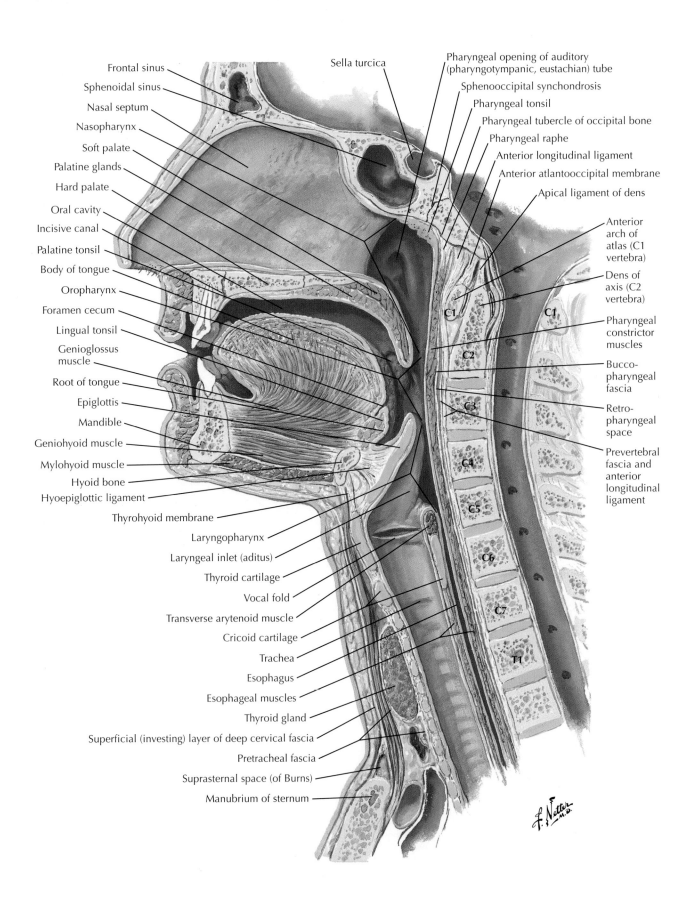

Frontal sinus

Sphenoidal sinus

Nasal septum

Nasopharynx

Soft palate

Palatine glands

Hard palate

Oral cavity

Incisive canal

Palatine tonsil

Body of tongue

Oropharynx

Foramen cecum

Lingual tonsil

Genioglossus muscle

Root of tongue

Epiglottis

Mandible

Geniohyoid muscle

Mylohyoid muscle

Hyoid bone

Hyoepiglottic ligament

Thyrohyoid membrane

Laryngopharynx

Laryngeal inlet (aditus)

Thyroid cartilage

Vocal fold

Transverse arytenoid muscle

Cricoid cartilage

Trachea

Esophagus

Esophageal muscles

Thyroid gland

Superficial (investing) layer of deep cervical fascia

Pretracheal fascia

Suprasternal space (of Burns)

Manubrium of sternum

Sella turcica

Pharyngeal opening of auditory (pharyngotympanic, eustachian) tube

Sphenooccipital synchondrosis

Pharyngeal tonsil

Pharyngeal tubercle of occipital bone

Pharyngeal raphe

Anterior longitudinal ligament

Anterior atlantooccipital membrane

Apical ligament of dens

Anterior arch of atlas (C1 vertebra)

Dens of axis (C2 vertebra)

Pharyngeal constrictor muscles

Bucco-pharyngeal fascia

Retro-pharyngeal space

Prevertebral fascia and anterior longitudinal ligament

C1

C2

C3

C4

C5

C6

C7

T1

C1

C1

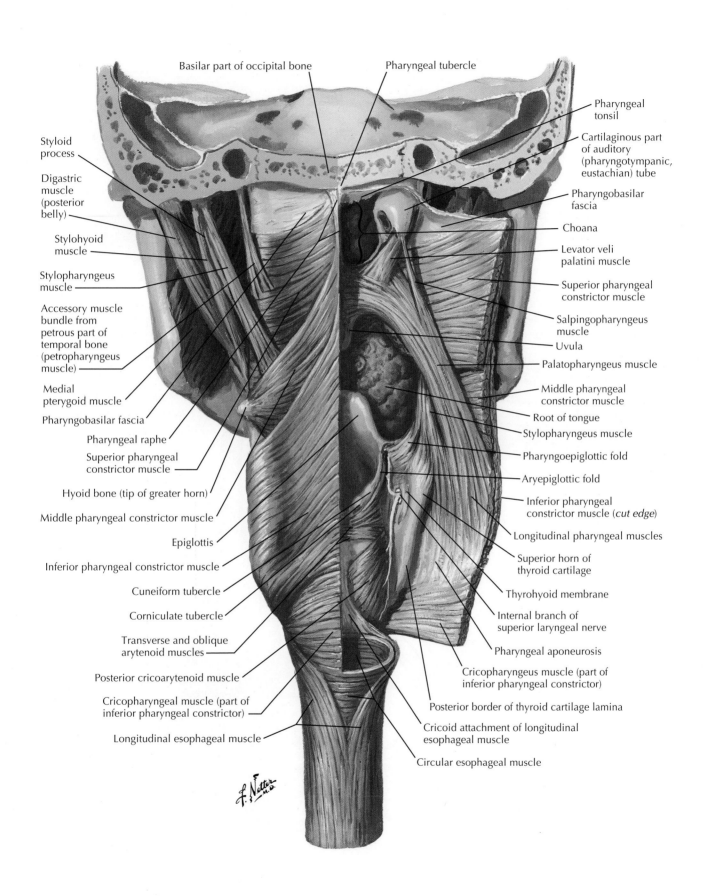

Basilar part of occipital bone

Pharyngeal tubercle

Pharyngeal tonsil

Styloid process

Cartilaginous part of auditory (pharyngotympanic, eustachian) tube

Digastric muscle (posterior belly)

Pharyngobasilar fascia

Stylohyoid muscle

Choana

Stylopharyngeus muscle

Levator veli palatini muscle

Superior pharyngeal constrictor muscle

Accessory muscle bundle from petrous part of temporal bone (petropharyngeus muscle)

Salpingopharyngeus muscle

Uvula

Palatopharyngeus muscle

Medial pterygoid muscle

Middle pharyngeal constrictor muscle

Pharyngobasilar fascia

Root of tongue

Pharyngeal raphe

Stylopharyngeus muscle

Superior pharyngeal constrictor muscle

Pharyngoepiglottic fold

Aryepiglottic fold

Hyoid bone (tip of greater horn)

Inferior pharyngeal constrictor muscle (cut edge)

Middle pharyngeal constrictor muscle

Longitudinal pharyngeal muscles

Epiglottis

Superior horn of thyroid cartilage

Inferior pharyngeal constrictor muscle

Thyrohyoid membrane

Cuneiform tubercle

Internal branch of superior laryngeal nerve

Corniculate tubercle

Pharyngeal aponeurosis

Transverse and oblique arytenoid muscles

Cricopharyngeus muscle (part of inferior pharyngeal constrictor)

Posterior cricoarytenoid muscle

Cricopharyngeal muscle (part of inferior pharyngeal constrictor)

Posterior border of thyroid cartilage lamina

Cricoid attachment of longitudinal esophageal muscle

Longitudinal esophageal muscle

Circular esophageal muscle

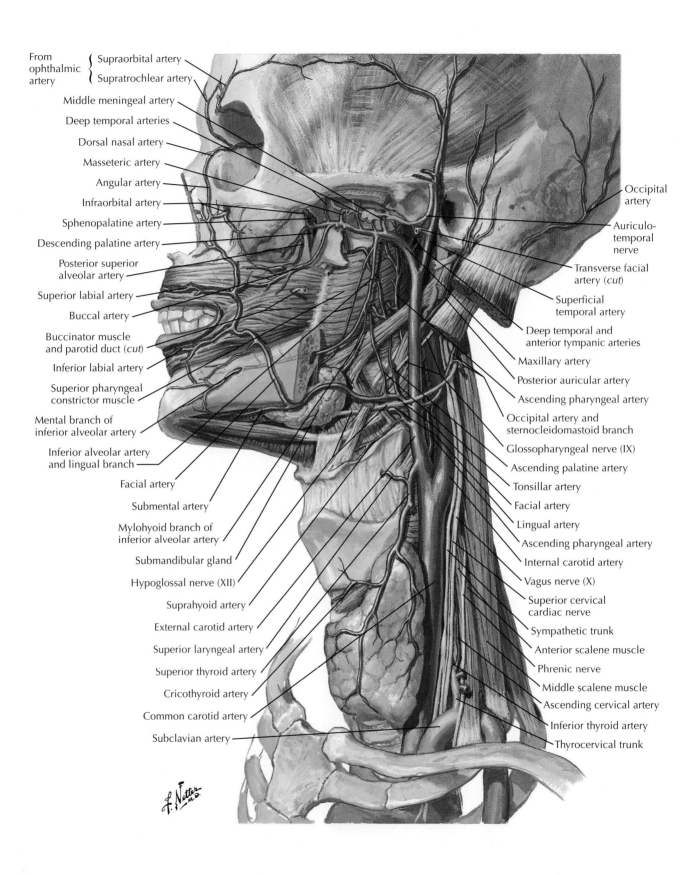

From ophthalmic artery {
Supraorbital artery
Supratrochlear artery

Middle meningeal artery

Deep temporal arteries

Dorsal nasal artery

Masseteric artery

Angular artery

Infraorbital artery

Sphenopalatine artery

Descending palatine artery

Posterior superior alveolar artery

Superior labial artery

Buccal artery

Buccinator muscle and parotid duct (cut)

Inferior labial artery

Superior pharyngeal constrictor muscle

Mental branch of inferior alveolar artery

Inferior alveolar artery and lingual branch

Facial artery

Submental artery

Mylohyoid branch of inferior alveolar artery

Submandibular gland

Hypoglossal nerve (XII)

Suprahyoid artery

External carotid artery

Superior laryngeal artery

Superior thyroid artery

Cricothyroid artery

Common carotid artery

Subclavian artery

Occipital artery

Auriculo-temporal nerve

Transverse facial artery (cut)

Superficial temporal artery

Deep temporal and anterior tympanic arteries

Maxillary artery

Posterior auricular artery

Ascending pharyngeal artery

Occipital artery and sternocleidomastoid branch

Glossopharyngeal nerve (IX)

Ascending palatine artery

Tonsillar artery

Facial artery

Lingual artery

Ascending pharyngeal artery

Internal carotid artery

Vagus nerve (X)

Superior cervical cardiac nerve

Sympathetic trunk

Anterior scalene muscle

Phrenic nerve

Middle scalene muscle

Ascending cervical artery

Inferior thyroid artery

Thyrocervical trunk

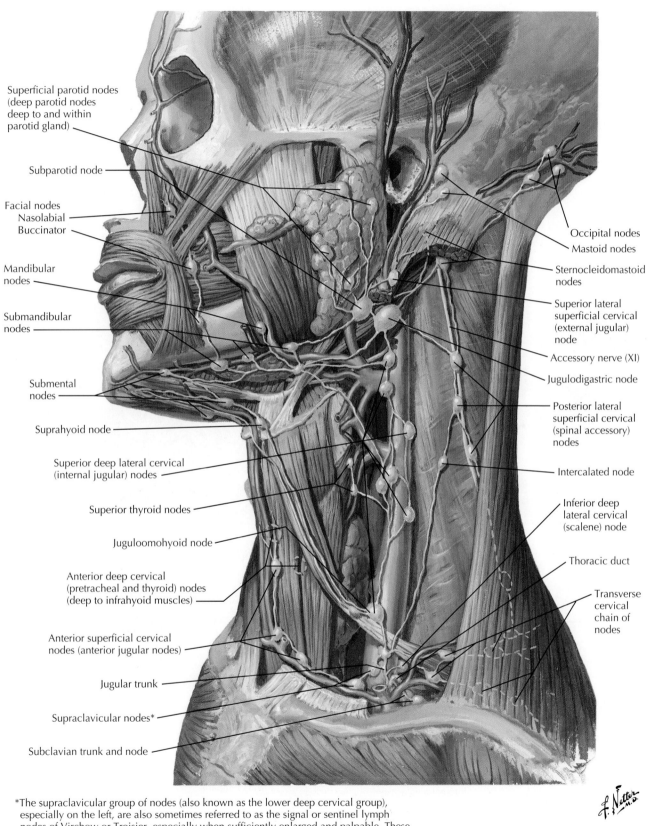

Superficial parotid nodes
(deep parotid nodes
deep to and within
parotid gland)

Subparotid node

Facial nodes
Nasolabial
Buccinator

Mandibular
nodes

Submandibular
nodes

Submental
nodes

Suprahyoid node

Superior deep lateral cervical
(internal jugular) nodes

Superior thyroid nodes

Juguloomohyoid node

Anterior deep cervical
(pretracheal and thyroid) nodes
(deep to infrahyoid muscles)

Anterior superficial cervical
nodes (anterior jugular nodes)

Jugular trunk

Supraclavicular nodes*

Subclavian trunk and node

Occipital nodes
Mastoid nodes

Sternocleidomastoid
nodes

Superior lateral
superficial cervical
(external jugular)
node

Accessory nerve (XI)

Jugulodigastric node

Posterior lateral
superficial cervical
(spinal accessory)
nodes

Intercalated node

Inferior deep
lateral cervical
(scalene) node

Thoracic duct

Transverse
cervical
chain of
nodes

*The supraclavicular group of nodes (also known as the lower deep cervical group),
especially on the left, are also sometimes referred to as the signal or sentinel lymph
nodes of Virchow or Troisier, especially when sufficiently enlarged and palpable. These
nodes (or a single node) are so termed because they may be the first recognized presumptive
evidence of malignant disease in the viscera.

Frontal section

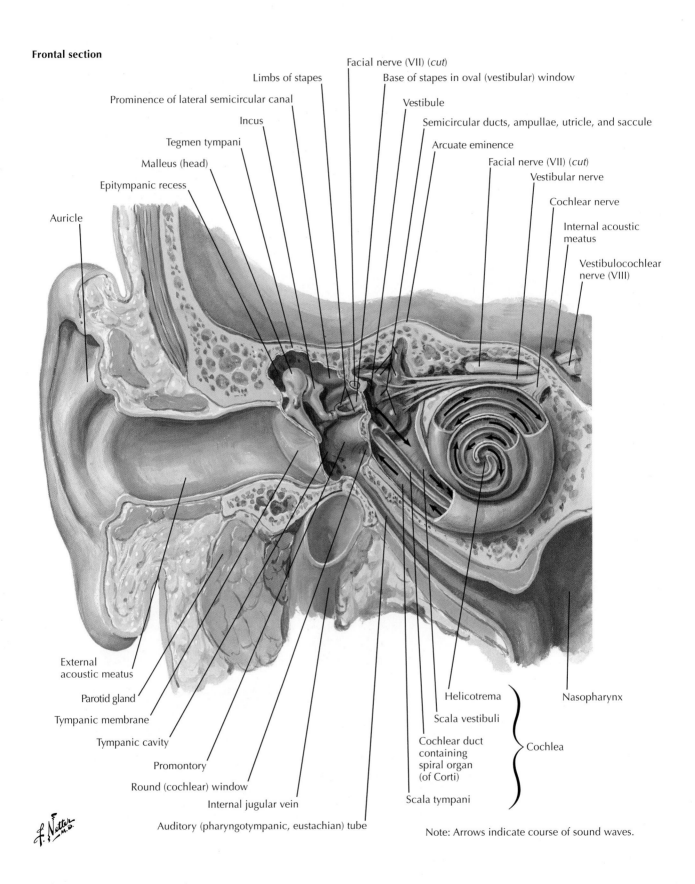

Facial nerve (VII) *(cut)*

Limbs of stapes

Base of stapes in oval (vestibular) window

Prominence of lateral semicircular canal

Vestibule

Incus

Semicircular ducts, ampullae, utricle, and saccule

Tegmen tympani

Arcuate eminence

Malleus (head)

Facial nerve (VII) *(cut)*

Epitympanic recess

Vestibular nerve

Cochlear nerve

Auricle

Internal acoustic meatus

Vestibulocochlear nerve (VIII)

External acoustic meatus

Parotid gland

Tympanic membrane

Tympanic cavity

Promontory

Round (cochlear) window

Internal jugular vein

Auditory (pharyngotympanic, eustachian) tube

Helicotrema

Scala vestibuli

Cochlear duct containing spiral organ (of Corti)

Scala tympani

Nasopharynx

Cochlea

Note: Arrows indicate course of sound waves.

Frontal view of 3D skull reformat

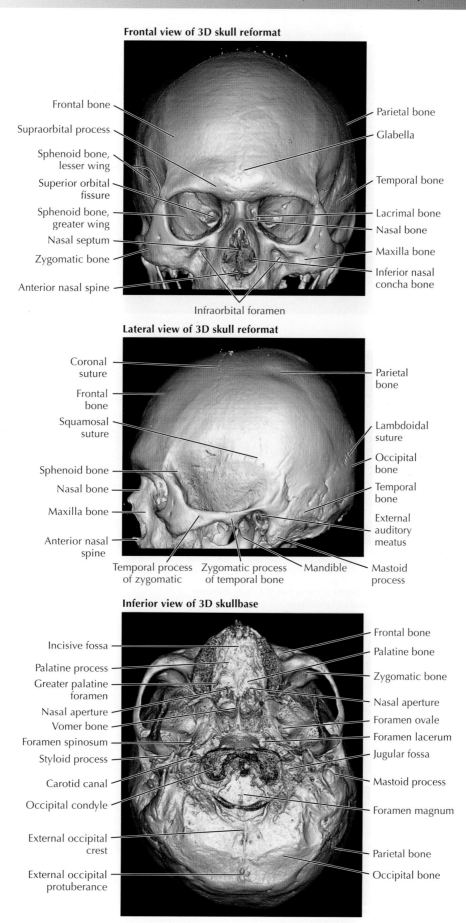

Frontal bone
Supraorbital process
Sphenoid bone, lesser wing
Superior orbital fissure
Sphenoid bone, greater wing
Nasal septum
Zygomatic bone
Anterior nasal spine

Parietal bone
Glabella
Temporal bone
Lacrimal bone
Nasal bone
Maxilla bone
Inferior nasal concha bone

Infraorbital foramen

Lateral view of 3D skull reformat

Coronal suture
Frontal bone
Squamosal suture
Sphenoid bone
Nasal bone
Maxilla bone
Anterior nasal spine

Parietal bone
Lambdoidal suture
Occipital bone
Temporal bone
External auditory meatus

Temporal process of zygomatic
Zygomatic process of temporal bone
Mandible
Mastoid process

Inferior view of 3D skullbase

Incisive fossa
Palatine process
Greater palatine foramen
Nasal aperture
Vomer bone
Foramen spinosum
Styloid process
Carotid canal
Occipital condyle
External occipital crest
External occipital protuberance

Frontal bone
Palatine bone
Zygomatic bone
Nasal aperture
Foramen ovale
Foramen lacerum
Jugular fossa
Mastoid process
Foramen magnum
Parietal bone
Occipital bone

Posterior view of 3D skull reformat

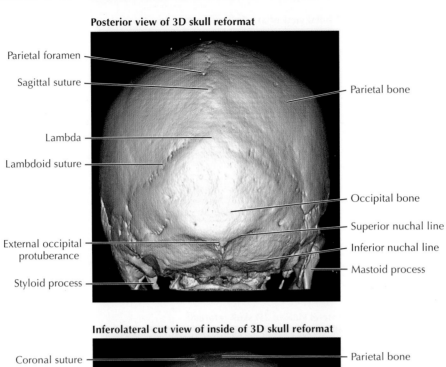

Parietal foramen

Sagittal suture

Lambda

Lambdoid suture

External occipital protuberance

Styloid process

Parietal bone

Occipital bone

Superior nuchal line

Inferior nuchal line

Mastoid process

Inferolateral cut view of inside of 3D skull reformat

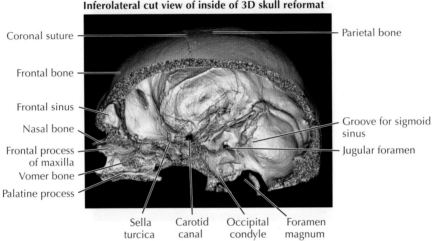

Coronal suture

Frontal bone

Frontal sinus

Nasal bone

Frontal process of maxilla

Vomer bone

Palatine process

Parietal bone

Groove for sigmoid sinus

Jugular foramen

Sella turcica   Carotid canal   Occipital condyle   Foramen magnum

Superior view of cut 3D skull showing inside of skullbase

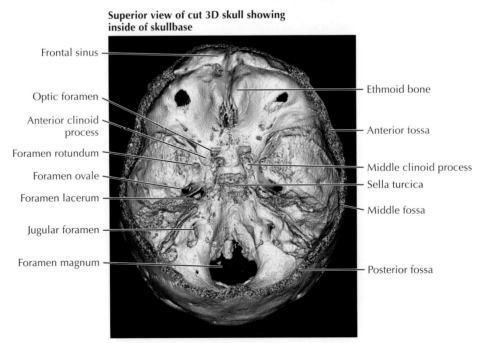

Frontal sinus

Optic foramen

Anterior clinoid process

Foramen rotundum

Foramen ovale

Foramen lacerum

Jugular foramen

Foramen magnum

Ethmoid bone

Anterior fossa

Middle clinoid process

Sella turcica

Middle fossa

Posterior fossa

Chapter 9 PARANASAL SINUSES

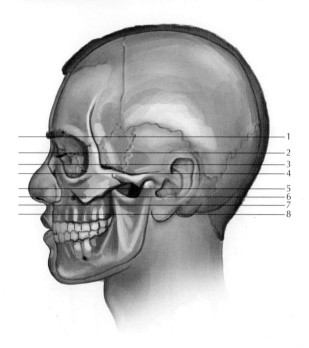

AXIAL   322

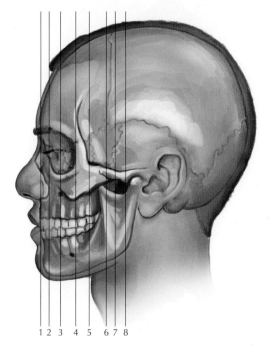

CORONAL   338

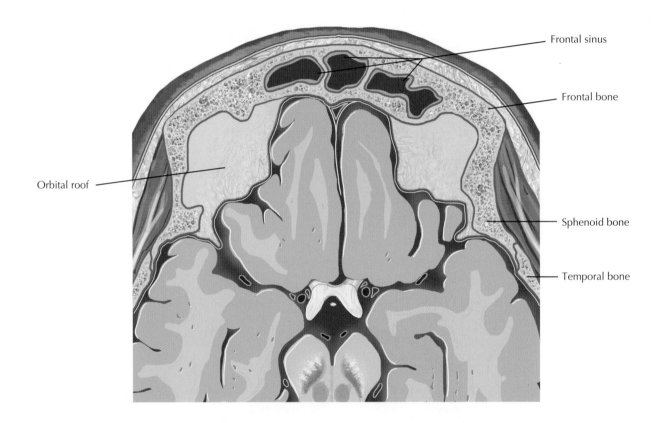

Frontal sinus

Frontal bone

Orbital roof

Sphenoid bone

Temporal bone

NORMAL ANATOMY

The paranasal sinuses are composed of the *frontal* sinuses, the *ethmoid* sinuses or ethmoid air cells, the *maxillary* sinuses or maxillary antra, and the *sphenoid* sinuses. The names are derived from the bones that form the walls of the sinuses.

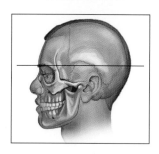

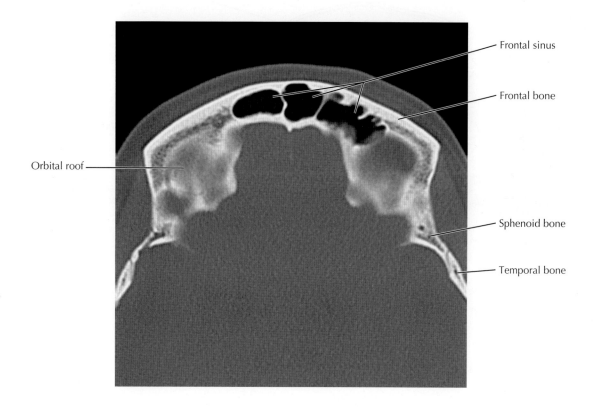

Frontal sinus

Frontal bone

Orbital roof

Sphenoid bone

Temporal bone

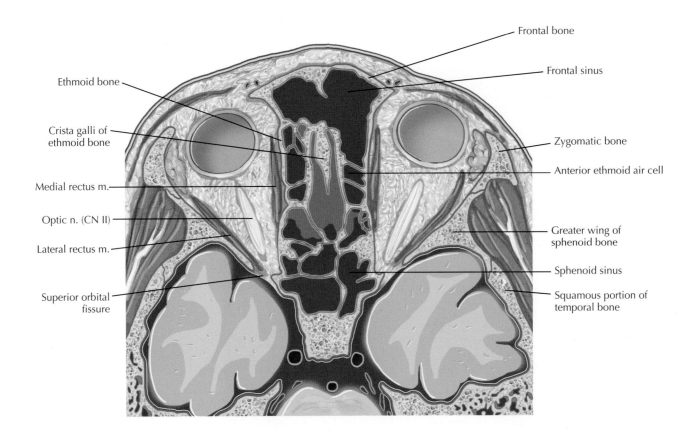

Frontal bone

Frontal sinus

Ethmoid bone

Crista galli of
ethmoid bone

Zygomatic bone

Medial rectus m.

Anterior ethmoid air cell

Optic n. (CN II)

Lateral rectus m.

Greater wing of
sphenoid bone

Superior orbital
fissure

Sphenoid sinus

Squamous portion of
temporal bone

NORMAL ANATOMY

The sphenoid sinuses are at the center of the skull base, immediately below the sella turcica (see Chapter 7). In ancient Egypt, mummification would involve driving a metal hook through the nasal passages and the sphenoid sinuses into the brain, which would be removed through the nostrils. This tract is used in modern days to pass a scope into the sella turcica to remove pituitary adenomas.

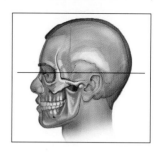

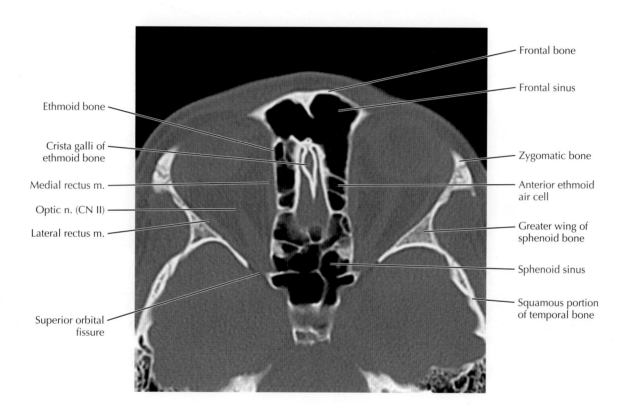

Frontal bone

Frontal sinus

Ethmoid bone

Crista galli of
ethmoid bone

Zygomatic bone

Medial rectus m.

Anterior ethmoid
air cell

Optic n. (CN II)

Greater wing of
sphenoid bone

Lateral rectus m.

Sphenoid sinus

Squamous portion
of temporal bone

Superior orbital
fissure

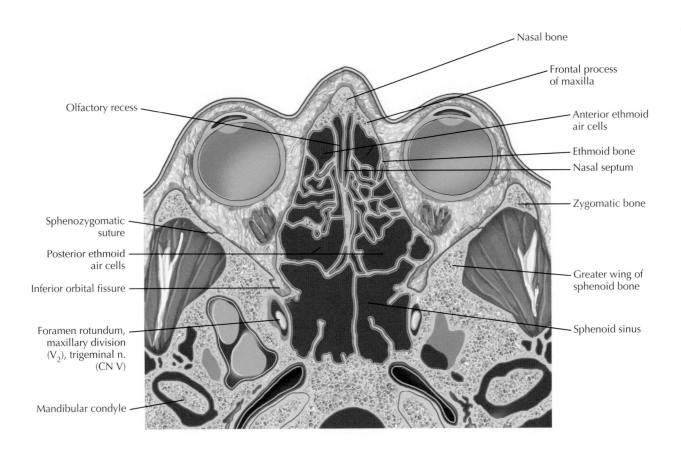

Nasal bone

Frontal process
of maxilla

Olfactory recess

Anterior ethmoid
air cells

Ethmoid bone

Nasal septum

Zygomatic bone

Sphenozygomatic
suture

Posterior ethmoid
air cells

Inferior orbital fissure

Greater wing of
sphenoid bone

Foramen rotundum,
maxillary division
(V₂), trigeminal n.
(CN V)

Sphenoid sinus

Mandibular condyle

DIAGNOSTIC CONSIDERATION

In the setting of trauma, careful evaluation of CT bone windows is important to identify fractures, particularly around critical structures such as the carotid canal. On MRI, subtle bone fractures may not be directly visible; therefore, secondary signs, such as the presence of a hemorrhagic fluid level in the paranasal sinuses may be the only indication of traumatic injury.

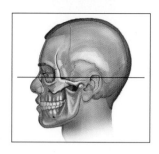

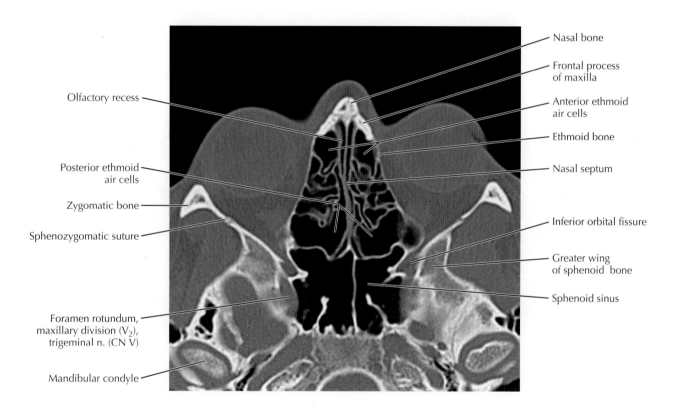

Olfactory recess

Posterior ethmoid air cells

Zygomatic bone

Sphenozygomatic suture

Foramen rotundum, maxillary division (V₂), trigeminal n. (CN V)

Mandibular condyle

Nasal bone

Frontal process of maxilla

Anterior ethmoid air cells

Ethmoid bone

Nasal septum

Inferior orbital fissure

Greater wing of sphenoid bone

Sphenoid sinus

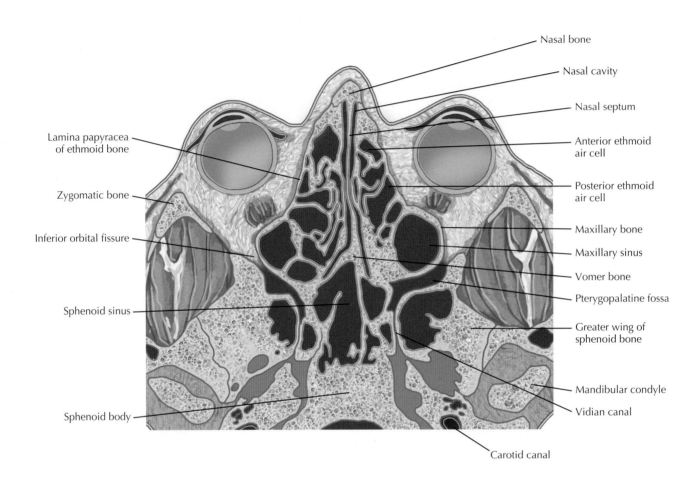

Nasal bone

Nasal cavity

Nasal septum

Anterior ethmoid air cell

Posterior ethmoid air cell

Maxillary bone

Maxillary sinus

Vomer bone

Pterygopalatine fossa

Greater wing of sphenoid bone

Mandibular condyle

Vidian canal

Carotid canal

Lamina papyracea of ethmoid bone

Zygomatic bone

Inferior orbital fissure

Sphenoid sinus

Sphenoid body

DIAGNOSTIC CONSIDERATION

Fracture of the *lamina papyracea*, the thin bone between the orbit and the ethmoid air cells (sinuses), can be subtle. Fat herniating into the ethmoid air cells is a sign of lamina papyracea fracture.

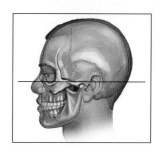

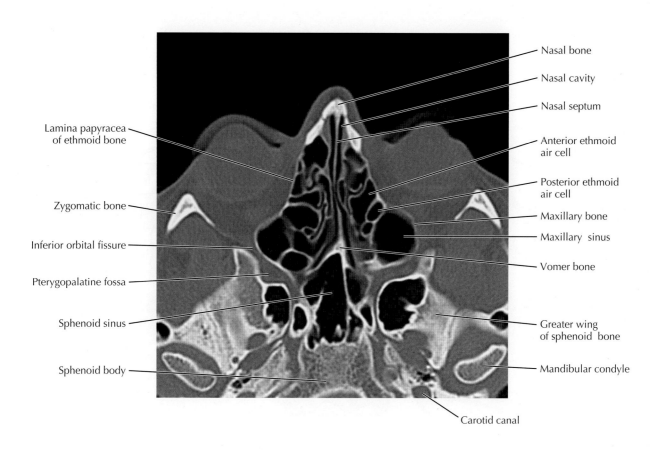

Nasal bone

Nasal cavity

Nasal septum

Anterior ethmoid air cell

Posterior ethmoid air cell

Maxillary bone

Maxillary sinus

Vomer bone

Greater wing of sphenoid bone

Mandibular condyle

Carotid canal

Lamina papyracea of ethmoid bone

Zygomatic bone

Inferior orbital fissure

Pterygopalatine fossa

Sphenoid sinus

Sphenoid body

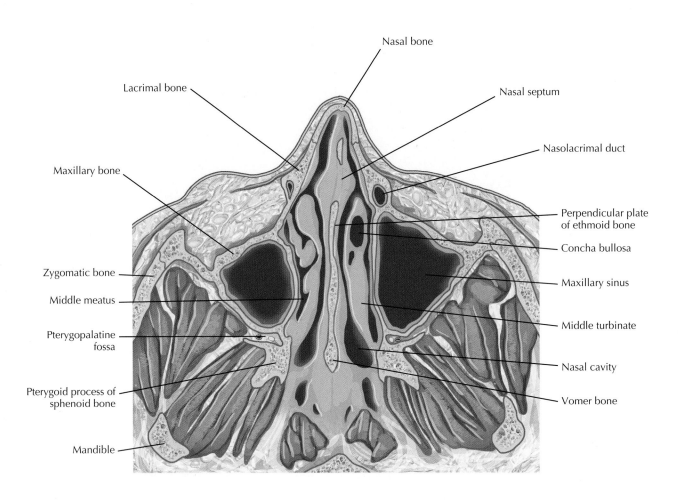

Nasal bone

Lacrimal bone

Nasal septum

Nasolacrimal duct

Maxillary bone

Perpendicular plate of ethmoid bone

Concha bullosa

Zygomatic bone

Maxillary sinus

Middle meatus

Pterygopalatine fossa

Middle turbinate

Pterygoid process of sphenoid bone

Nasal cavity

Mandible

Vomer bone

NORMAL ANATOMY

The *pterygopalatine fossa* houses the second division of the fifth cranial nerve (CN V), the maxillary nerve (V$_2$). The ganglion associated with V$_2$ lying in this fossa is known as *Meckel's* (pterygopalatine) ganglion, whereas the *Gasserian* (trigeminal) ganglion lies in Meckel's cave. Loss of the fat surrounding the nerve and ganglion is seen in perineural infiltration by malignancy.

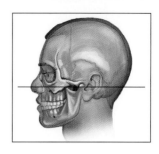

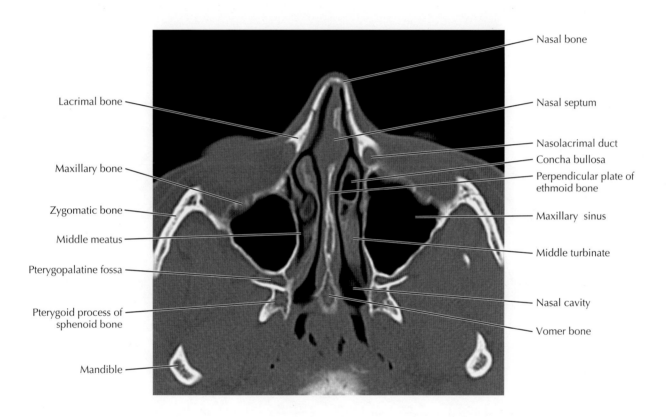

Nasal bone

Nasal septum

Lacrimal bone

Nasolacrimal duct

Concha bullosa

Maxillary bone

Perpendicular plate of
ethmoid bone

Zygomatic bone

Maxillary sinus

Middle meatus

Middle turbinate

Pterygopalatine fossa

Pterygoid process of
sphenoid bone

Nasal cavity

Vomer bone

Mandible

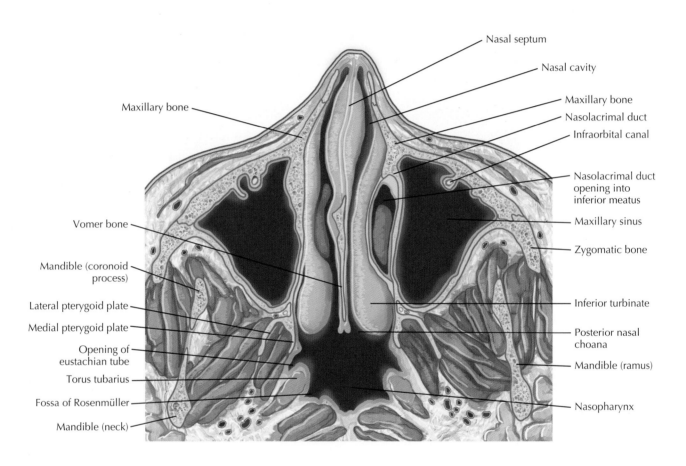

Nasal septum

Nasal cavity

Maxillary bone

Maxillary bone

Nasolacrimal duct

Infraorbital canal

Nasolacrimal duct opening into inferior meatus

Maxillary sinus

Vomer bone

Zygomatic bone

Mandible (coronoid process)

Lateral pterygoid plate

Medial pterygoid plate

Inferior turbinate

Opening of eustachian tube

Posterior nasal choana

Torus tubarius

Mandible (ramus)

Fossa of Rosenmüller

Nasopharynx

Mandible (neck)

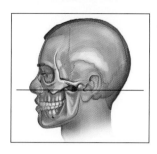

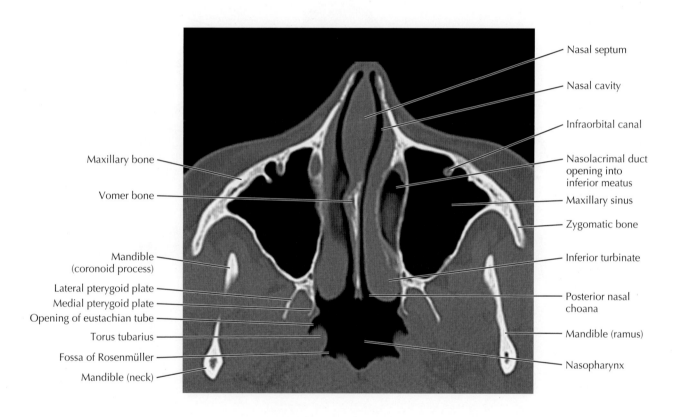

Nasal septum

Nasal cavity

Infraorbital canal

Nasolacrimal duct opening into inferior meatus

Maxillary sinus

Zygomatic bone

Inferior turbinate

Posterior nasal choana

Mandible (ramus)

Nasopharynx

Maxillary bone

Vomer bone

Mandible (coronoid process)

Lateral pterygoid plate

Medial pterygoid plate

Opening of eustachian tube

Torus tubarius

Fossa of Rosenmüller

Mandible (neck)

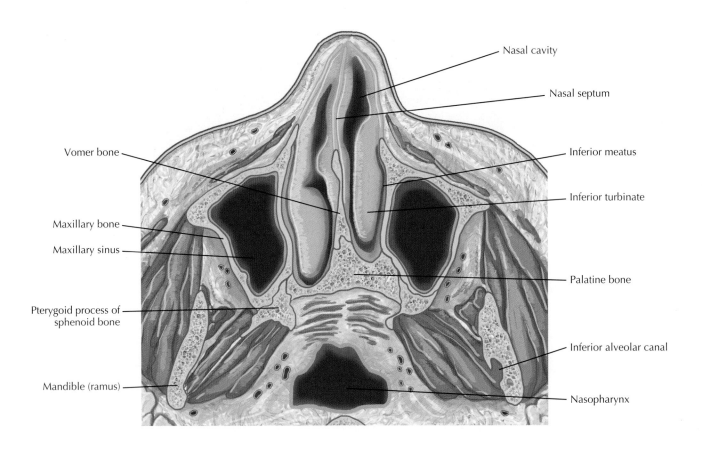

Nasal cavity

Nasal septum

Vomer bone

Inferior meatus

Inferior turbinate

Maxillary bone

Maxillary sinus

Palatine bone

Pterygoid process of sphenoid bone

Inferior alveolar canal

Mandible (ramus)

Nasopharynx

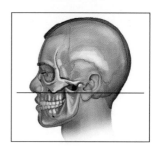

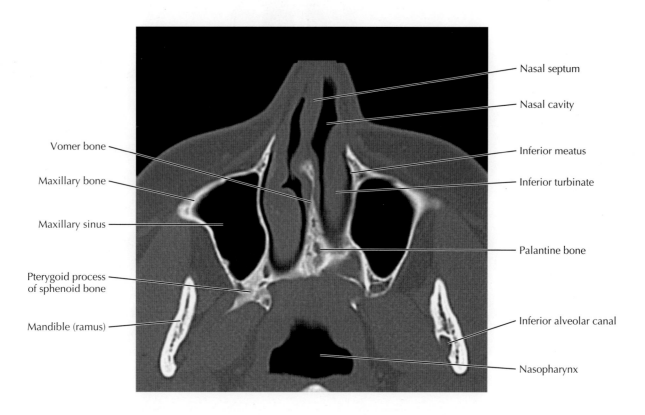

Nasal septum

Nasal cavity

Inferior meatus

Inferior turbinate

Vomer bone

Maxillary bone

Maxillary sinus

Palantine bone

Pterygoid process
of sphenoid bone

Mandible (ramus)

Inferior alveolar canal

Nasopharynx

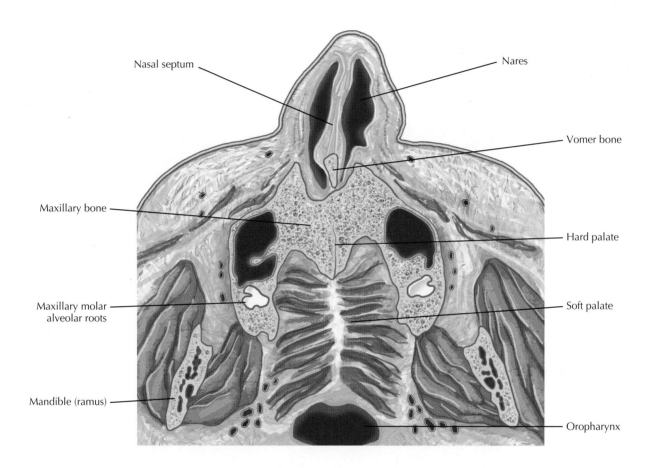

Nasal septum

Nares

Vomer bone

Maxillary bone

Hard palate

Maxillary molar alveolar roots

Soft palate

Mandible (ramus)

Oropharynx

NORMAL ANATOMY

Note that no true boundary exists between the nasopharynx and the oropharynx on axial images. The teeth can provide a helpful anatomic landmark. When the teeth are clearly in view, the lumen is likely that of the oropharynx. On this image, where the alveolar roots of the maxillary molar teeth are visible, along with part of the hard palate and much of the soft palate, the lumen in view is likely junctional between the nasopharynx and the oropharynx.

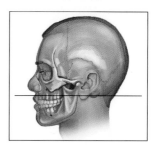

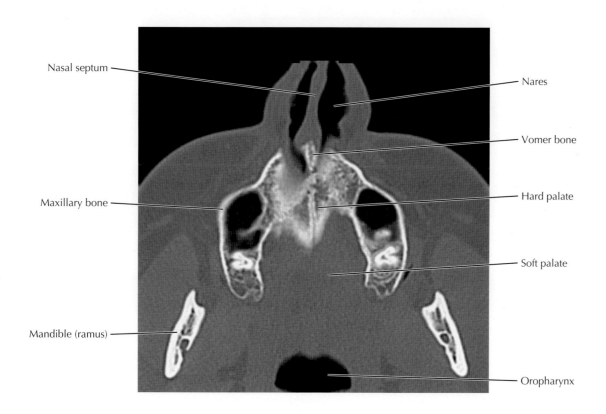

Nasal septum

Nares

Vomer bone

Maxillary bone

Hard palate

Soft palate

Mandible (ramus)

Oropharynx

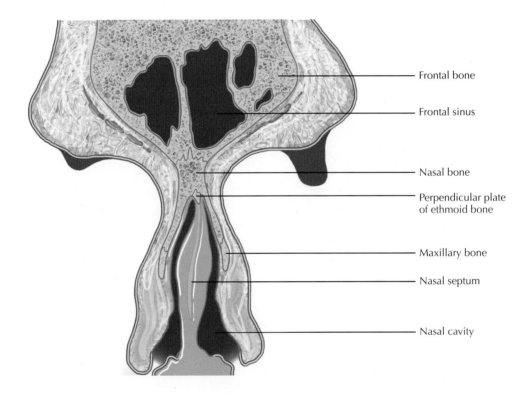

Frontal bone

Frontal sinus

Nasal bone

Perpendicular plate of ethmoid bone

Maxillary bone

Nasal septum

Nasal cavity

NORMAL ANATOMY

The frontal bone above the level of the sinuses is extremely hard. More inferiorly, however, where the frontal sinuses are located, the walls can be relatively thin.

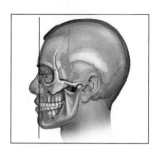

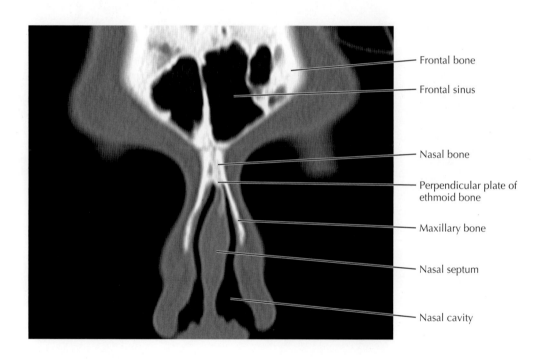

Frontal bone

Frontal sinus

Nasal bone

Perpendicular plate of ethmoid bone

Maxillary bone

Nasal septum

Nasal cavity

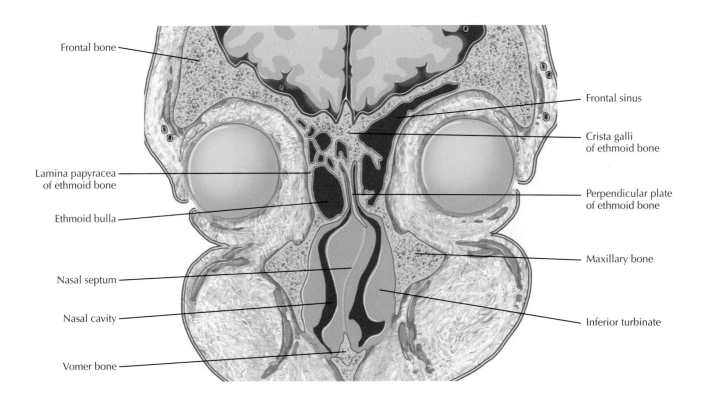

Frontal bone

Frontal sinus

Crista galli of ethmoid bone

Lamina papyracea of ethmoid bone

Perpendicular plate of ethmoid bone

Ethmoid bulla

Maxillary bone

Nasal septum

Nasal cavity

Inferior turbinate

Vomer bone

SURGICAL CONSIDERATION

Functional endoscopic sinus surgery can be performed to open the nasal passages when the nasal septum is significantly deviated to one side.

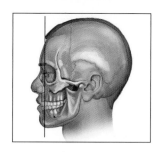

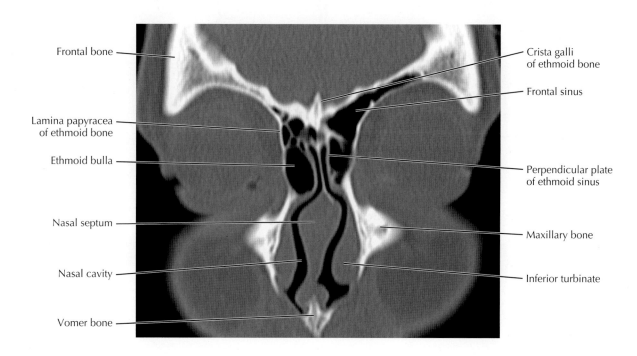

Frontal bone

Lamina papyracea
of ethmoid bone

Ethmoid bulla

Nasal septum

Nasal cavity

Vomer bone

Crista galli
of ethmoid bone

Frontal sinus

Perpendicular plate
of ethmoid sinus

Maxillary bone

Inferior turbinate

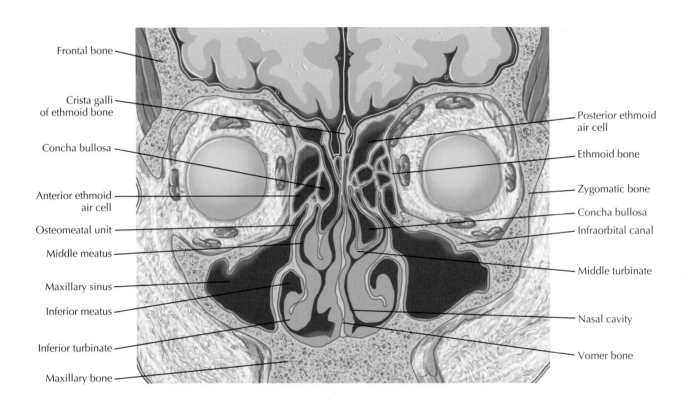

Frontal bone

Crista galli
of ethmoid bone

Concha bullosa

Anterior ethmoid
air cell

Osteomeatal unit

Middle meatus

Maxillary sinus

Inferior meatus

Inferior turbinate

Maxillary bone

Posterior ethmoid
air cell

Ethmoid bone

Zygomatic bone

Concha bullosa

Infraorbital canal

Middle turbinate

Nasal cavity

Vomer bone

NORMAL ANATOMY

The Coronal 3 view gives the best visualization of the *osteomeatal unit*. The osteomeatal complex is part of the middle meatus, which drains the frontal and maxillary sinuses and the anterior two thirds of the ethmoid air cells. When the osteomeatal unit is obstructed, these sinuses become inflamed and opacified with mucosal thickening and fluid.

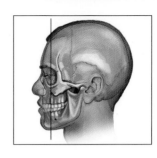

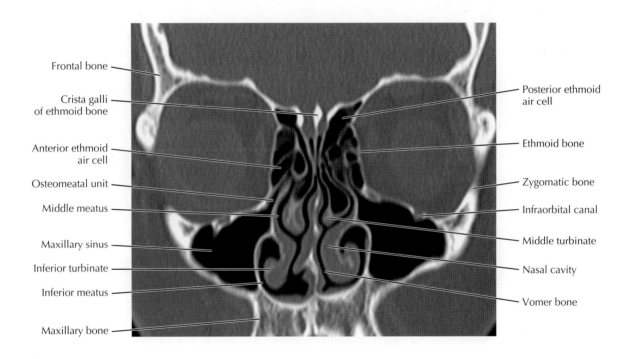

Frontal bone

Crista galli
of ethmoid bone

Anterior ethmoid
air cell

Osteomeatal unit

Middle meatus

Maxillary sinus

Inferior turbinate

Inferior meatus

Maxillary bone

Posterior ethmoid
air cell

Ethmoid bone

Zygomatic bone

Infraorbital canal

Middle turbinate

Nasal cavity

Vomer bone

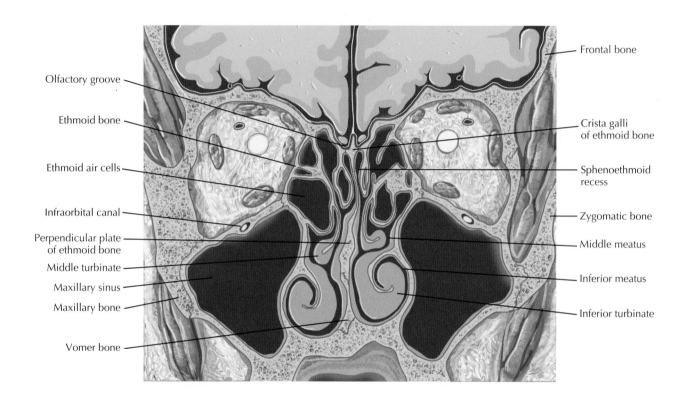

Olfactory groove

Ethmoid bone

Ethmoid air cells

Infraorbital canal

Perpendicular plate
of ethmoid bone

Middle turbinate

Maxillary sinus

Maxillary bone

Vomer bone

Frontal bone

Crista galli
of ethmoid bone

Sphenoethmoid
recess

Zygomatic bone

Middle meatus

Inferior meatus

Inferior turbinate

NORMAL ANATOMY

Note the paired olfactory grooves housing the olfactory nerves (cranial nerve I). An asymmetrically low olfactory groove can be important to note in patients who will undergo endoscopic sinus surgery.

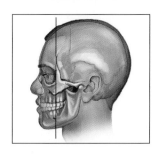

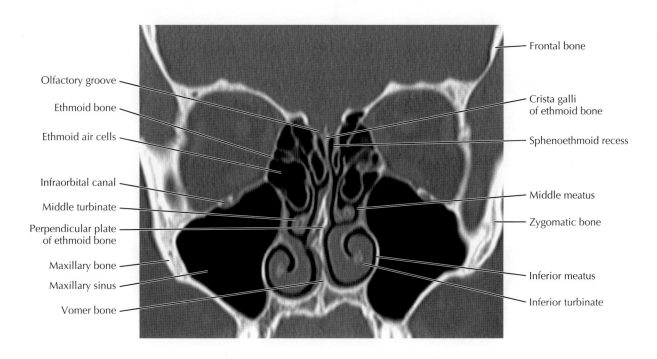

Olfactory groove

Ethmoid bone

Ethmoid air cells

Infraorbital canal

Middle turbinate

Perpendicular plate of ethmoid bone

Maxillary bone

Maxillary sinus

Vomer bone

Frontal bone

Crista galli of ethmoid bone

Sphenoethmoid recess

Middle meatus

Zygomatic bone

Inferior meatus

Inferior turbinate

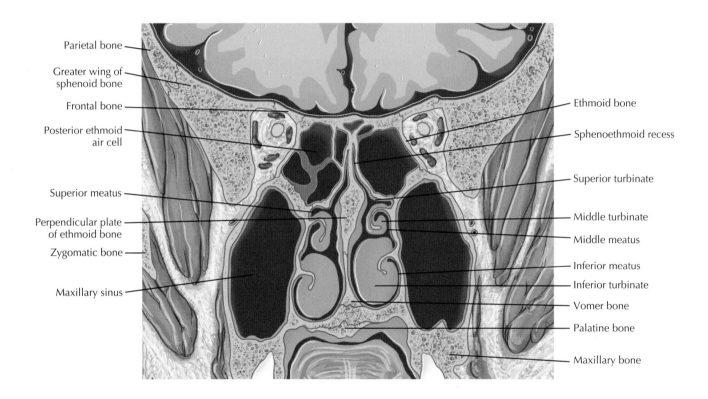

Parietal bone

Greater wing of sphenoid bone

Frontal bone

Posterior ethmoid air cell

Superior meatus

Perpendicular plate of ethmoid bone

Zygomatic bone

Maxillary sinus

Ethmoid bone

Sphenoethmoid recess

Superior turbinate

Middle turbinate

Middle meatus

Inferior meatus

Inferior turbinate

Vomer bone

Palatine bone

Maxillary bone

PATHOLOGIC PROCESS

The alveolar roots of the maxillary teeth are just underneath the maxillary sinuses. Inflammation or opacification within the inferior maxillary sinuses may be caused by periodontal disease.

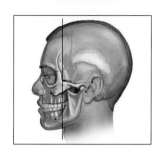

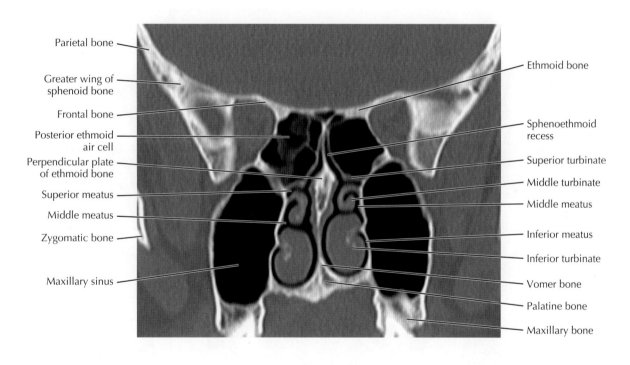

Parietal bone

Greater wing of sphenoid bone

Frontal bone

Posterior ethmoid air cell

Perpendicular plate of ethmoid bone

Superior meatus

Middle meatus

Zygomatic bone

Maxillary sinus

Ethmoid bone

Sphenoethmoid recess

Superior turbinate

Middle turbinate

Middle meatus

Inferior meatus

Inferior turbinate

Vomer bone

Palatine bone

Maxillary bone

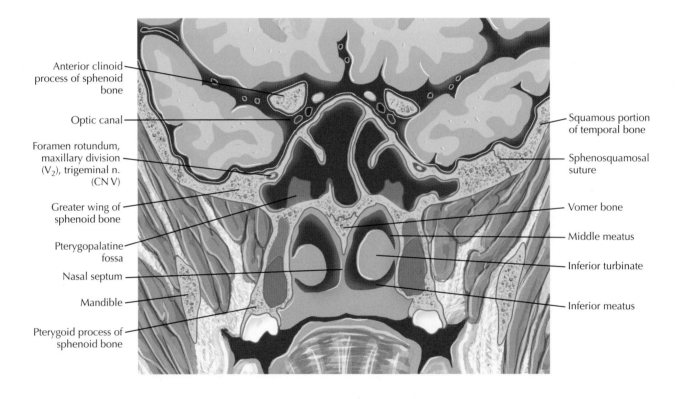

Anterior clinoid process of sphenoid bone

Optic canal

Foramen rotundum, maxillary division (V₂), trigeminal n. (CN V)

Greater wing of sphenoid bone

Pterygopalatine fossa

Nasal septum

Mandible

Pterygoid process of sphenoid bone

Squamous portion of temporal bone

Sphenosquamosal suture

Vomer bone

Middle meatus

Inferior turbinate

Inferior meatus

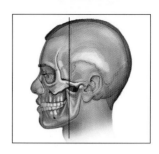

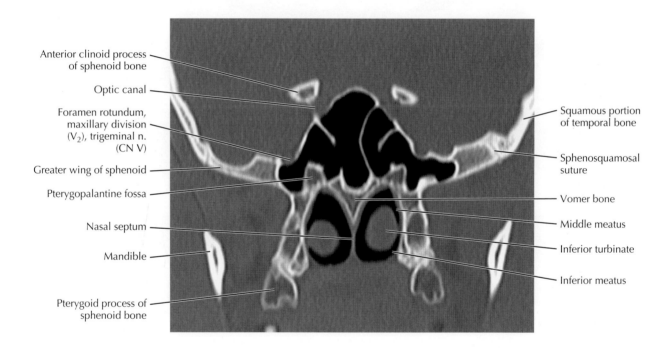

Anterior clinoid process of sphenoid bone

Optic canal

Foramen rotundum, maxillary division (V_2), trigeminal n. (CN V)

Greater wing of sphenoid

Pterygopalantine fossa

Nasal septum

Mandible

Pterygoid process of sphenoid bone

Squamous portion of temporal bone

Sphenosquamosal suture

Vomer bone

Middle meatus

Inferior turbinate

Inferior meatus

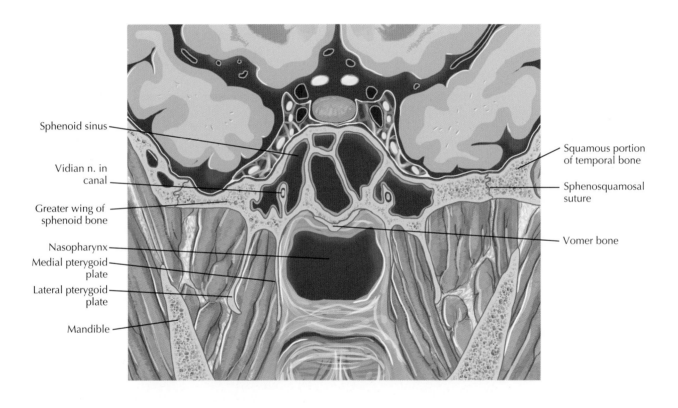

Sphenoid sinus

Vidian n. in canal

Greater wing of sphenoid bone

Nasopharynx

Medial pterygoid plate

Lateral pterygoid plate

Mandible

Squamous portion of temporal bone

Sphenosquamosal suture

Vomer bone

NORMAL ANATOMY

Note that the vidian nerve may often protrude into the sphenoid sinuses, resembling a stalk on coronal images.

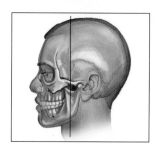

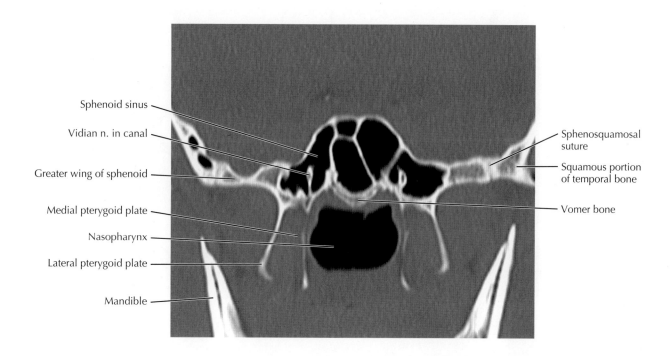

Sphenoid sinus

Vidian n. in canal

Greater wing of sphenoid

Medial pterygoid plate

Nasopharynx

Lateral pterygoid plate

Mandible

Sphenosquamosal suture

Squamous portion of temporal bone

Vomer bone

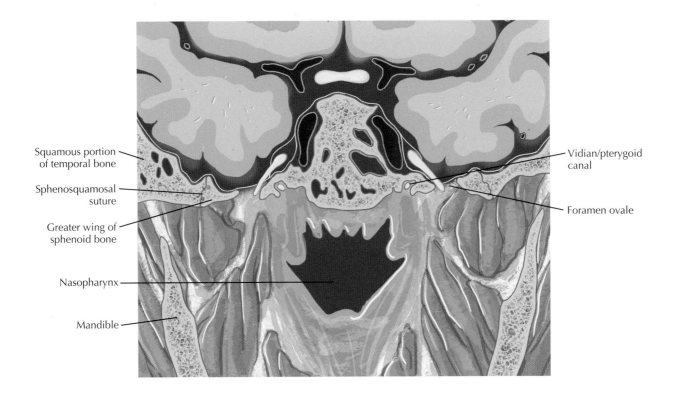

Squamous portion of temporal bone

Sphenosquamosal suture

Greater wing of sphenoid bone

Nasopharynx

Mandible

Vidian/pterygoid canal

Foramen ovale

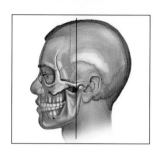

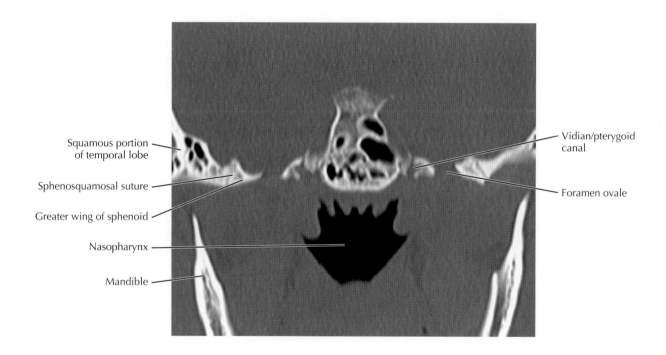

Squamous portion of temporal lobe

Sphenosquamosal suture

Greater wing of sphenoid

Nasopharynx

Mandible

Vidian/pterygoid canal

Foramen ovale

Chapter 10 ORBITS

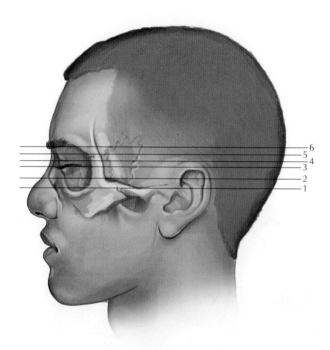

AXIAL   356

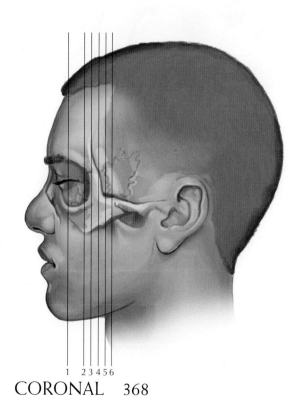

CORONAL   368

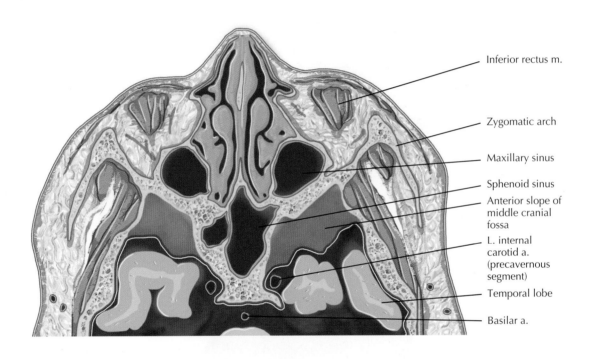

Inferior rectus m.

Zygomatic arch

Maxillary sinus

Sphenoid sinus

Anterior slope of middle cranial fossa

L. internal carotid a. (precavernous segment)

Temporal lobe

Basilar a.

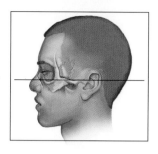

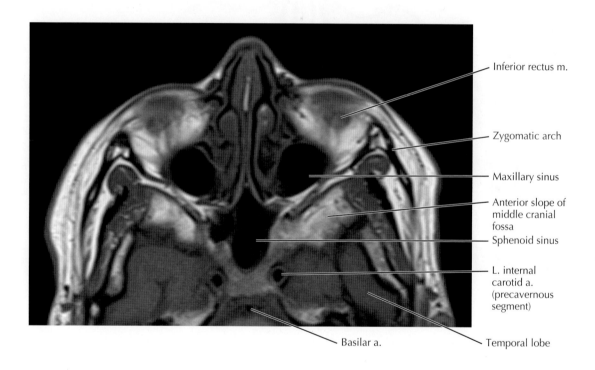

Inferior rectus m.

Zygomatic arch

Maxillary sinus

Anterior slope of middle cranial fossa

Sphenoid sinus

L. internal carotid a. (precavernous segment)

Basilar a.

Temporal lobe

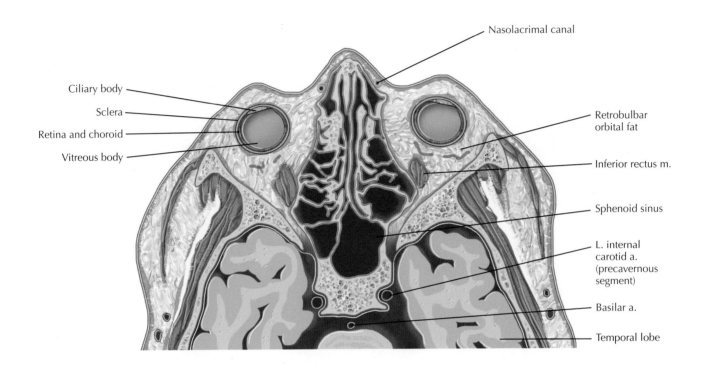

Nasolacrimal canal

Ciliary body

Sclera

Retina and choroid

Vitreous body

Retrobulbar orbital fat

Inferior rectus m.

Sphenoid sinus

L. internal carotid a. (precavernous segment)

Basilar a.

Temporal lobe

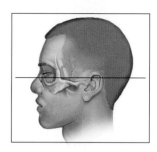

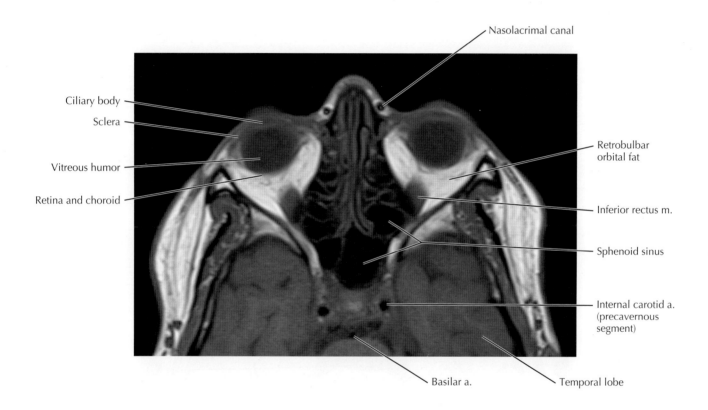

Nasolacrimal canal

Ciliary body

Sclera

Vitreous humor

Retina and choroid

Retrobulbar orbital fat

Inferior rectus m.

Sphenoid sinus

Internal carotid a. (precavernous segment)

Basilar a.

Temporal lobe

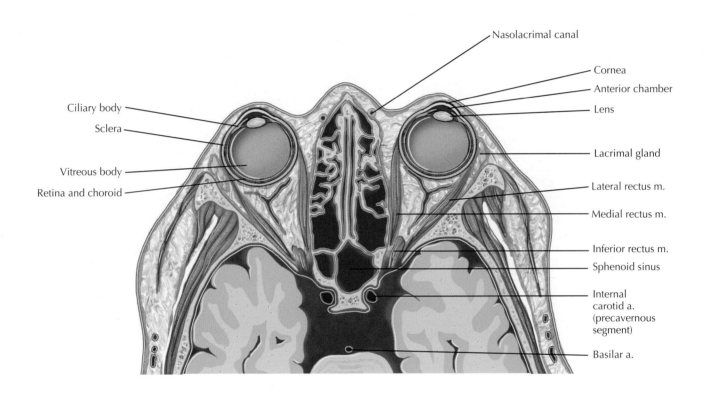

Nasolacrimal canal

Cornea

Anterior chamber

Lens

Ciliary body

Sclera

Lacrimal gland

Vitreous body

Lateral rectus m.

Retina and choroid

Medial rectus m.

Inferior rectus m.

Sphenoid sinus

Internal
carotid a.
(precavernous
segment)

Basilar a.

NORMAL ANATOMY

The lenses are normally biconvex in shape. If this configuration is replaced by a thin line, the patient likely has had the lens removed because of cataracts and replaced with an artificial lens.

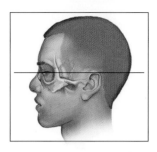

Nasolacrimal canal

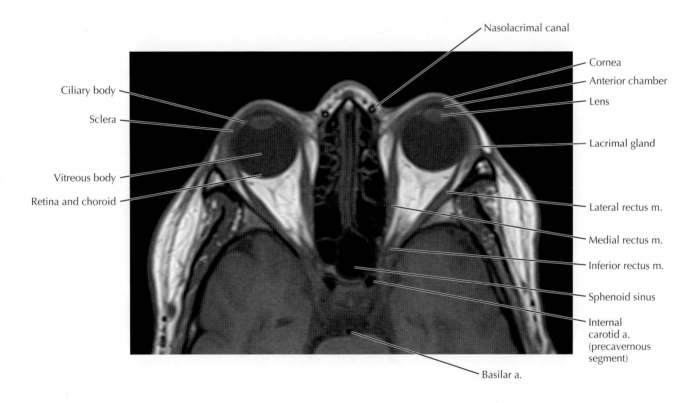

Ciliary body

Sclera

Vitreous body

Retina and choroid

Cornea

Anterior chamber

Lens

Lacrimal gland

Lateral rectus m.

Medial rectus m.

Inferior rectus m.

Sphenoid sinus

Internal
carotid a.
(precavernous
segment)

Basilar a.

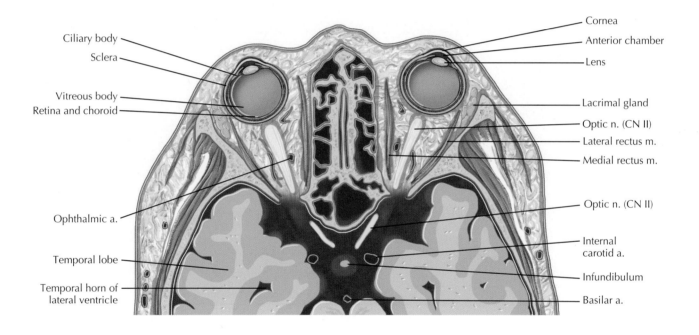

Ciliary body

Sclera

Vitreous body

Retina and choroid

Ophthalmic a.

Temporal lobe

Temporal horn of
lateral ventricle

Cornea

Anterior chamber

Lens

Lacrimal gland

Optic n. (CN II)

Lateral rectus m.

Medial rectus m.

Optic n. (CN II)

Internal
carotid a.

Infundibulum

Basilar a.

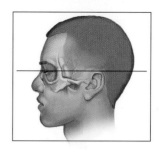

Ciliary body

Sclera

Retina and choroid

Vitreous body

R. superior
ophthalmic vv.
and branches

R. inferior
ophthalmic vv.
and branches

R. ophthalmic a.

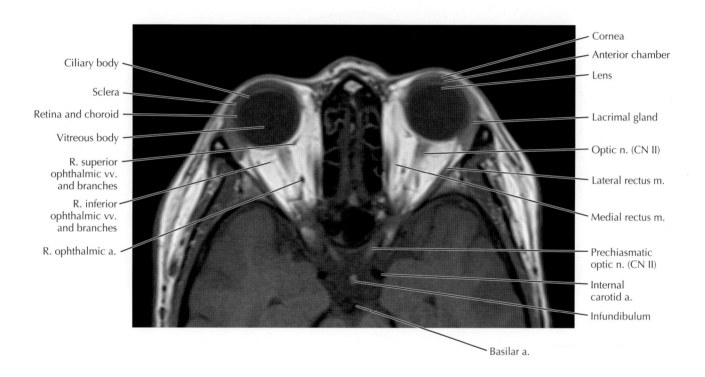

Cornea

Anterior chamber

Lens

Lacrimal gland

Optic n. (CN II)

Lateral rectus m.

Medial rectus m.

Prechiasmatic
optic n. (CN II)

Internal
carotid a.

Infundibulum

Basilar a.

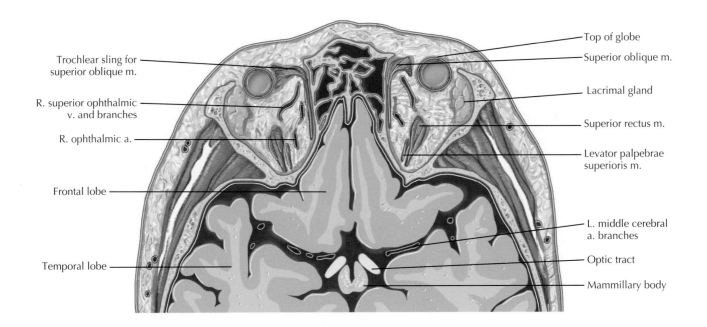

Trochlear sling for superior oblique m.

R. superior ophthalmic v. and branches

R. ophthalmic a.

Frontal lobe

Temporal lobe

Top of globe

Superior oblique m.

Lacrimal gland

Superior rectus m.

Levator palpebrae superioris m.

L. middle cerebral a. branches

Optic tract

Mammillary body

PATHOLOGIC PROCESS

Note the thin superior ophthalmic vein (SOV). Dilatation should lead to consideration of increased pressure within the cavernous sinus, as in carotid cavernous fistula (CCF) following trauma. Early, asymmetric filling of the cavernous sinus in the arterial phase confirms the diagnosis of CCF (see also Orbits Coronal 1).

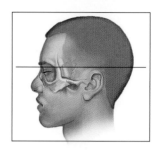

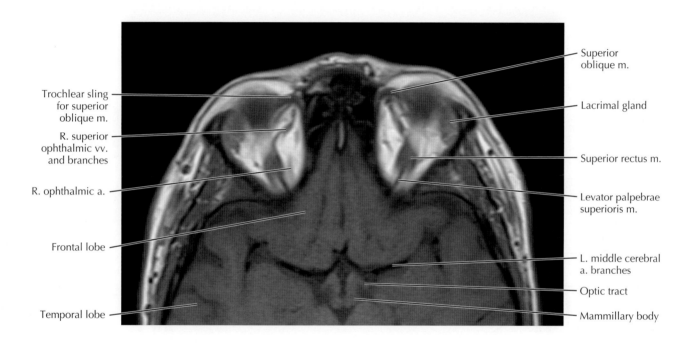

Trochlear sling
for superior
oblique m.

R. superior
ophthalmic vv.
and branches

R. ophthalmic a.

Frontal lobe

Temporal lobe

Superior
oblique m.

Lacrimal gland

Superior rectus m.

Levator palpebrae
superioris m.

L. middle cerebral
a. branches

Optic tract

Mammillary body

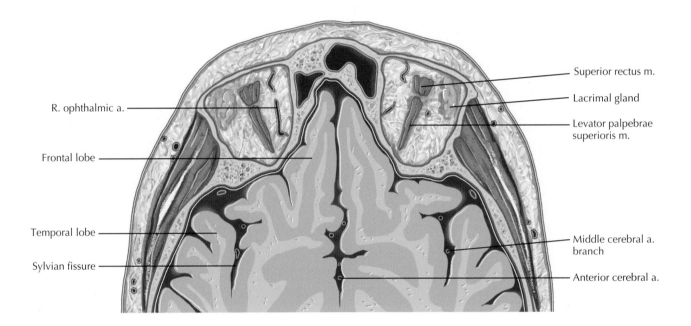

R. ophthalmic a.

Frontal lobe

Temporal lobe

Sylvian fissure

Superior rectus m.

Lacrimal gland

Levator palpebrae superioris m.

Middle cerebral a. branch

Anterior cerebral a.

NORMAL ANATOMY

The lacrimal gland is located in the upper outer aspect of the orbit. It produces tears, which coat the eye in a superolateral to inferomedial direction, eventually being drained through the two lacrimal puncta leading to the canaliculi and then the nasolacrimal duct.

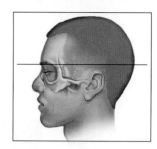

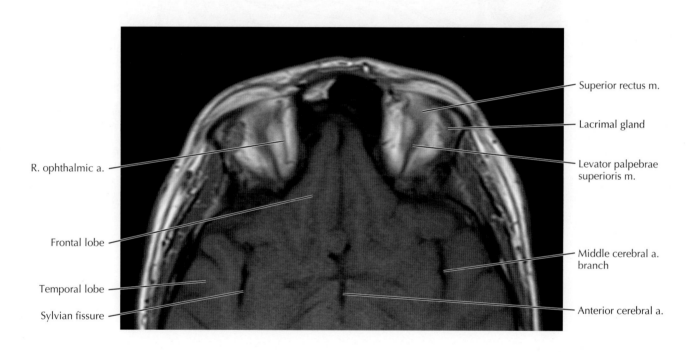

Superior rectus m.

Lacrimal gland

R. ophthalmic a.

Levator palpebrae
superioris m.

Frontal lobe

Middle cerebral a.
branch

Temporal lobe

Sylvian fissure

Anterior cerebral a.

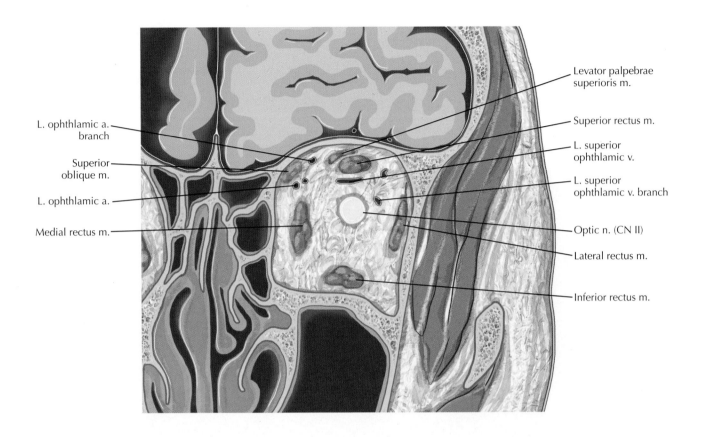

Levator palpebrae superioris m.

Superior rectus m.

L. superior ophthlamic v.

L. superior ophthlamic v. branch

Optic n. (CN II)

Lateral rectus m.

Inferior rectus m.

L. ophthlamic a. branch

Superior oblique m.

L. ophthlamic a.

Medial rectus m.

NORMAL ANATOMY

The optic nerve, cranial nerve (CN) II, is the only cranial nerve that is part of the central nervous system in that, like the brain and spinal cord, it has no ability to regenerate, unlike peripheral nerves. CN II is a direct extension of the brain and is surrounded by cerebrospinal fluid (CSF) and dura.

PATHOLOGIC PROCESS

If the normally thin and flat superior ophthalmic vein (SOV) is dilated, rounded, and tortuous, increased pressure within the cavernous sinus should be suspected, as with post-trauma carotid-cavernous fistula (CCF; see also Axial 5).

IMAGING TECHNIQUE CONSIDERATION

Note that in the bottom MR image of Coronal 1, the white matter is brighter than the gray matter; thus this sequence must be T1 weighted (think of "fatty" myelin being bright on T1). The subcutaneous fat is dark, so this must be a fat-saturated sequence, and the vessels and mucosa are both bright, so contrast has been administered.

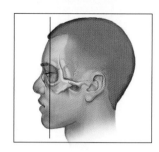

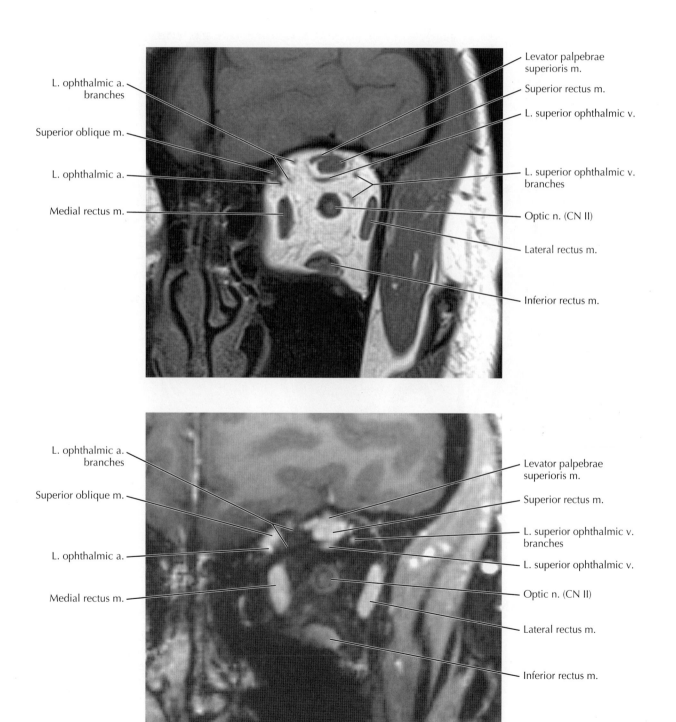

L. ophthalmic a. branches

Superior oblique m.

L. ophthalmic a.

Medial rectus m.

Levator palpebrae superioris m.

Superior rectus m.

L. superior ophthalmic v.

L. superior ophthalmic v. branches

Optic n. (CN II)

Lateral rectus m.

Inferior rectus m.

L. ophthalmic a. branches

Superior oblique m.

L. ophthalmic a.

Medial rectus m.

Levator palpebrae superioris m.

Superior rectus m.

L. superior ophthalmic v. branches

L. superior ophthalmic v.

Optic n. (CN II)

Lateral rectus m.

Inferior rectus m.

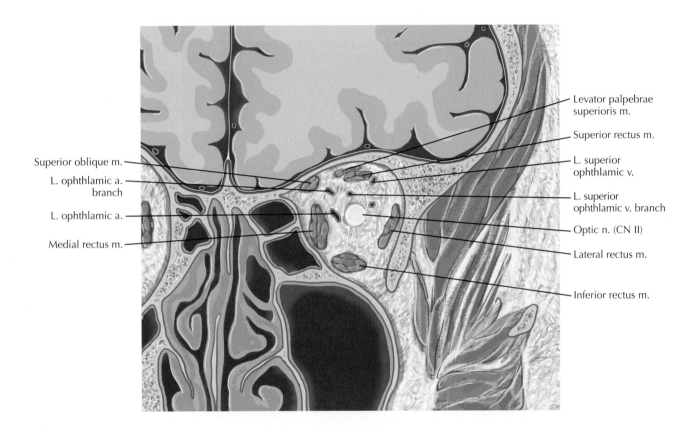

Superior oblique m.
L. ophthlamic a. branch
L. ophthlamic a.
Medial rectus m.

Levator palpebrae superioris m.
Superior rectus m.
L. superior ophthlamic v.
L. superior ophthlamic v. branch
Optic n. (CN II)
Lateral rectus m.
Inferior rectus m.

NORMAL ANATOMY

There are five intraorbital muscles that contribute to the annulus of Zinn (the inferior oblique muscle does not). The superior oblique muscle is supplied by the trochlear nerve (CN IV) and causes the eye to point downward and medially toward the tip of the nose. The lateral rectus muscle is supplied by the abucens nerve (CN VI) and points the eye medially. The oculomotor nerve (CN III) supplies the inferior rectus, medial rectus, superior rectus, levator palpebrae superioris, and inferior oblique muscles. When there is diplopia with unilateral palsy of CN III causing the eye to point "down and out," the clinician must consider aneurysm of the posterior communicating artery compressing the oculomotor nerve.

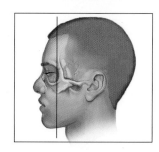

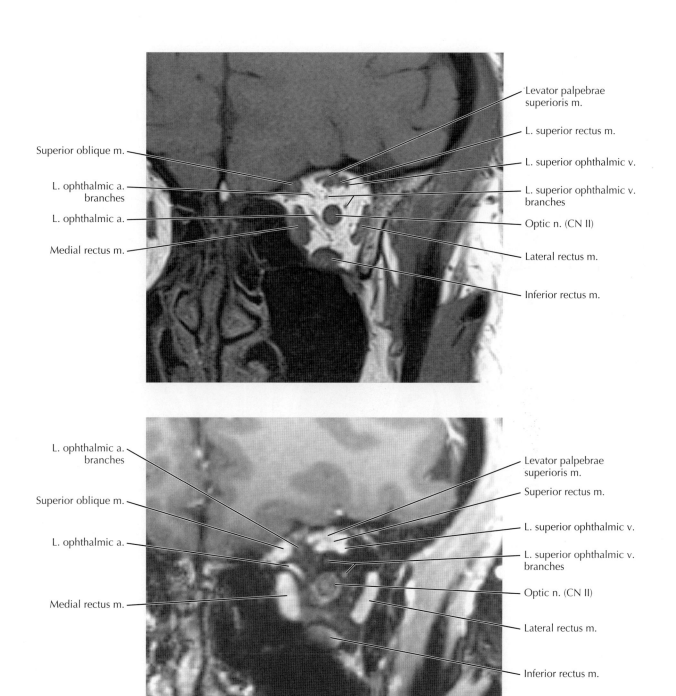

Superior oblique m.

L. ophthalmic a.
branches

L. ophthalmic a.

Medial rectus m.

Levator palpebrae
superioris m.

L. superior rectus m.

L. superior ophthalmic v.

L. superior ophthalmic v.
branches

Optic n. (CN II)

Lateral rectus m.

Inferior rectus m.

L. ophthalmic a.
branches

Superior oblique m.

L. ophthalmic a.

Medial rectus m.

Levator palpebrae
superioris m.

Superior rectus m.

L. superior ophthalmic v.

L. superior ophthalmic v.
branches

Optic n. (CN II)

Lateral rectus m.

Inferior rectus m.

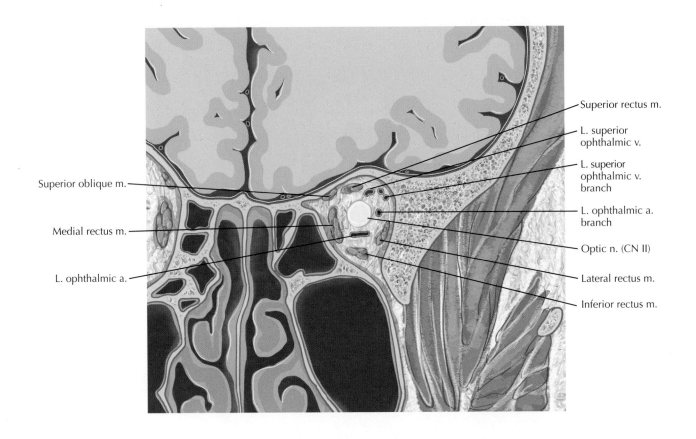

Superior oblique m.

Medial rectus m.

L. ophthalmic a.

Superior rectus m.

L. superior
ophthalmic v.

L. superior
ophthalmic v.
branch

L. ophthalmic a.
branch

Optic n. (CN II)

Lateral rectus m.

Inferior rectus m.

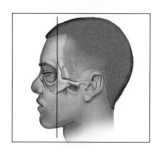

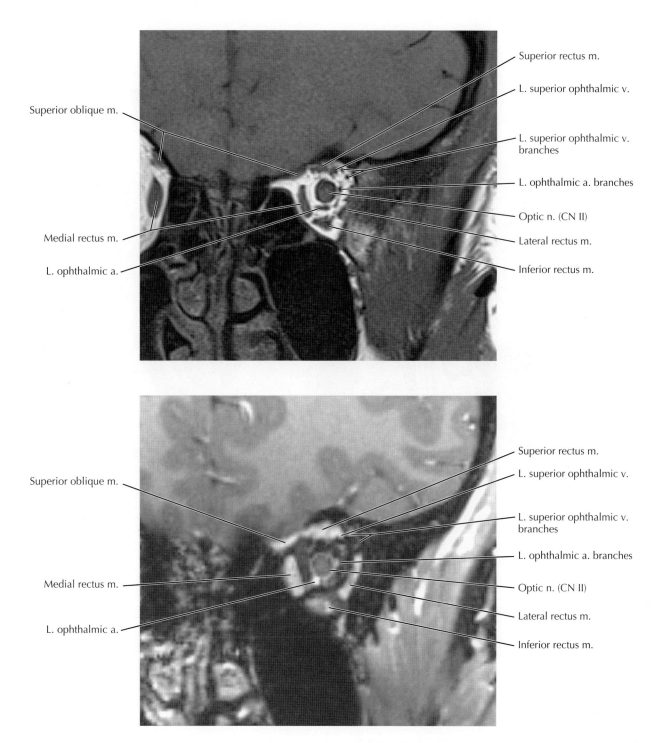

Superior rectus m.

L. superior ophthalmic v.

L. superior ophthalmic v. branches

L. ophthalmic a. branches

Optic n. (CN II)

Lateral rectus m.

Inferior rectus m.

Superior oblique m.

Medial rectus m.

L. ophthalmic a.

Superior rectus m.

L. superior ophthalmic v.

L. superior ophthalmic v. branches

L. ophthalmic a. branches

Optic n. (CN II)

Lateral rectus m.

Inferior rectus m.

Superior oblique m.

Medial rectus m.

L. ophthalmic a.

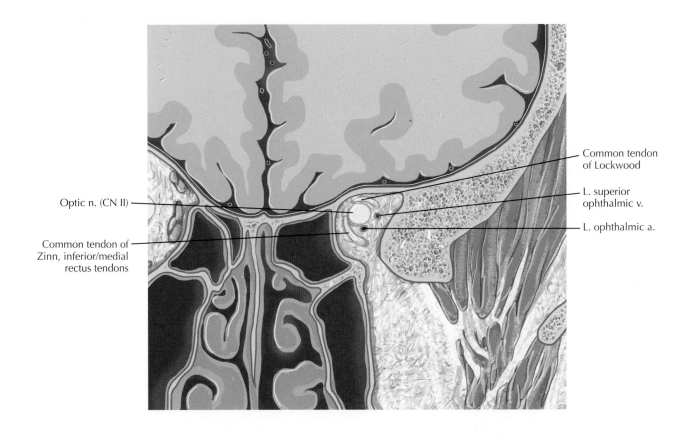

Common tendon
of Lockwood

L. superior
ophthalmic v.

Optic n. (CN II)

L. ophthalmic a.

Common tendon of
Zinn, inferior/medial
rectus tendons

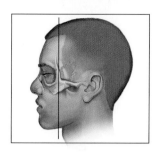

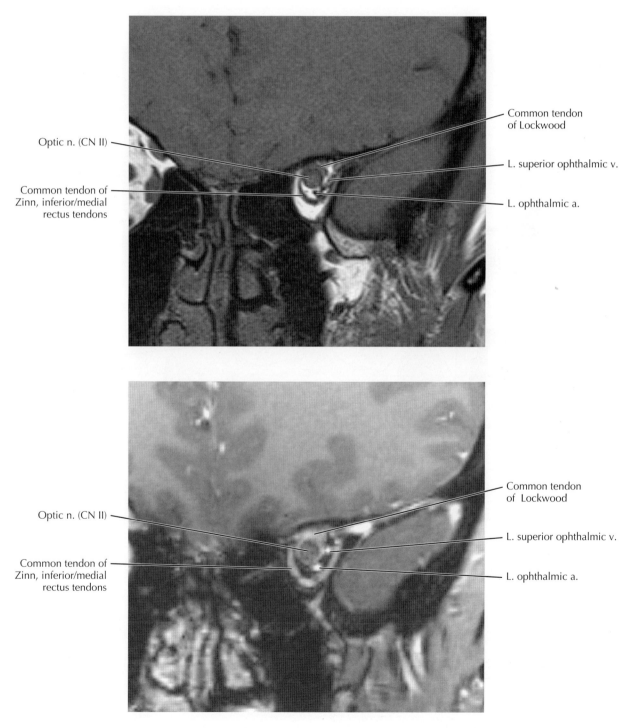

Optic n. (CN II)

Common tendon of Zinn, inferior/medial rectus tendons

Common tendon of Lockwood

L. superior ophthalmic v.

L. ophthalmic a.

Optic n. (CN II)

Common tendon of Zinn, inferior/medial rectus tendons

Common tendon of Lockwood

L. superior ophthalmic v.

L. ophthalmic a.

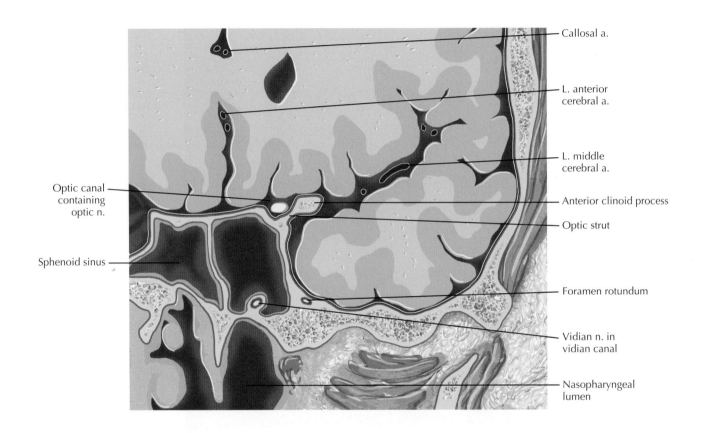

Callosal a.

L. anterior
cerebral a.

L. middle
cerebral a.

Anterior clinoid process

Optic strut

Foramen rotundum

Vidian n. in
vidian canal

Nasopharyngeal
lumen

Optic canal
containing
optic n.

Sphenoid sinus

NORMAL ANATOMY

The *optic strut* is a precise landmark between intradural and extradural/intracavernous aneurysms involving the paraclinoid segment of the internal carotid artery.

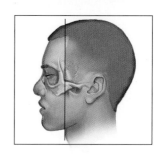

Callosal a.

L. anterior cerebral a.

L. middle cerebral a.

Anterior clinoid process

Optic canal
containing optic n.

Optic strut

Sphenoid sinus

Foramen rotundum

Nasopharyngeal lumen

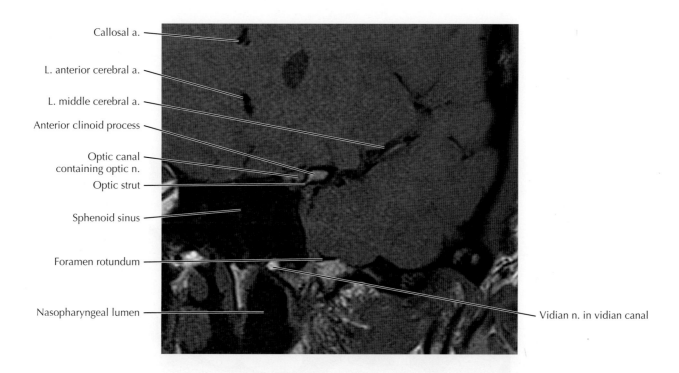

Vidian n. in vidian canal

Callosal a.

L. anterior cerebral a.

L. middle cerebral a.

Anterior clinoid process

Optic canal
containing optic n.

Optic strut

Sphenoid sinus

Foramen rotundum

Nasopharyngeal lumen

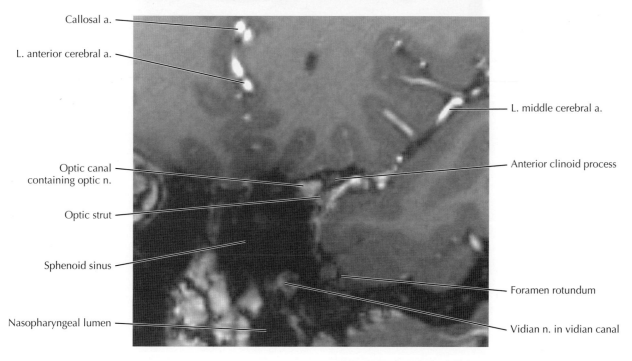

Vidian n. in vidian canal

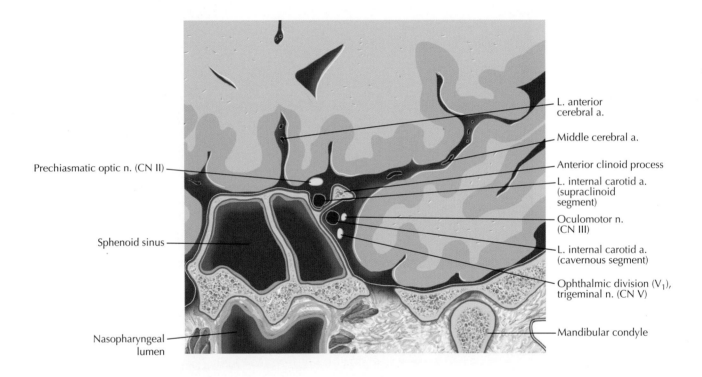

Prechiasmatic optic n. (CN II)

Sphenoid sinus

Nasopharyngeal lumen

L. anterior cerebral a.

Middle cerebral a.

Anterior clinoid process

L. internal carotid a. (supraclinoid segment)

Oculomotor n. (CN III)

L. internal carotid a. (cavernous segment)

Ophthalmic division (V_1), trigeminal n. (CN V)

Mandibular condyle

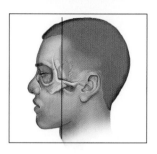

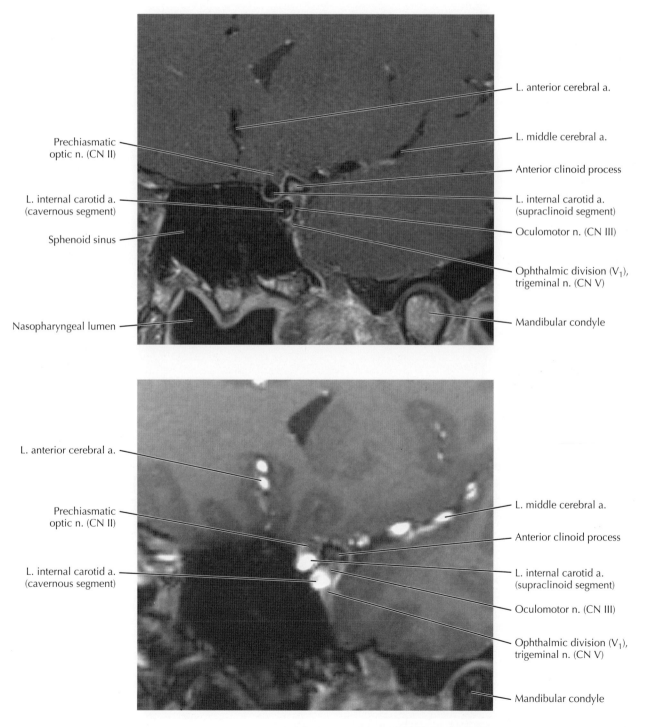

Prechiasmatic optic n. (CN II)

L. internal carotid a. (cavernous segment)

Sphenoid sinus

Nasopharyngeal lumen

L. anterior cerebral a.

L. middle cerebral a.

Anterior clinoid process

L. internal carotid a. (supraclinoid segment)

Oculomotor n. (CN III)

Ophthalmic division (V₁), trigeminal n. (CN V)

Mandibular condyle

L. anterior cerebral a.

Prechiasmatic optic n. (CN II)

L. internal carotid a. (cavernous segment)

L. middle cerebral a.

Anterior clinoid process

L. internal carotid a. (supraclinoid segment)

Oculomotor n. (CN III)

Ophthalmic division (V₁), trigeminal n. (CN V)

Mandibular condyle

Chapter 11 MANDIBLE AND MUSCLES OF MASTICATION

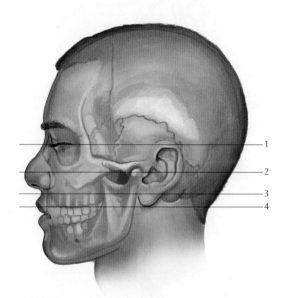

AXIAL 382

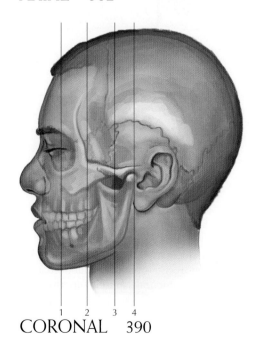

CORONAL 390

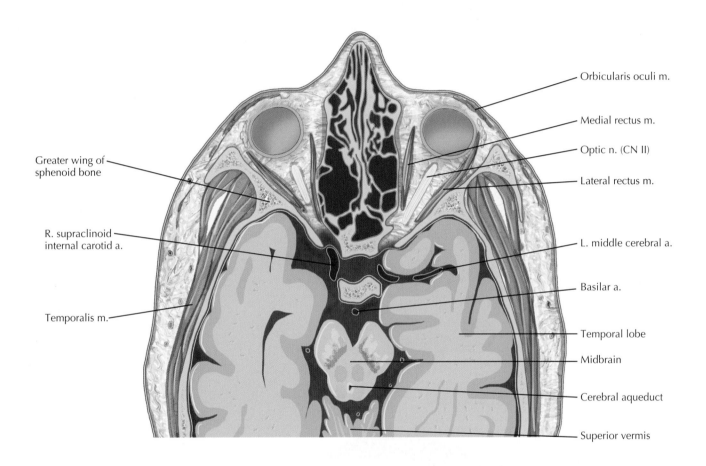

Orbicularis oculi m.

Medial rectus m.

Optic n. (CN II)

Lateral rectus m.

Greater wing of sphenoid bone

R. supraclinoid internal carotid a.

L. middle cerebral a.

Basilar a.

Temporalis m.

Temporal lobe

Midbrain

Cerebral aqueduct

Superior vermis

NORMAL ANATOMY

Four paired muscles—temporalis, masseter, medial pterygoid, and lateral pterygoid—are the primary muscles of mastication, responsible for adduction and lateral motion. In the axial MR image on the next page, note the temporalis muscle superficial to the temporal lobe of the brain.

These muscles are innervated by the mandibular branch (V_3) of the trigeminal nerve, cranial nerve (CN) V (see Axial 2). The lateral pterygoid helps open the mouth, and the medial pterygoid helps close the mouth ("lateral lowers and medial munches").

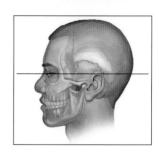

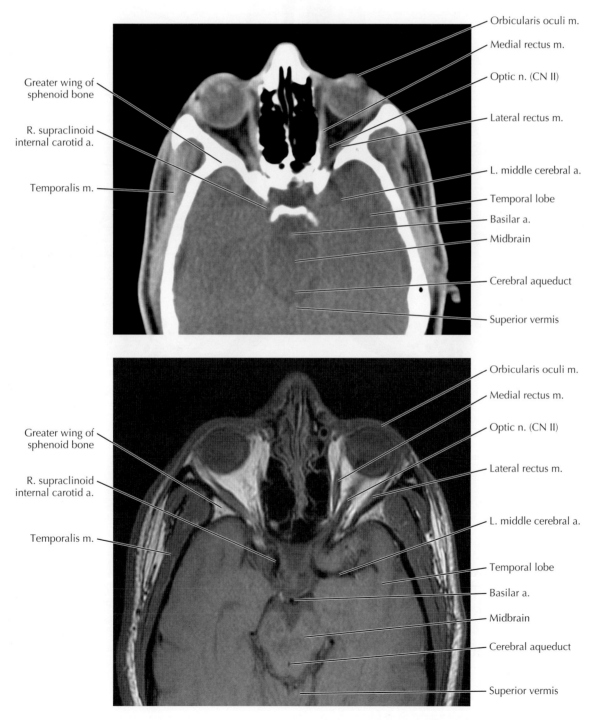

Orbicularis oculi m.

Medial rectus m.

Optic n. (CN II)

Greater wing of sphenoid bone

Lateral rectus m.

R. supraclinoid internal carotid a.

L. middle cerebral a.

Temporal lobe

Temporalis m.

Basilar a.

Midbrain

Cerebral aqueduct

Superior vermis

Orbicularis oculi m.

Medial rectus m.

Optic n. (CN II)

Greater wing of sphenoid bone

Lateral rectus m.

R. supraclinoid internal carotid a.

L. middle cerebral a.

Temporalis m.

Temporal lobe

Basilar a.

Midbrain

Cerebral aqueduct

Superior vermis

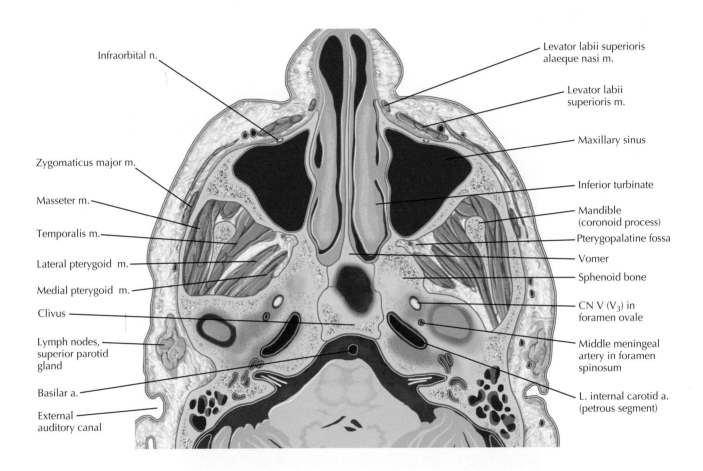

Infraorbital n.

Levator labii superioris alaeque nasi m.

Levator labii superioris m.

Maxillary sinus

Zygomaticus major m.

Inferior turbinate

Masseter m.

Mandible (coronoid process)

Temporalis m.

Pterygopalatine fossa

Lateral pterygoid m.

Vomer

Medial pterygoid m.

Sphenoid bone

Clivus

CN V (V_3) in foramen ovale

Lymph nodes, superior parotid gland

Middle meningeal artery in foramen spinosum

Basilar a.

External auditory canal

L. internal carotid a. (petrous segment)

NORMAL ANATOMY

Note that from superficial to deep, the muscles are zygomaticus major, masseter, temporalis, and lateral pterygoid. The medial pterygoid muscle is located deeper and more caudal.

PATHOLOGIC PROCESS

Denervation of the V_3 branch of the trigeminal nerve can lead to atrophy of the ipsilateral muscles of mastication.

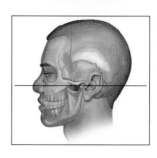

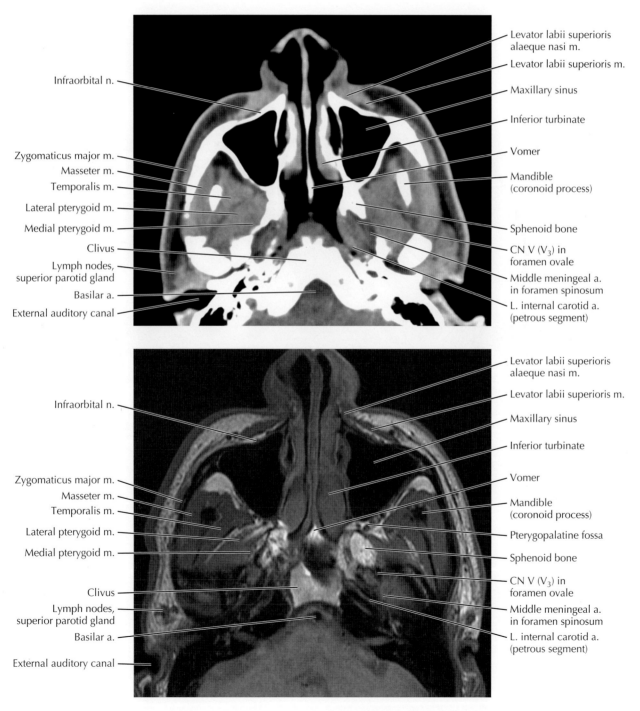

Levator labii superioris alaeque nasi m.

Levator labii superioris m.

Maxillary sinus

Inferior turbinate

Vomer

Mandible (coronoid process)

Sphenoid bone

CN V (V₃) in foramen ovale

Middle meningeal a. in foramen spinosum

L. internal carotid a. (petrous segment)

Infraorbital n.

Zygomaticus major m.
Masseter m.
Temporalis m.
Lateral pterygoid m.
Medial pterygoid m.
Clivus
Lymph nodes, superior parotid gland
Basilar a.
External auditory canal

Levator labii superioris alaeque nasi m.

Levator labii superioris m.

Maxillary sinus

Inferior turbinate

Vomer

Mandible (coronoid process)

Pterygopalatine fossa

Sphenoid bone

CN V (V₃) in foramen ovale

Middle meningeal a. in foramen spinosum

L. internal carotid a. (petrous segment)

Infraorbital n.

Zygomaticus major m.
Masseter m.
Temporalis m.
Lateral pterygoid m.
Medial pterygoid m.
Clivus
Lymph nodes, superior parotid gland
Basilar a.
External auditory canal

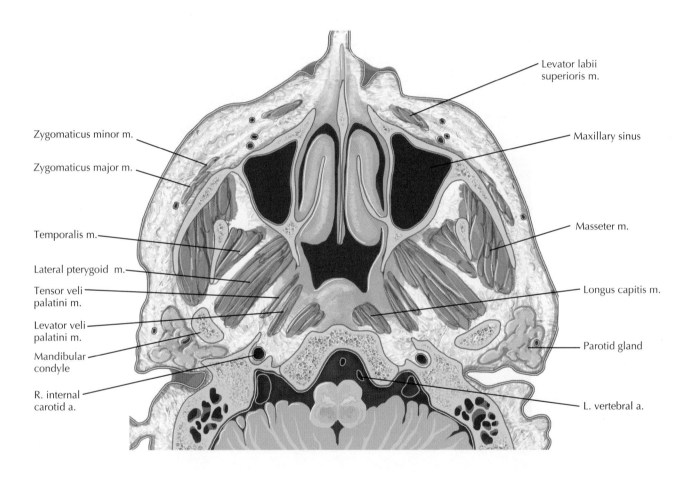

Levator labii
superioris m.

Zygomaticus minor m.

Zygomaticus major m.

Temporalis m.

Lateral pterygoid m.

Tensor veli
palatini m.

Levator veli
palatini m.

Mandibular
condyle

R. internal
carotid a.

Maxillary sinus

Masseter m.

Longus capitis m.

Parotid gland

L. vertebral a.

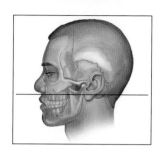

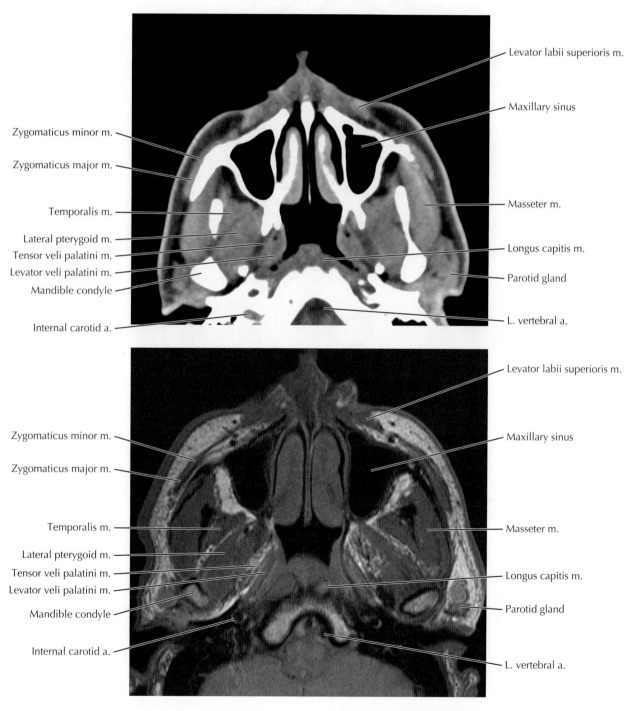

Levator labii superioris m.

Maxillary sinus

Zygomaticus minor m.

Zygomaticus major m.

Temporalis m.

Lateral pterygoid m.
Tensor veli palatini m.
Levator veli palatini m.
Mandible condyle

Masseter m.

Longus capitis m.

Parotid gland

Internal carotid a.

L. vertebral a.

Levator labii superioris m.

Maxillary sinus

Zygomaticus minor m.

Zygomaticus major m.

Temporalis m.

Lateral pterygoid m.
Tensor veli palatini m.
Levator veli palatini m.
Mandible condyle

Masseter m.

Longus capitis m.

Parotid gland

Internal carotid a.

L. vertebral a.

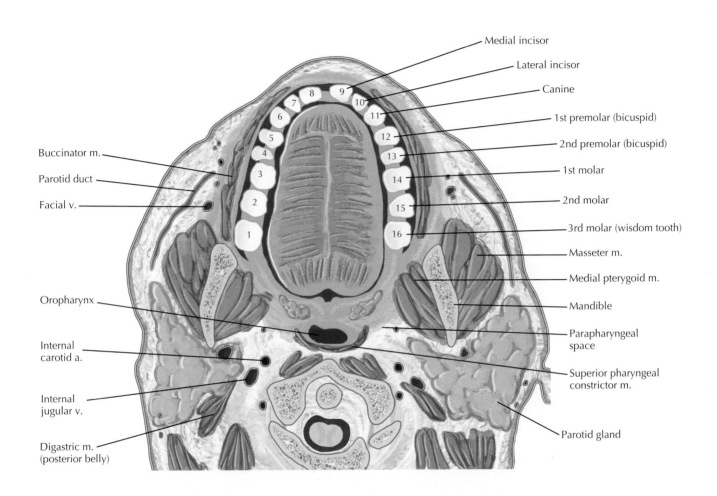

Medial incisor
Lateral incisor
Canine
1st premolar (bicuspid)
2nd premolar (bicuspid)
1st molar
2nd molar
3rd molar (wisdom tooth)
Masseter m.
Medial pterygoid m.
Mandible
Parapharyngeal space
Superior pharyngeal constrictor m.
Parotid gland

Buccinator m.
Parotid duct
Facial v.
Oropharynx
Internal carotid a.
Internal jugular v.
Digastric m. (posterior belly)

NOMENCLATURE

The two most common dental notation systems are the International Dental Association (Fédération Dentaire Internationale, FDI) notation and the Universal numbering system (dental). The FDI system uses a two-digit numbering system in which the first number represents a tooth's quadrant and the second number represents the number of the tooth from the midline of the face. For permanent teeth, the upper-right teeth begin with 1, the upper-left teeth with 2, the lower-left teeth with 3, and the lower-right teeth with 4. For primary teeth the sequence of numbers is 5, 6, 7, and 8 for the teeth in the upper right, upper left, lower left, and lower right, respectively.

The Universal number system (dental) is used in the United States and begins labeling at the upper-right maxillary wisdom tooth as 1 and continues clockwise (see Axial 4), when viewing the open mouth from a dentist's perspective, up to 32 at the right mandibular wisdom tooth.

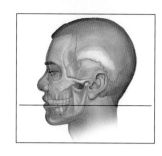

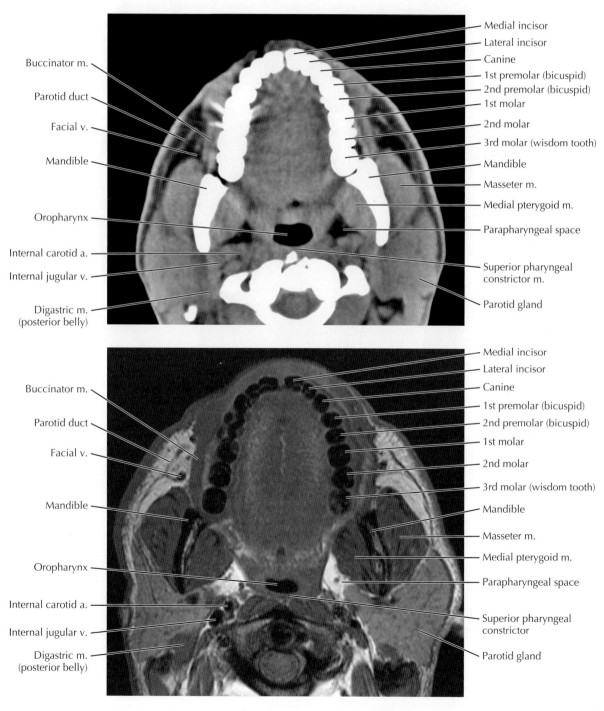

Buccinator m.

Parotid duct

Facial v.

Mandible

Oropharynx

Internal carotid a.

Internal jugular v.

Digastric m.
(posterior belly)

Medial incisor

Lateral incisor

Canine

1st premolar (bicuspid)

2nd premolar (bicuspid)

1st molar

2nd molar

3rd molar (wisdom tooth)

Mandible

Masseter m.

Medial pterygoid m.

Parapharyngeal space

Superior pharyngeal
constrictor m.

Parotid gland

Buccinator m.

Parotid duct

Facial v.

Mandible

Oropharynx

Internal carotid a.

Internal jugular v.

Digastric m.
(posterior belly)

Medial incisor

Lateral incisor

Canine

1st premolar (bicuspid)

2nd premolar (bicuspid)

1st molar

2nd molar

3rd molar (wisdom tooth)

Mandible

Masseter m.

Medial pterygoid m.

Parapharyngeal space

Superior pharyngeal
constrictor

Parotid gland

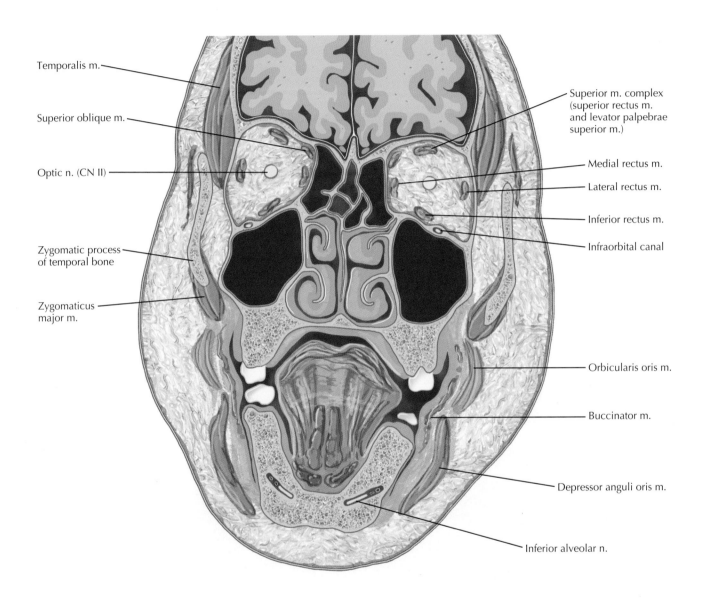

Temporalis m.

Superior oblique m.

Optic n. (CN II)

Zygomatic process of temporal bone

Zygomaticus major m.

Superior m. complex (superior rectus m. and levator palpebrae superior m.)

Medial rectus m.

Lateral rectus m.

Inferior rectus m.

Infraorbital canal

Orbicularis oris m.

Buccinator m.

Depressor anguli oris m.

Inferior alveolar n.

PATHOLOGIC PROCESS

The inferior alveolar nerves course through the mandible in the inferior alveolar canals, exiting superficially at the mental foramina. Squamous cell carcinoma of the mandible can invade the mandible and track perineurally along the inferior alveolar nerve, back to the V_3 branch of the trigeminal nerve and Meckel's cave.

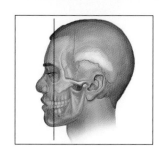

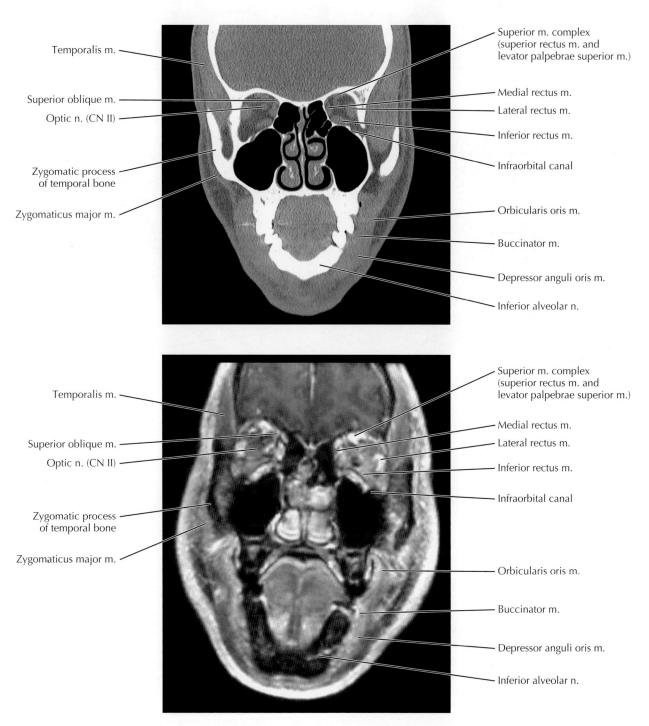

Temporalis m.

Superior oblique m.

Optic n. (CN II)

Zygomatic process
of temporal bone

Zygomaticus major m.

Superior m. complex
(superior rectus m. and
levator palpebrae superior m.)

Medial rectus m.

Lateral rectus m.

Inferior rectus m.

Infraorbital canal

Orbicularis oris m.

Buccinator m.

Depressor anguli oris m.

Inferior alveolar n.

Temporalis m.

Superior oblique m.

Optic n. (CN II)

Zygomatic process
of temporal bone

Zygomaticus major m.

Superior m. complex
(superior rectus m. and
levator palpebrae superior m.)

Medial rectus m.

Lateral rectus m.

Inferior rectus m.

Infraorbital canal

Orbicularis oris m.

Buccinator m.

Depressor anguli oris m.

Inferior alveolar n.

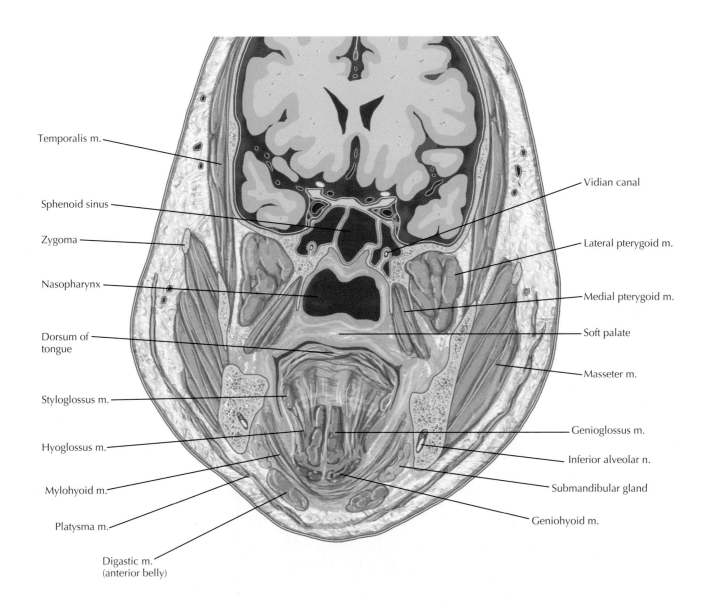

Temporalis m.

Sphenoid sinus

Zygoma

Nasopharynx

Dorsum of tongue

Styloglossus m.

Hyoglossus m.

Mylohyoid m.

Platysma m.

Digastic m. (anterior belly)

Vidian canal

Lateral pterygoid m.

Medial pterygoid m.

Soft palate

Masseter m.

Genioglossus m.

Inferior alveolar n.

Submandibular gland

Geniohyoid m.

NORMAL ANATOMY

The temporalis muscle has a broad origin from the outer temporal fossa, passes deep to the zygomatic arch, and inserts onto the coronoid process of the mandible to pull back and elevate the mandible. The temporalis muscle can be felt at the temples and can be seen and felt contracting as a person bites down.

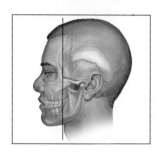

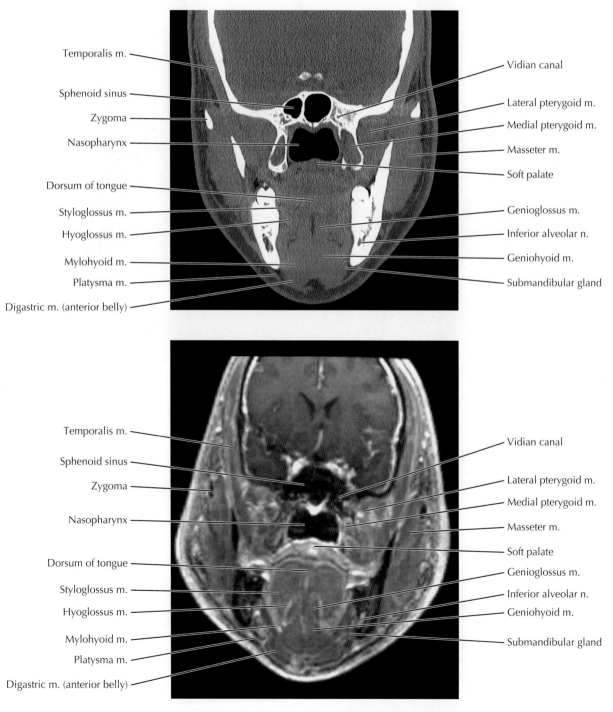

Temporalis m.

Sphenoid sinus

Zygoma

Nasopharynx

Dorsum of tongue

Styloglossus m.

Hyoglossus m.

Mylohyoid m.

Platysma m.

Digastric m. (anterior belly)

Vidian canal

Lateral pterygoid m.

Medial pterygoid m.

Masseter m.

Soft palate

Genioglossus m.

Inferior alveolar n.

Geniohyoid m.

Submandibular gland

Temporalis m.

Sphenoid sinus

Zygoma

Nasopharynx

Dorsum of tongue

Styloglossus m.

Hyoglossus m.

Mylohyoid m.

Platysma m.

Digastric m. (anterior belly)

Vidian canal

Lateral pterygoid m.

Medial pterygoid m.

Masseter m.

Soft palate

Genioglossus m.

Inferior alveolar n.

Geniohyoid m.

Submandibular gland

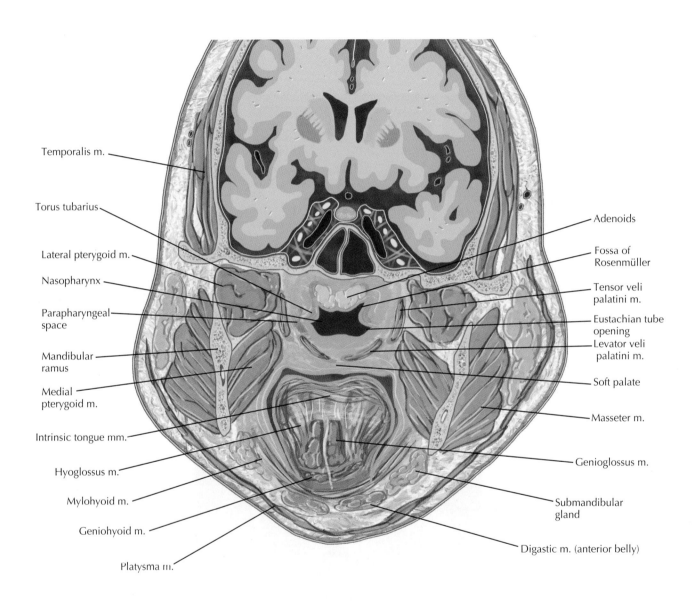

Temporalis m.

Torus tubarius

Lateral pterygoid m.

Nasopharynx

Parapharyngeal space

Mandibular ramus

Medial pterygoid m.

Intrinsic tongue mm.

Hyoglossus m.

Mylohyoid m.

Geniohyoid m.

Platysma m.

Adenoids

Fossa of Rosenmüller

Tensor veli palatini m.

Eustachian tube opening

Levator veli palatini m.

Soft palate

Masseter m.

Genioglossus m.

Submandibular gland

Digastic m. (anterior belly)

NORMAL ANATOMY

The medial and lateral pterygoid muscles originate from the respective medial and lateral pterygoid bone plates and pass inferiorly and laterally to insert on the inner mandible.

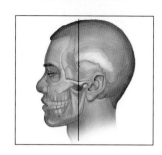

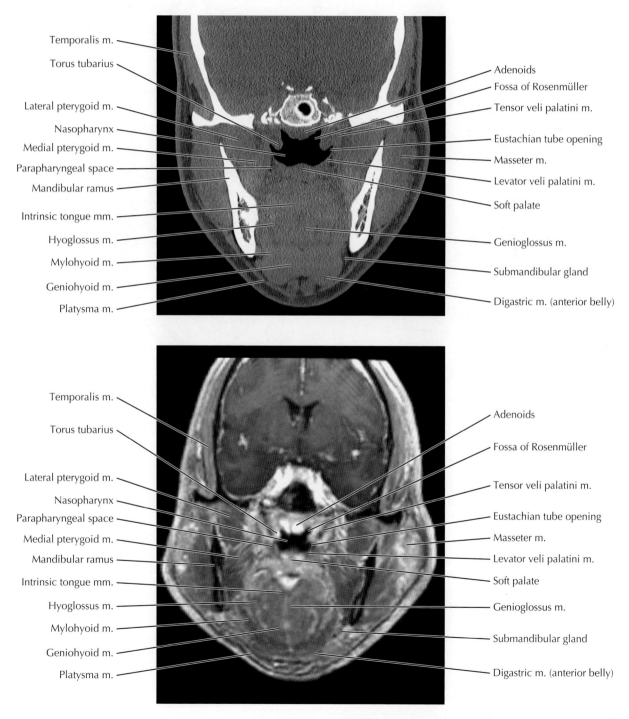

Temporalis m.

Torus tubarius

Lateral pterygoid m.

Nasopharynx

Medial pterygoid m.

Parapharyngeal space

Mandibular ramus

Intrinsic tongue mm.

Hyoglossus m.

Mylohyoid m.

Geniohyoid m.

Platysma m.

Adenoids

Fossa of Rosenmüller

Tensor veli palatini m.

Eustachian tube opening

Masseter m.

Levator veli palatini m.

Soft palate

Genioglossus m.

Submandibular gland

Digastric m. (anterior belly)

Temporalis m.

Torus tubarius

Lateral pterygoid m.

Nasopharynx

Parapharyngeal space

Medial pterygoid m.

Mandibular ramus

Intrinsic tongue mm.

Hyoglossus m.

Mylohyoid m.

Geniohyoid m.

Platysma m.

Adenoids

Fossa of Rosenmüller

Tensor veli palatini m.

Eustachian tube opening

Masseter m.

Levator veli palatini m.

Soft palate

Genioglossus m.

Submandibular gland

Digastric m. (anterior belly)

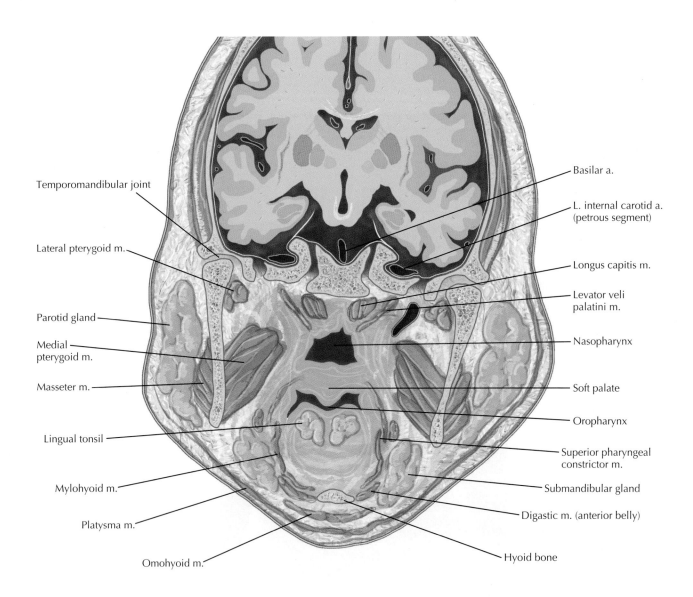

Temporomandibular joint

Lateral pterygoid m.

Parotid gland

Medial pterygoid m.

Masseter m.

Lingual tonsil

Mylohyoid m.

Platysma m.

Omohyoid m.

Basilar a.

L. internal carotid a. (petrous segment)

Longus capitis m.

Levator veli palatini m.

Nasopharynx

Soft palate

Oropharynx

Superior pharyngeal constrictor m.

Submandibular gland

Digastic m. (anterior belly)

Hyoid bone

IMAGING TECHNIQUE CONSIDERATION

The temporomandibular joint (TMJ) is formed by two bones, the condyle of the mandible and the glenoid fossa of the temporal bone. The space between these bones contains an articular disc. The TMJ is one of the few synovial joints in the human body with a disc. MR images of different jaw positions can show whether the disc is torn or fails to recapture into normal position between the bones.

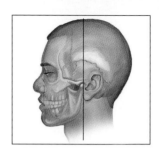

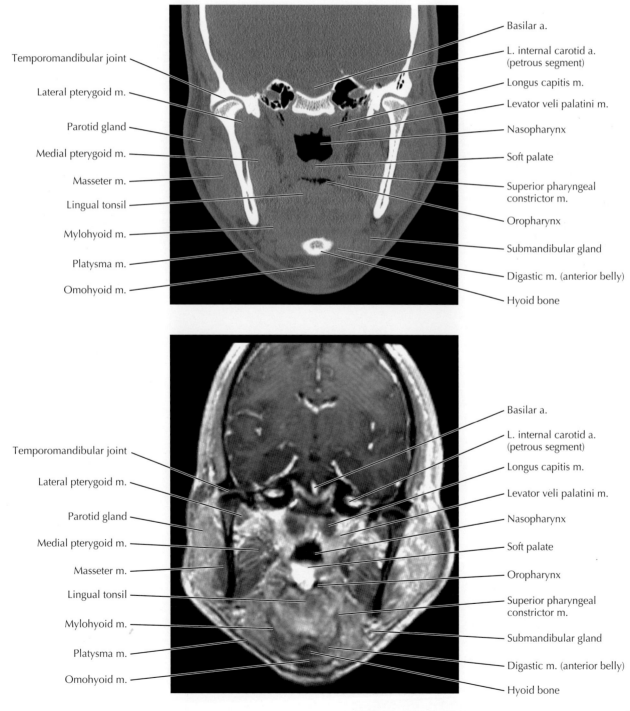

Temporomandibular joint

Lateral pterygoid m.

Parotid gland

Medial pterygoid m.

Masseter m.

Lingual tonsil

Mylohyoid m.

Platysma m.

Omohyoid m.

Basilar a.

L. internal carotid a. (petrous segment)

Longus capitis m.

Levator veli palatini m.

Nasopharynx

Soft palate

Superior pharyngeal constrictor m.

Oropharynx

Submandibular gland

Digastic m. (anterior belly)

Hyoid bone

Temporomandibular joint

Lateral pterygoid m.

Parotid gland

Medial pterygoid m.

Masseter m.

Lingual tonsil

Mylohyoid m.

Platysma m.

Omohyoid m.

Basilar a.

L. internal carotid a. (petrous segment)

Longus capitis m.

Levator veli palatini m.

Nasopharynx

Soft palate

Oropharynx

Superior pharyngeal constrictor m.

Submandibular gland

Digastic m. (anterior belly)

Hyoid bone

12 TEMPORAL BONE (MIDDLE EAR, COCHLEA, VESTIBULAR SYSTEM)

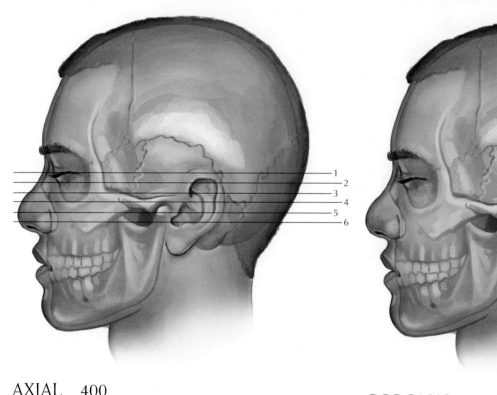

AXIAL 400

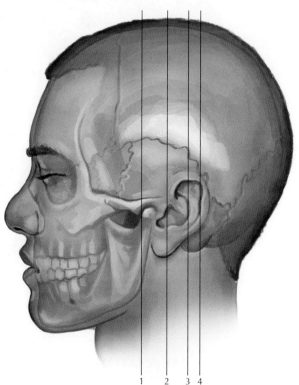

CORONAL 412

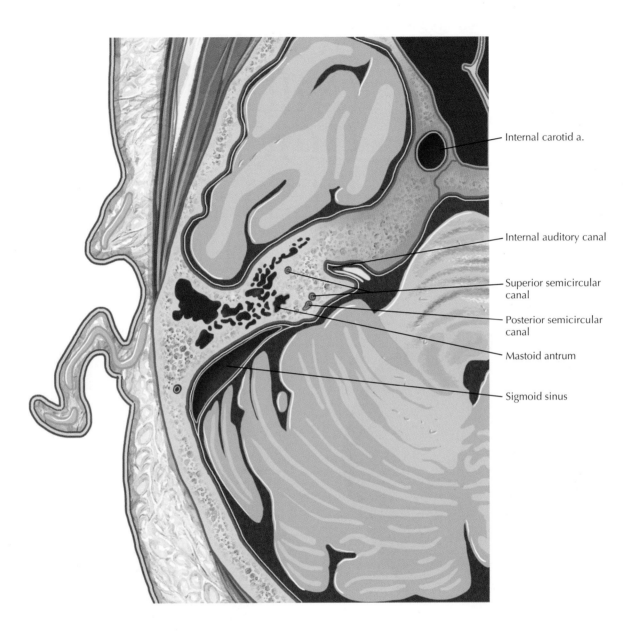

- Internal carotid a.
- Internal auditory canal
- Superior semicircular canal
- Posterior semicircular canal
- Mastoid antrum
- Sigmoid sinus

NORMAL ANATOMY

The temporal bone initially may seem a daunting area for magnetic resonance imaging because of the apparent structural complexity. To understand the temporal region better, trace the hearing pathway from auricle through external auditory canal, to tympanic membrane attached to small bones (ossicles; malleus, incus, and stapes) in the middle ear cavity, through stapes stirrup on oval window, then vestibule to cochlea to inner auditory canal (IAC). The vestibulocochlear nerve (cranial nerve [CN] VIII) also provides balance with superior and inferior vestibular branches in the IAC, leading to the semicircular canals. Finally, the nearby facial nerve (CN VII) provides motor innervation to the face.

These nerves can be tracked easily on computed tomography (CT) by the corresponding bony canals, although the nerves themselves are best seen on MRI (see also Chapter 5).

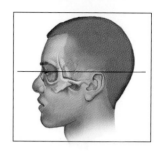

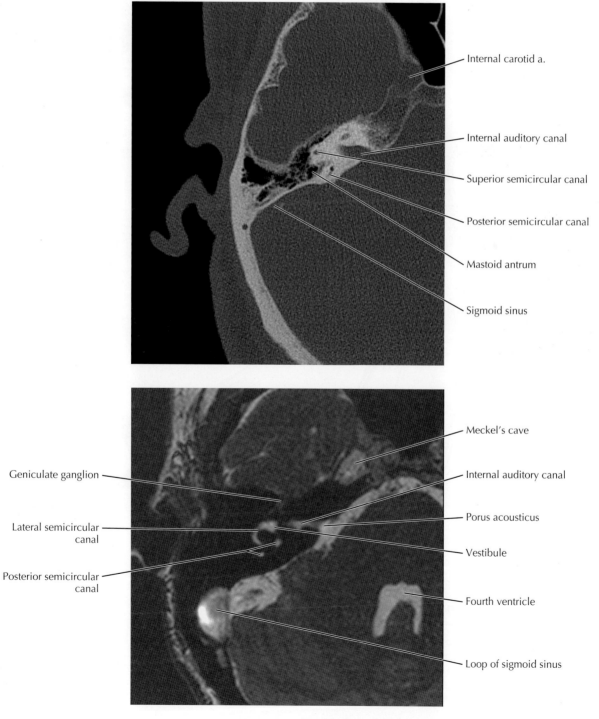

Internal carotid a.

Internal auditory canal

Superior semicircular canal

Posterior semicircular canal

Mastoid antrum

Sigmoid sinus

Geniculate ganglion

Lateral semicircular canal

Posterior semicircular canal

Meckel's cave

Internal auditory canal

Porus acousticus

Vestibule

Fourth ventricle

Loop of sigmoid sinus

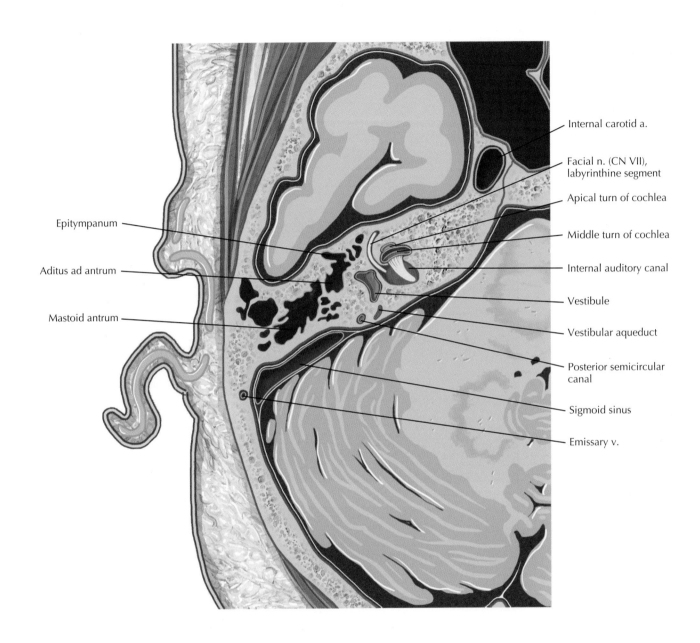

Internal carotid a.

Facial n. (CN VII), labyrinthine segment

Apical turn of cochlea

Middle turn of cochlea

Internal auditory canal

Vestibule

Vestibular aqueduct

Posterior semicircular canal

Sigmoid sinus

Emissary v.

Epitympanum

Aditus ad antrum

Mastoid antrum

PATHOLOGIC PROCESS

Note the fan-shaped appearance of the labyrinthine segment of the facial nerve connecting the intracanalicular segment with the geniculate ganglion more anteriorly. Damage to the facial nerve, as occurs with trauma and temporal bone fracture, leads to loss of motor control on the ipsilateral side of the face, mimicking a stroke, with profound social impact given the sensitivity to facial expression. (See facial nerve [CN VII] images in Chapter 5.)

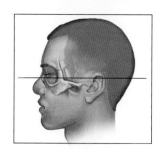

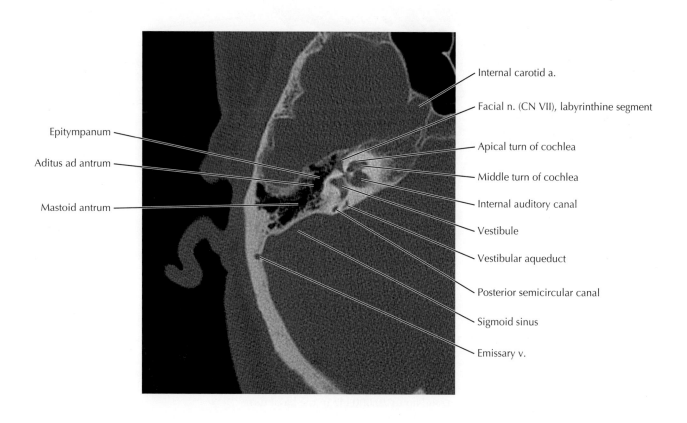

Epitympanum

Aditus ad antrum

Mastoid antrum

Internal carotid a.

Facial n. (CN VII), labyrinthine segment

Apical turn of cochlea

Middle turn of cochlea

Internal auditory canal

Vestibule

Vestibular aqueduct

Posterior semicircular canal

Sigmoid sinus

Emissary v.

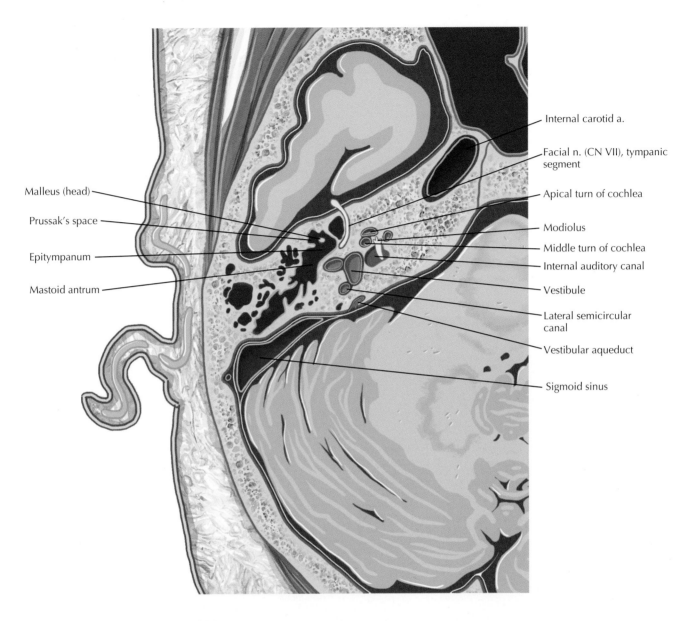

Internal carotid a.

Facial n. (CN VII), tympanic segment

Apical turn of cochlea

Modiolus

Middle turn of cochlea

Internal auditory canal

Vestibule

Lateral semicircular canal

Vestibular aqueduct

Sigmoid sinus

Malleus (head)

Prussak's space

Epitympanum

Mastoid antrum

NORMAL ANATOMY

Note the apical and middle turns of the cochlea. Counterintuitively, the tip of the cochlea (the apex) is sensitive to lower frequencies, down to 20 Hz, moving to higher frequencies in the middle turn, and up to 20,000 Hz in the basal turn.

Note also the very thin vestibular aqueduct, which connects the inner ear to a balloon-shaped structure called the *endolymphatic sac.* Although its function is not clearly known, the endolymphatic sac may help to ensure that fluid in the inner ear contains the correct ion concentration. The vestibular aqueduct is normally less than 1 mm in diameter, or smaller than the adjacent medial limb of the superior semicircular canal (a good anatomic reference). Enlarged vestibular aqueducts, associated with hearing loss in children, are thought to be related to the same underlying defect.

PATHOLOGIC PROCESS

Damage to the cochlear nerve, as in trauma with temporal bone fracture, is more classically seen with *transverse* fractures perpendicular to the long axis of the temporal bone, from auricle to petrous apex. Transverse fractures are more frequently associated with sensorineural hearing loss. Practically, however, many fractures combine both conditions.

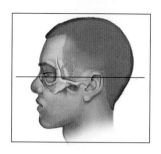

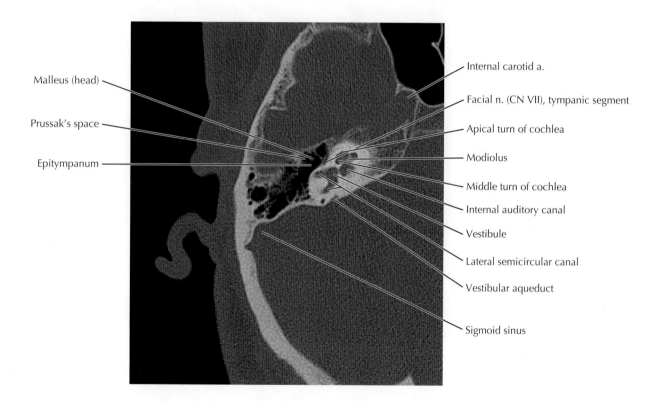

Malleus (head)

Prussak's space

Epitympanum

Internal carotid a.

Facial n. (CN VII), tympanic segment

Apical turn of cochlea

Modiolus

Middle turn of cochlea

Internal auditory canal

Vestibule

Lateral semicircular canal

Vestibular aqueduct

Sigmoid sinus

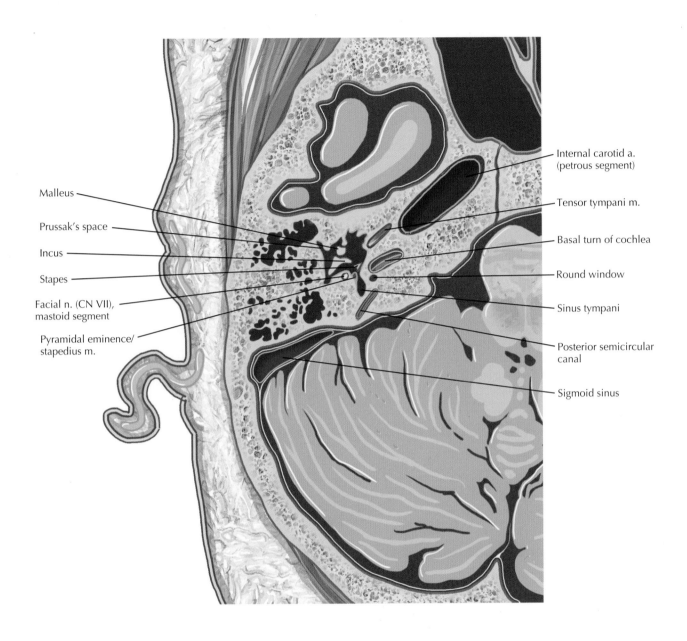

Malleus

Prussak's space

Incus

Stapes

Facial n. (CN VII),
mastoid segment

Pyramidal eminence/
stapedius m.

Internal carotid a.
(petrous segment)

Tensor tympani m.

Basal turn of cochlea

Round window

Sinus tympani

Posterior semicircular
canal

Sigmoid sinus

NORMAL ANATOMY

The basal turn of the cochlea is connected to the stapes stirrup through the oval window. Immediately anterior to the oval window is the *fissula ante fenestram*, a small, connective tissue–filled cleft where the tendon of the tensor tympani muscle turns laterally toward the malleus. In otosclerosis, the most common cause of hearing loss in people age 15 to 50, a small lytic lesion often develops at the fissula ante fenestram.

DIAGNOSTIC CONSIDERATION

The head of the malleus forms a "scoop of ice cream" on the cone-shaped incus. Loss of this ice cream cone appearance indicates ossicular dislocation.

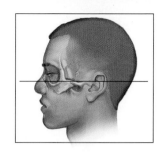

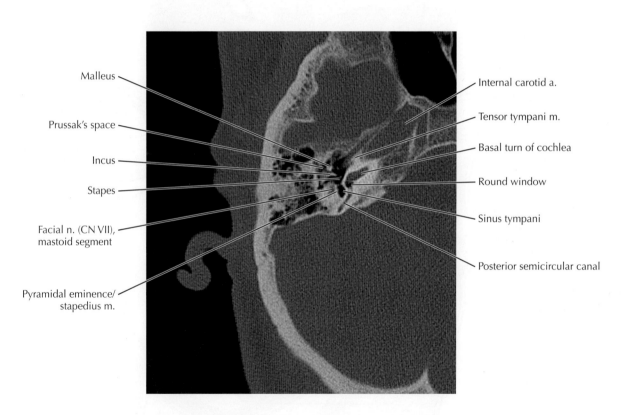

Malleus

Prussak's space

Incus

Stapes

Facial n. (CN VII),
mastoid segment

Pyramidal eminence/
stapedius m.

Internal carotid a.

Tensor tympani m.

Basal turn of cochlea

Round window

Sinus tympani

Posterior semicircular canal

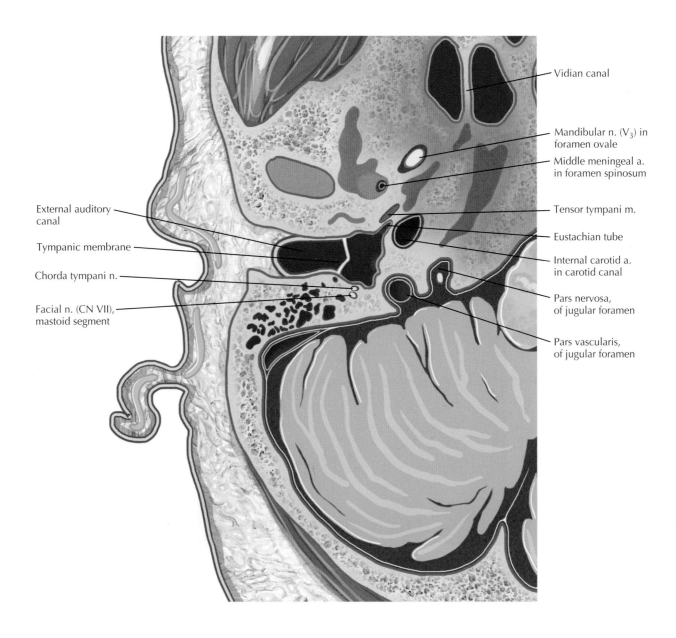

Vidian canal

Mandibular n. (V₃) in
foramen ovale

Middle meningeal a.
in foramen spinosum

External auditory
canal

Tympanic membrane

Chorda tympani n.

Facial n. (CN VII),
mastoid segment

Tensor tympani m.

Eustachian tube

Internal carotid a.
in carotid canal

Pars nervosa,
of jugular foramen

Pars vascularis,
of jugular foramen

PATHOLOGIC PROCESS

The tympanic membrane separating the external auditory canal from the middle ear cavity
is normally extremely thin and barely perceptible on CT. Thickening can often be caused by
inflammatory or infectious conditons such as otitis media.

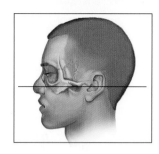

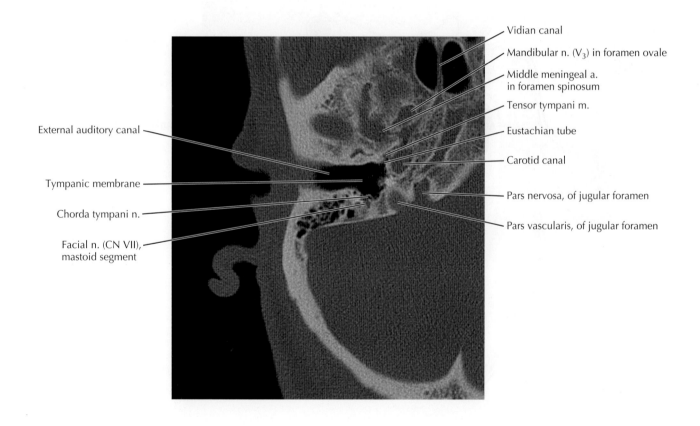

Vidian canal

Mandibular n. (V₃) in foramen ovale

Middle meningeal a. in foramen spinosum

Tensor tympani m.

Eustachian tube

Carotid canal

Pars nervosa, of jugular foramen

Pars vascularis, of jugular foramen

External auditory canal

Tympanic membrane

Chorda tympani n.

Facial n. (CN VII), mastoid segment

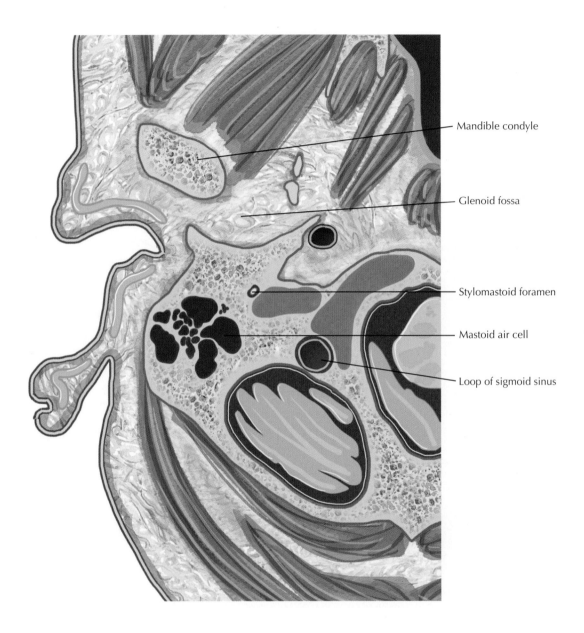

Mandible condyle

Glenoid fossa

Stylomastoid foramen

Mastoid air cell

Loop of sigmoid sinus

NORMAL ANATOMY

At the bottom of the temporal bone, the only nerve canal visible is the mastoid segment of the facial nerve. The mastoid segment descends vertically from the tympanic segment to the stylomastoid foramen at the skull base, between the styloid process and inferior aspect of the mastoid air cells.

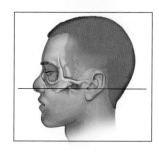

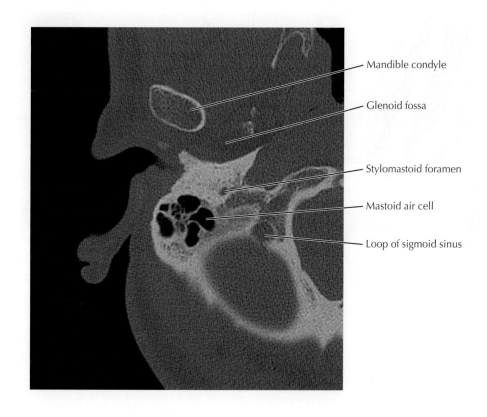

- Mandible condyle
- Glenoid fossa
- Stylomastoid foramen
- Mastoid air cell
- Loop of sigmoid sinus

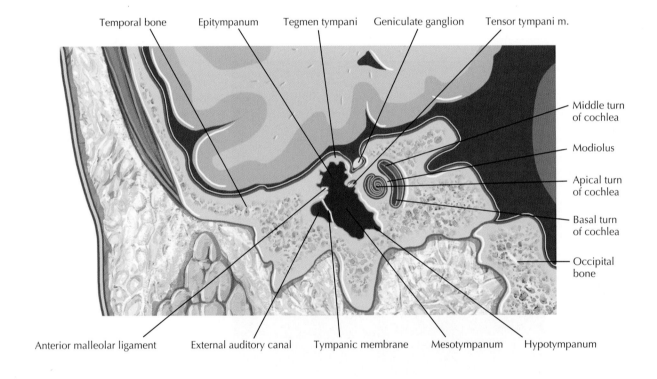

Temporal bone   Epitympanum   Tegmen tympani   Geniculate ganglion   Tensor tympani m.

Middle turn of cochlea

Modiolus

Apical turn of cochlea

Basal turn of cochlea

Occipital bone

Anterior malleolar ligament   External auditory canal   Tympanic membrane   Mesotympanum   Hypotympanum

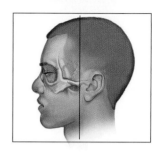

Temporal bone   Epitympanum   Tegmen tympani   Geniculate ganglion

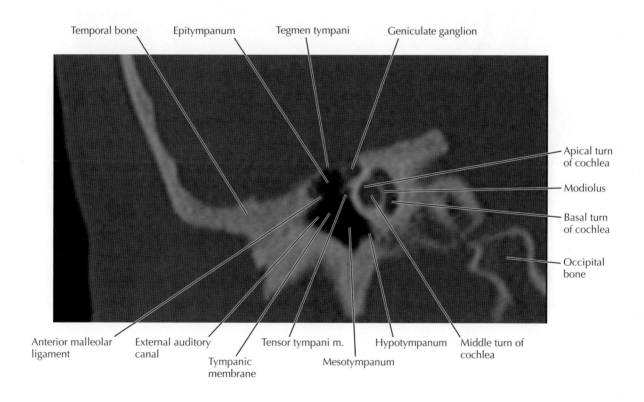

Apical turn of cochlea

Modiolus

Basal turn of cochlea

Occipital bone

Anterior malleolar ligament   External auditory canal   Tensor tympani m.   Hypotympanum   Middle turn of cochlea

Tympanic membrane   Mesotympanum

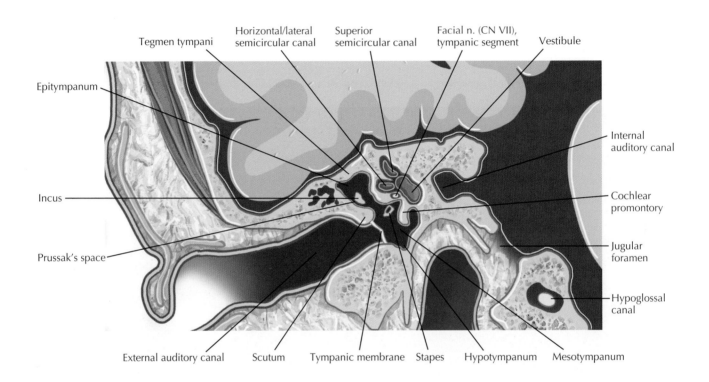

Tegmen tympani
Horizontal/lateral semicircular canal
Superior semicircular canal
Facial n. (CN VII), tympanic segment
Vestibule
Epitympanum
Internal auditory canal
Incus
Cochlear promontory
Prussak's space
Jugular foramen
Hypoglossal canal
External auditory canal
Scutum
Tympanic membrane
Stapes
Hypotympanum
Mesotympanum

PATHOLOGIC PROCESS

The air space lateral to the neck of the malleus is known as *Prussak's space* (superior recess of tympanic membrane). This space is important because cholesteatoma can occur there. A *cholesteatoma* forms when there is a deep retraction pocket in the tympanic membrane. The lining of the tympanic membrane is shed like skin, but if the membrane is retracted, the dead cells are trapped and can enlarge. This cholesteatoma can eventually erode the surrounding bony structures. One of the early signs differentiating simple middle ear fluid from a cholesteatoma is erosion of the scutum (bony plate) lateral to the Prussak's space at the upper edge of the tympanic membrane. Coronal is the best imaging plane on MRI to evaluate this scutum (tympanic scute).

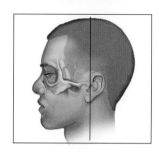

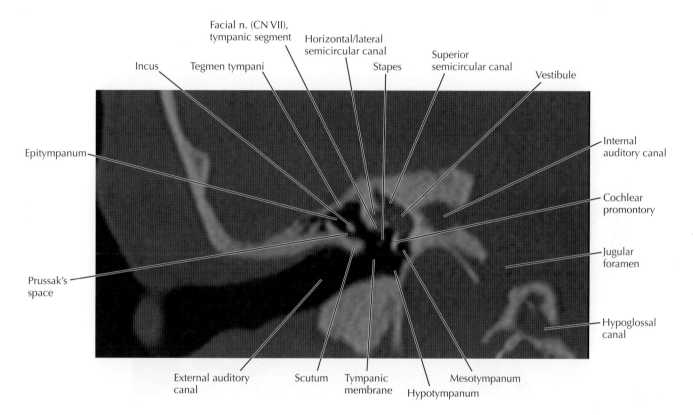

Facial n. (CN VII),
tympanic segment

Horizontal/lateral
semicircular canal

Incus

Tegmen tympani

Stapes

Superior
semicircular canal

Vestibule

Epitympanum

Internal
auditory canal

Cochlear
promontory

Jugular
foramen

Prussak's
space

Hypoglossal
canal

External auditory
canal

Scutum

Tympanic
membrane

Hypotympanum

Mesotympanum

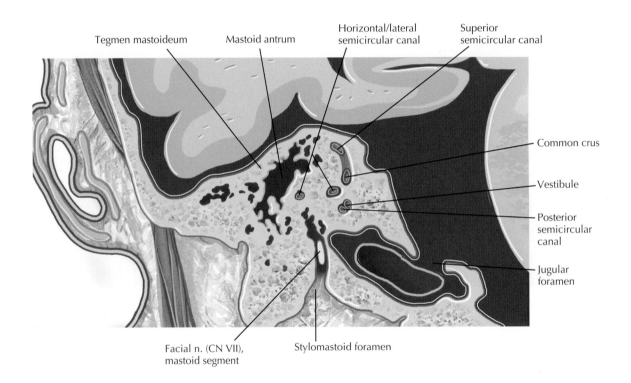

Tegmen mastoideum

Mastoid antrum

Horizontal/lateral semicircular canal

Superior semicircular canal

Common crus

Vestibule

Posterior semicircular canal

Jugular foramen

Facial n. (CN VII), mastoid segment

Stylomastoid foramen

NORMAL ANATOMY

Coronal MR images are useful for assessing the bony roof (tegmen) of the superior semicircular canal. Loss of this roof, or semicircular canal dehiscence and communication with the cerebrospinal fluid around the brain, can lead to disruption of vestibulocochlear nerve function.

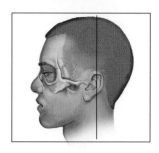

Tegmen mastoideum   Mastoid antrum   Horizontal/lateral semicircular canal   Superior semicircular canal

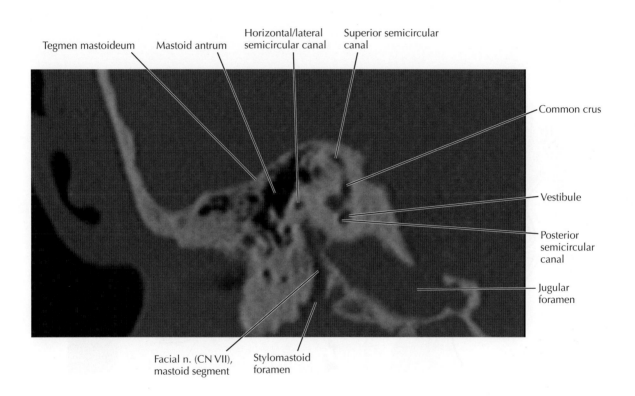

Common crus

Vestibule

Posterior semicircular canal

Jugular foramen

Facial n. (CN VII), mastoid segment   Stylomastoid foramen

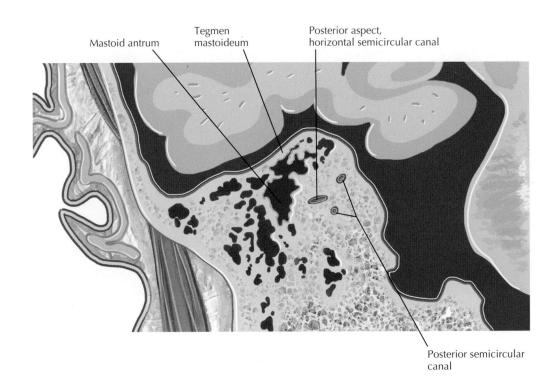

Mastoid antrum

Tegmen
mastoideum

Posterior aspect,
horizontal semicircular canal

Posterior semicircular
canal

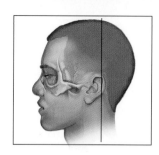

Mastoid antrum   Tegmen mastoideum   Posterior aspect, horizontal semicircular canal   Common crus

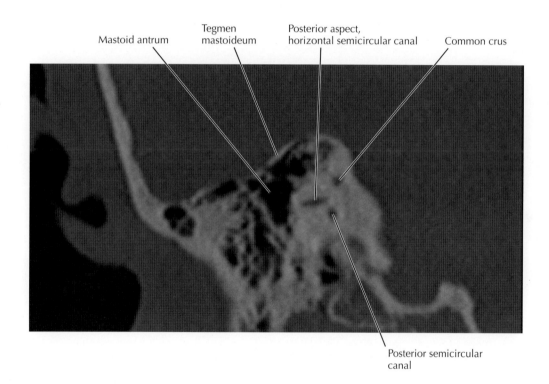

Posterior semicircular canal

Chapter 13 ORAL CAVITY, PHARYNX, AND SUPRAHYOID NECK

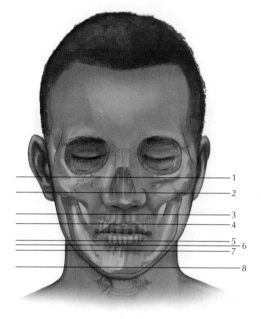

1
2
3
4
5
6
7
8

AXIAL   422

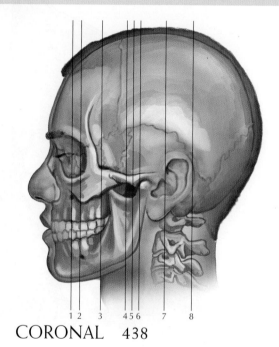

1 2 3   4 5 6   7   8

CORONAL   438

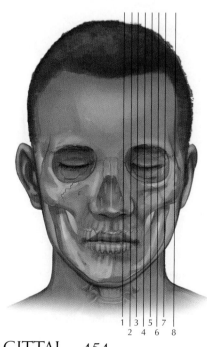

1 3 5 7
 2 4 6 8

SAGITTAL   454

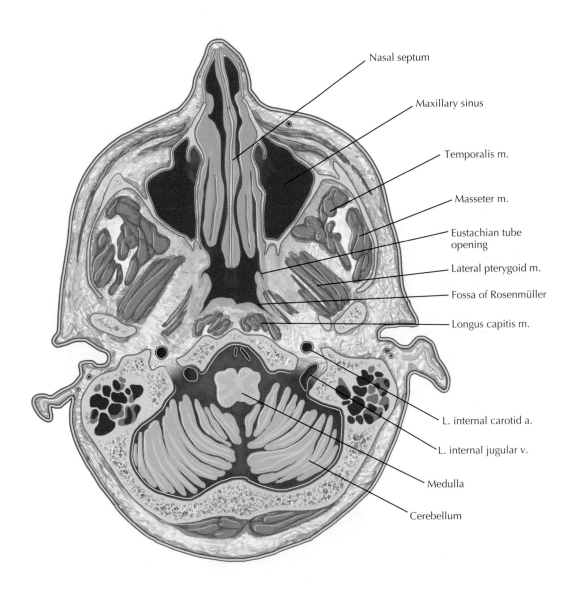

Nasal septum

Maxillary sinus

Temporalis m.

Masseter m.

Eustachian tube opening

Lateral pterygoid m.

Fossa of Rosenmüller

Longus capitis m.

L. internal carotid a.

L. internal jugular v.

Medulla

Cerebellum

NORMAL ANATOMY

Note the enhancement of the mucosal surfaces of the aerodigestive tract on the lower magnetic resonance (MR) image in Axial 1 after gadolinium contrast administration. The subcutaneous adipose tissue and the adipose planes between the structures in the neck are visible on both the upper pre-contrast T1-weighted MR image and the lower post-contrast T1-weighted MR image.

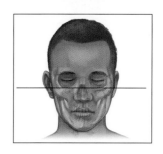

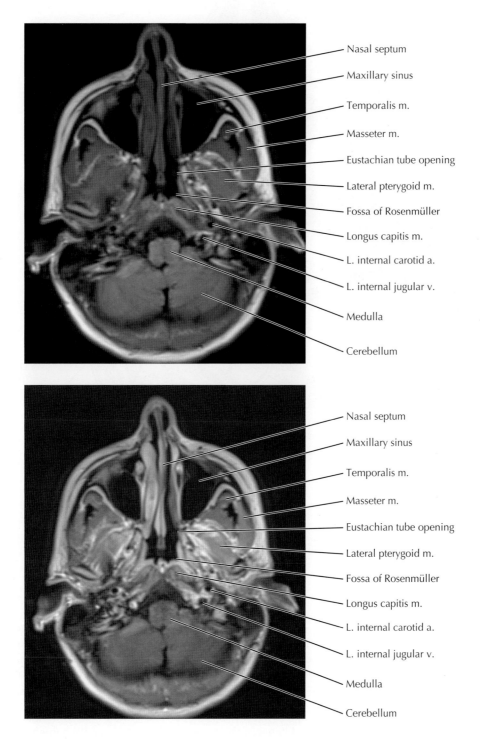

— Nasal septum

— Maxillary sinus

— Temporalis m.

— Masseter m.

— Eustachian tube opening

— Lateral pterygoid m.

— Fossa of Rosenmüller

— Longus capitis m.

— L. internal carotid a.

— L. internal jugular v.

— Medulla

— Cerebellum

— Nasal septum

— Maxillary sinus

— Temporalis m.

— Masseter m.

— Eustachian tube opening

— Lateral pterygoid m.

— Fossa of Rosenmüller

— Longus capitis m.

— L. internal carotid a.

— L. internal jugular v.

— Medulla

— Cerebellum

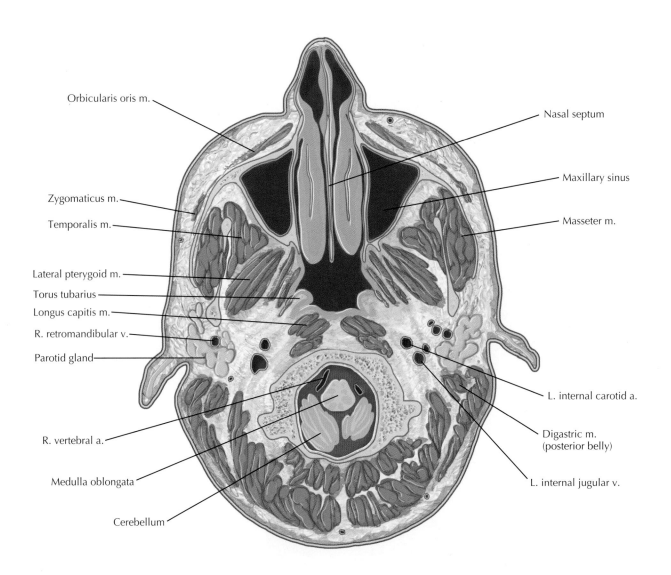

Orbicularis oris m.

Nasal septum

Zygomaticus m.

Maxillary sinus

Temporalis m.

Masseter m.

Lateral pterygoid m.

Torus tubarius

Longus capitis m.

R. retromandibular v.

Parotid gland

L. internal carotid a.

R. vertebral a.

Digastric m.
(posterior belly)

Medulla oblongata

L. internal jugular v.

Cerebellum

PATHOLOGIC PROCESS

An axial image of the nasopharynx at the level of the foramen magnum is visible on typically every brain study. Fluid in the mastoid air cells on one side may indicate a mass obstructing the Eustachian canal opening anterior to the *torus tubarius* (posterior protuberance of pharyngeal opening of auditory tube). The *fossa of Rosenmüller* is a blind-ending divot between the torus tubarius and the longus capitis muscle more posteriorly. Asymmetric loss of this fossa may be the first sign of a nasopharyngeal lesion. Malignant spread of a nasopharyngeal carcinoma may first reach the retropharyngeal lymph node. This lymph node is normally less than 8 mm in long axis and located between the longus capitis muscle and the internal carotid artery more posterolaterally.

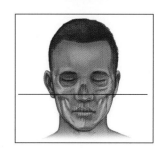

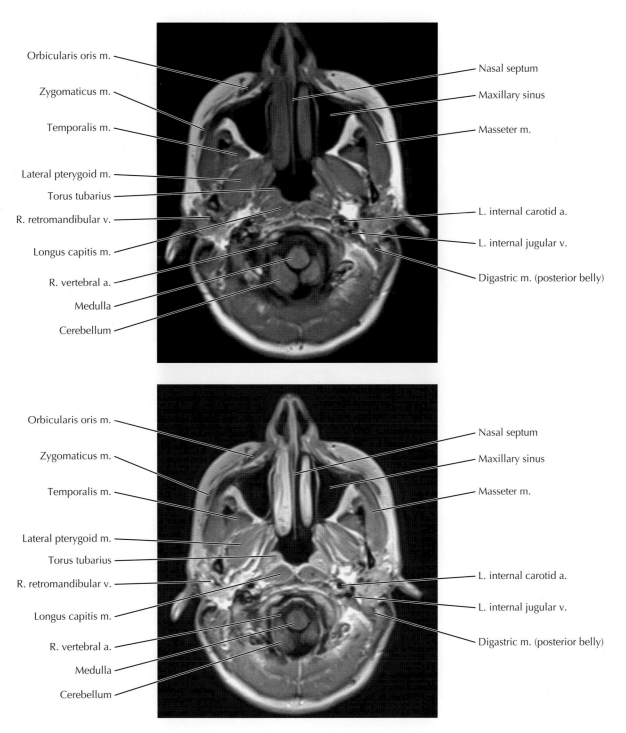

Orbicularis oris m.

Zygomaticus m.

Temporalis m.

Lateral pterygoid m.

Torus tubarius

R. retromandibular v.

Longus capitis m.

R. vertebral a.

Medulla

Cerebellum

Nasal septum

Maxillary sinus

Masseter m.

L. internal carotid a.

L. internal jugular v.

Digastric m. (posterior belly)

Orbicularis oris m.

Zygomaticus m.

Temporalis m.

Lateral pterygoid m.

Torus tubarius

R. retromandibular v.

Longus capitis m.

R. vertebral a.

Medulla

Cerebellum

Nasal septum

Maxillary sinus

Masseter m.

L. internal carotid a.

L. internal jugular v.

Digastric m. (posterior belly)

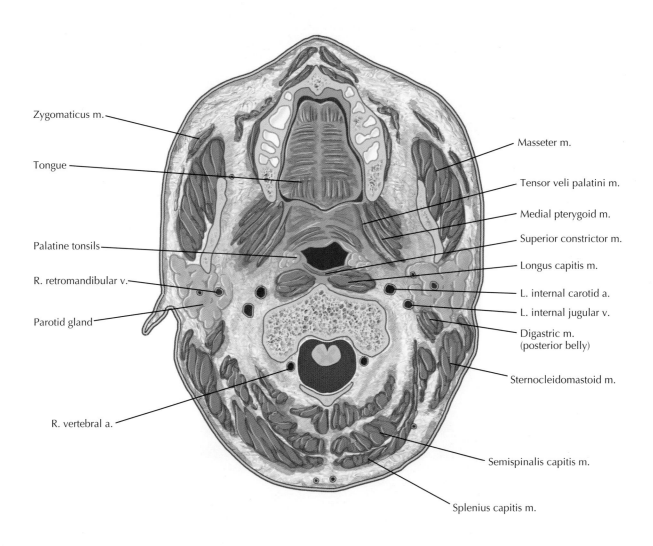

Zygomaticus m.

Tongue

Palatine tonsils

R. retromandibular v.

Parotid gland

R. vertebral a.

Masseter m.

Tensor veli palatini m.

Medial pterygoid m.

Superior constrictor m.

Longus capitis m.

L. internal carotid a.

L. internal jugular v.

Digastric m. (posterior belly)

Sternocleidomastoid m.

Semispinalis capitis m.

Splenius capitis m.

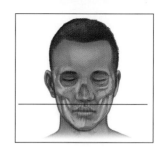

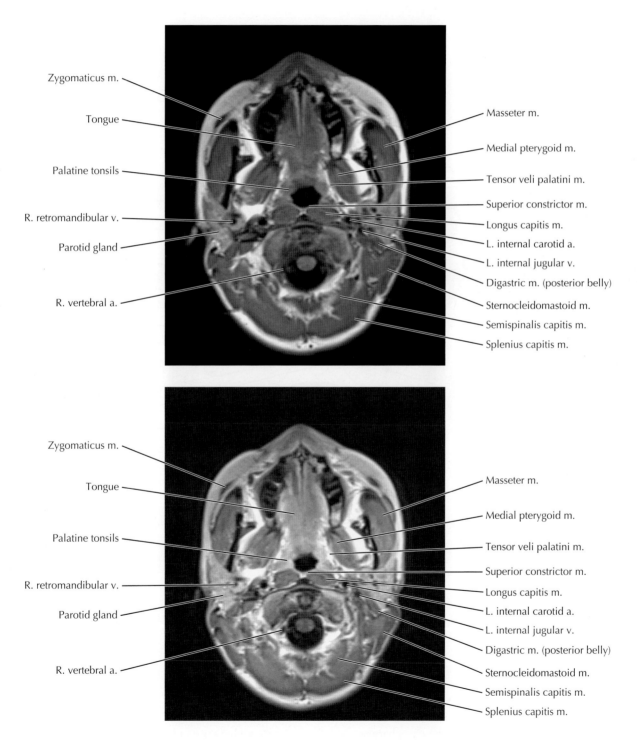

Zygomaticus m.

Tongue

Palatine tonsils

R. retromandibular v.

Parotid gland

R. vertebral a.

Masseter m.

Medial pterygoid m.

Tensor veli palatini m.

Superior constrictor m.

Longus capitis m.

L. internal carotid a.

L. internal jugular v.

Digastric m. (posterior belly)

Sternocleidomastoid m.

Semispinalis capitis m.

Splenius capitis m.

Zygomaticus m.

Tongue

Palatine tonsils

R. retromandibular v.

Parotid gland

R. vertebral a.

Masseter m.

Medial pterygoid m.

Tensor veli palatini m.

Superior constrictor m.

Longus capitis m.

L. internal carotid a.

L. internal jugular v.

Digastric m. (posterior belly)

Sternocleidomastoid m.

Semispinalis capitis m.

Splenius capitis m.

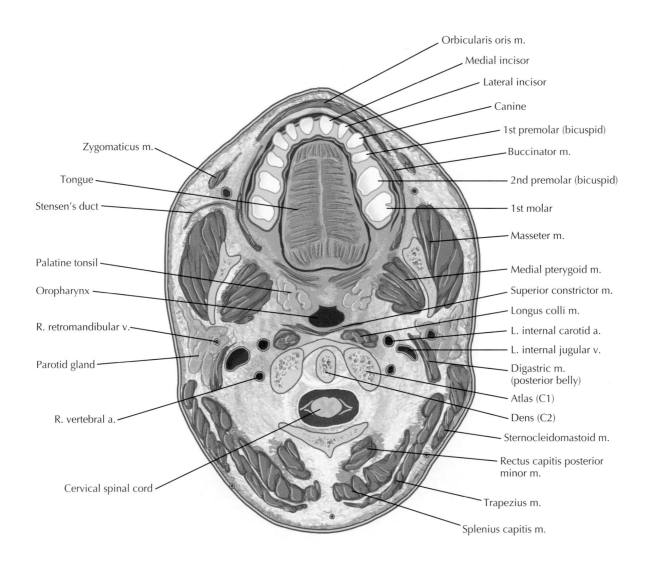

Orbicularis oris m.
Medial incisor
Lateral incisor
Canine
1st premolar (bicuspid)
Buccinator m.
2nd premolar (bicuspid)
1st molar
Masseter m.
Medial pterygoid m.
Superior constrictor m.
Longus colli m.
L. internal carotid a.
L. internal jugular v.
Digastric m. (posterior belly)
Atlas (C1)
Dens (C2)
Sternocleidomastoid m.
Rectus capitis posterior minor m.
Trapezius m.
Splenius capitis m.

Zygomaticus m.
Tongue
Stensen's duct
Palatine tonsil
Oropharynx
R. retromandibular v.
Parotid gland
R. vertebral a.
Cervical spinal cord

NORMAL ANATOMY

Unlike the nasopharynx cranially or the hypopharynx caudally, the lumen of the oropharynx can be grossly identified on axial MR images by visualization of teeth.

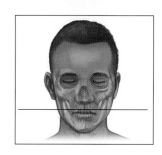

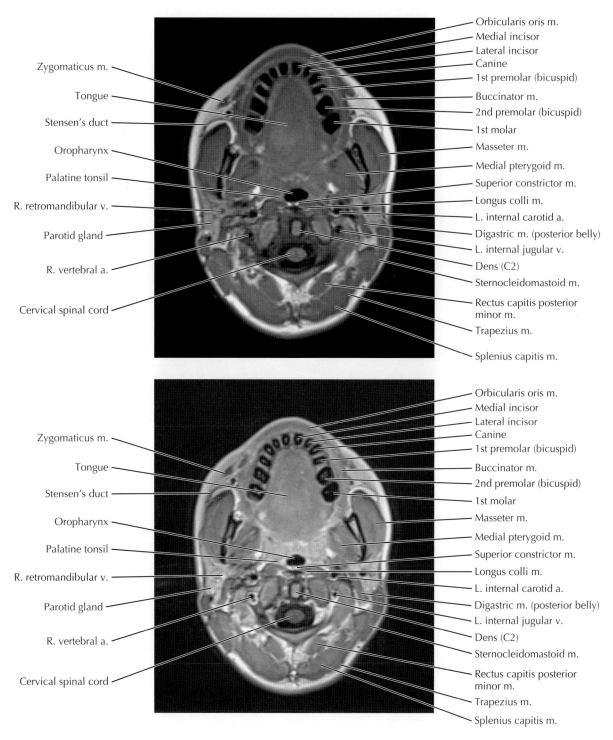

Zygomaticus m.
Tongue
Stensen's duct
Oropharynx
Palatine tonsil
R. retromandibular v.
Parotid gland
R. vertebral a.
Cervical spinal cord

Orbicularis oris m.
Medial incisor
Lateral incisor
Canine
1st premolar (bicuspid)
Buccinator m.
2nd premolar (bicuspid)
1st molar
Masseter m.
Medial pterygoid m.
Superior constrictor m.
Longus colli m.
L. internal carotid a.
Digastric m. (posterior belly)
L. internal jugular v.
Dens (C2)
Sternocleidomastoid m.
Rectus capitis posterior minor m.
Trapezius m.
Splenius capitis m.

Zygomaticus m.
Tongue
Stensen's duct
Oropharynx
Palatine tonsil
R. retromandibular v.
Parotid gland
R. vertebral a.
Cervical spinal cord

Orbicularis oris m.
Medial incisor
Lateral incisor
Canine
1st premolar (bicuspid)
Buccinator m.
2nd premolar (bicuspid)
1st molar
Masseter m.
Medial pterygoid m.
Superior constrictor m.
Longus colli m.
L. internal carotid a.
Digastric m. (posterior belly)
L. internal jugular v.
Dens (C2)
Sternocleidomastoid m.
Rectus capitis posterior minor m.
Trapezius m.
Splenius capitis m.

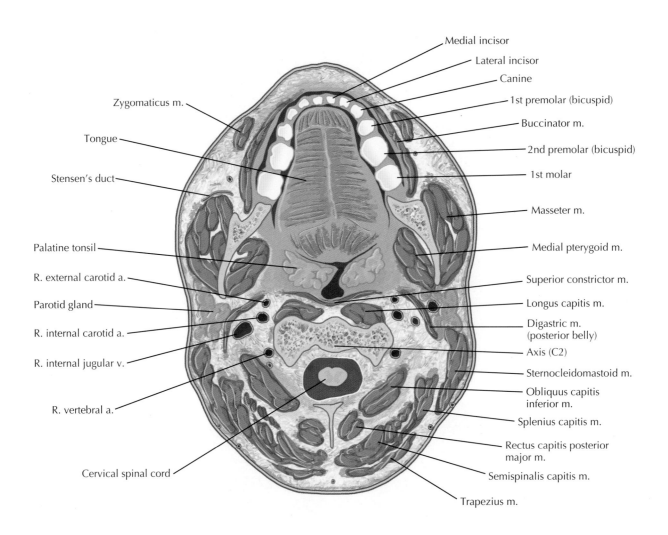

Medial incisor
Lateral incisor
Canine
1st premolar (bicuspid)
Buccinator m.
2nd premolar (bicuspid)
1st molar
Masseter m.
Medial pterygoid m.
Superior constrictor m.
Longus capitis m.
Digastric m. (posterior belly)
Axis (C2)
Sternocleidomastoid m.
Obliquus capitis inferior m.
Splenius capitis m.
Rectus capitis posterior major m.
Semispinalis capitis m.
Trapezius m.

Zygomaticus m.
Tongue
Stensen's duct
Palatine tonsil
R. external carotid a.
Parotid gland
R. internal carotid a.
R. internal jugular v.
R. vertebral a.
Cervical spinal cord

PATHOLOGIC PROCESS

Lesions of the head and neck are often most easily detected by loss of normal fat planes. On these T1-weighted precontrast (upper) and postcontrast (lower) MR images, note the fat within the *retromolar trigone* (retromandibular triangle) located posterior to the third molar. Once a malignancy or infection has reached the parapharyngeal fat located more posteriorly, it has an easy route of spread craniocaudally from the skull base down to the inferior pericardial recess.

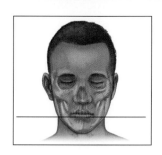

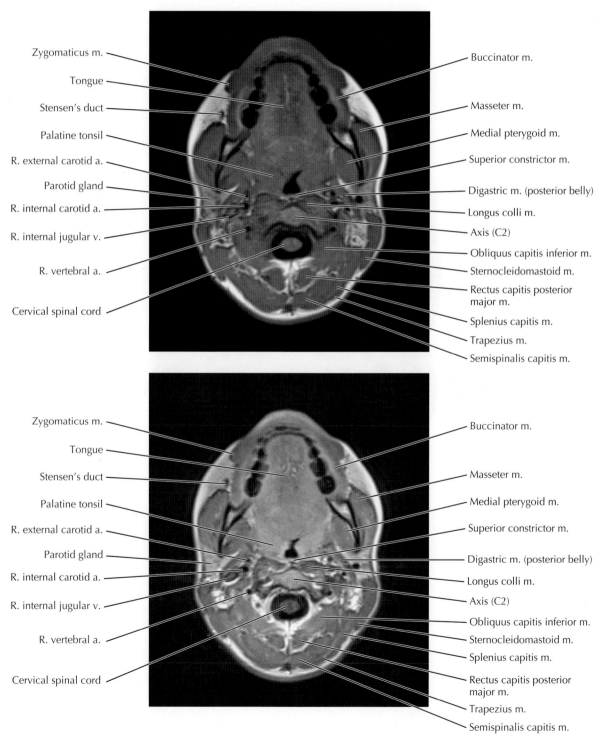

Zygomaticus m. — Buccinator m.

Tongue —

Stensen's duct — Masseter m.

Palatine tonsil — Medial pterygoid m.

R. external carotid a. — Superior constrictor m.

Parotid gland — Digastric m. (posterior belly)

R. internal carotid a. — Longus colli m.

R. internal jugular v. — Axis (C2)

— Obliquus capitis inferior m.

R. vertebral a. — Sternocleidomastoid m.

— Rectus capitis posterior major m.

Cervical spinal cord — Splenius capitis m.

— Trapezius m.

— Semispinalis capitis m.

Zygomaticus m. — Buccinator m.

Tongue —

Stensen's duct — Masseter m.

Palatine tonsil — Medial pterygoid m.

R. external carotid a. — Superior constrictor m.

Parotid gland — Digastric m. (posterior belly)

R. internal carotid a. — Longus colli m.

R. internal jugular v. — Axis (C2)

— Obliquus capitis inferior m.

R. vertebral a. — Sternocleidomastoid m.

— Splenius capitis m.

Cervical spinal cord — Rectus capitis posterior major m.

— Trapezius m.

— Semispinalis capitis m.

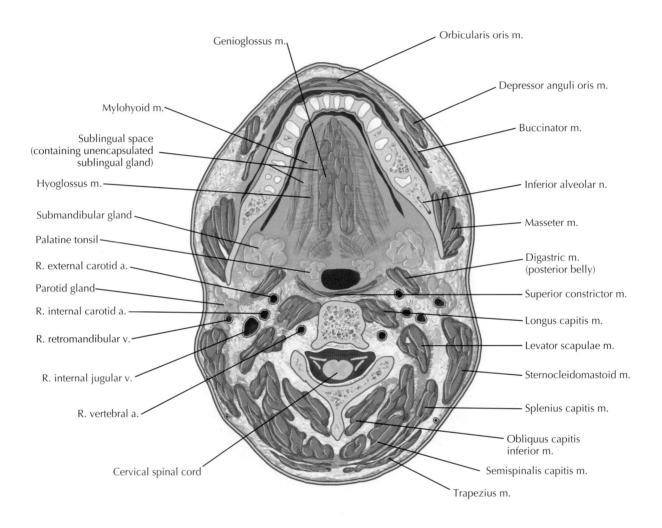

Genioglossus m.

Orbicularis oris m.

Depressor anguli oris m.

Mylohyoid m.

Buccinator m.

Sublingual space
(containing unencapsulated
sublingual gland)

Inferior alveolar n.

Hyoglossus m.

Submandibular gland

Masseter m.

Palatine tonsil

Digastric m.
(posterior belly)

R. external carotid a.

Superior constrictor m.

Parotid gland

Longus capitis m.

R. internal carotid a.

Levator scapulae m.

R. retromandibular v.

Sternocleidomastoid m.

R. internal jugular v.

Splenius capitis m.

R. vertebral a.

Obliquus capitis
inferior m.

Cervical spinal cord

Semispinalis capitis m.

Trapezius m.

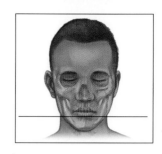

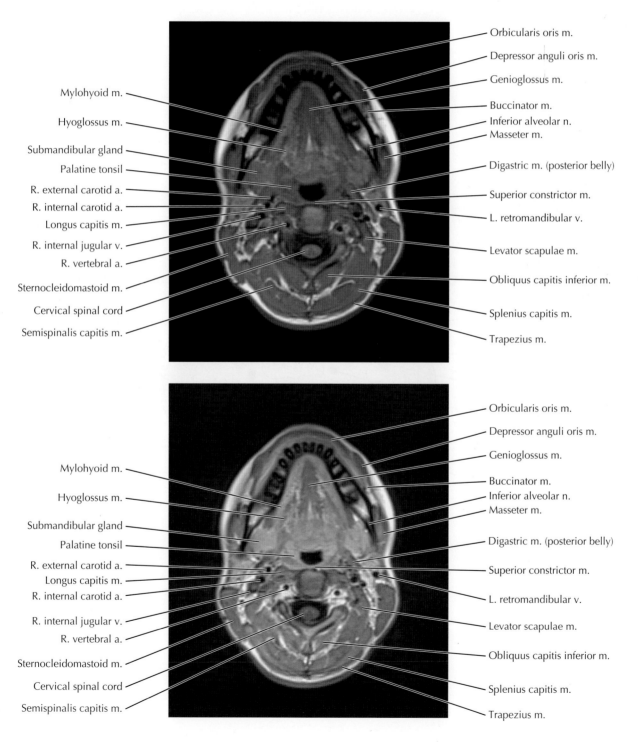

Mylohyoid m.

Hyoglossus m.

Submandibular gland

Palatine tonsil

R. external carotid a.

R. internal carotid a.

Longus capitis m.

R. internal jugular v.

R. vertebral a.

Sternocleidomastoid m.

Cervical spinal cord

Semispinalis capitis m.

Orbicularis oris m.

Depressor anguli oris m.

Genioglossus m.

Buccinator m.

Inferior alveolar n.

Masseter m.

Digastric m. (posterior belly)

Superior constrictor m.

L. retromandibular v.

Levator scapulae m.

Obliquus capitis inferior m.

Splenius capitis m.

Trapezius m.

Mylohyoid m.

Hyoglossus m.

Submandibular gland

Palatine tonsil

R. external carotid a.

Longus capitis m.

R. internal carotid a.

R. internal jugular v.

R. vertebral a.

Sternocleidomastoid m.

Cervical spinal cord

Semispinalis capitis m.

Orbicularis oris m.

Depressor anguli oris m.

Genioglossus m.

Buccinator m.

Inferior alveolar n.

Masseter m.

Digastric m. (posterior belly)

Superior constrictor m.

L. retromandibular v.

Levator scapulae m.

Obliquus capitis inferior m.

Splenius capitis m.

Trapezius m.

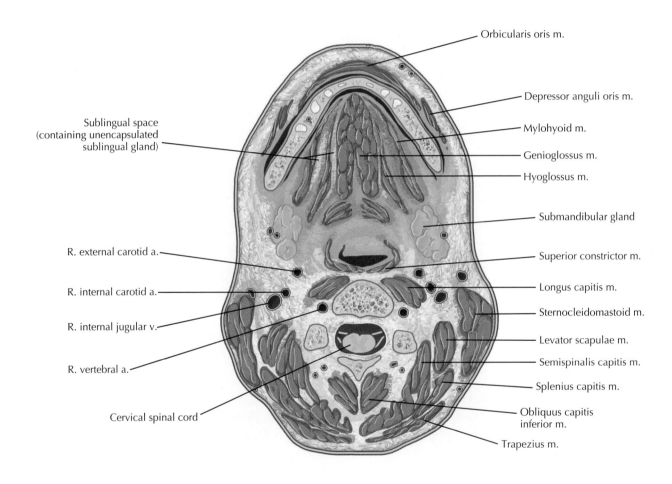

Orbicularis oris m.

Depressor anguli oris m.

Mylohyoid m.

Genioglossus m.

Hyoglossus m.

Submandibular gland

Superior constrictor m.

Longus capitis m.

Sternocleidomastoid m.

Levator scapulae m.

Semispinalis capitis m.

Splenius capitis m.

Obliquus capitis inferior m.

Trapezius m.

Sublingual space (containing unencapsulated sublingual gland)

R. external carotid a.

R. internal carotid a.

R. internal jugular v.

R. vertebral a.

Cervical spinal cord

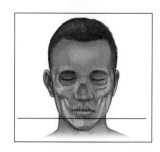

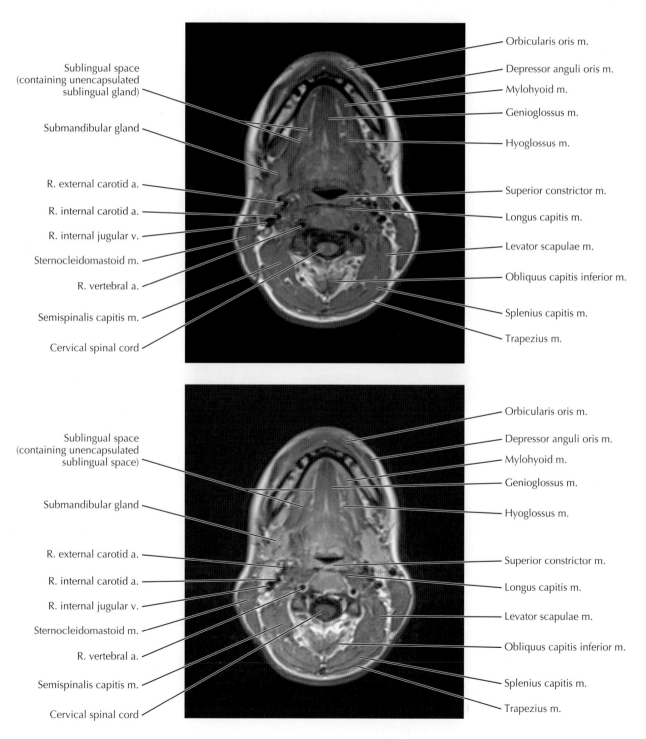

Sublingual space (containing unencapsulated sublingual gland)

Submandibular gland

R. external carotid a.

R. internal carotid a.

R. internal jugular v.

Sternocleidomastoid m.

R. vertebral a.

Semispinalis capitis m.

Cervical spinal cord

Orbicularis oris m.

Depressor anguli oris m.

Mylohyoid m.

Genioglossus m.

Hyoglossus m.

Superior constrictor m.

Longus capitis m.

Levator scapulae m.

Obliquus capitis inferior m.

Splenius capitis m.

Trapezius m.

Sublingual space (containing unencapsulated sublingual space)

Submandibular gland

R. external carotid a.

R. internal carotid a.

R. internal jugular v.

Sternocleidomastoid m.

R. vertebral a.

Semispinalis capitis m.

Cervical spinal cord

Orbicularis oris m.

Depressor anguli oris m.

Mylohyoid m.

Genioglossus m.

Hyoglossus m.

Superior constrictor m.

Longus capitis m.

Levator scapulae m.

Obliquus capitis inferior m.

Splenius capitis m.

Trapezius m.

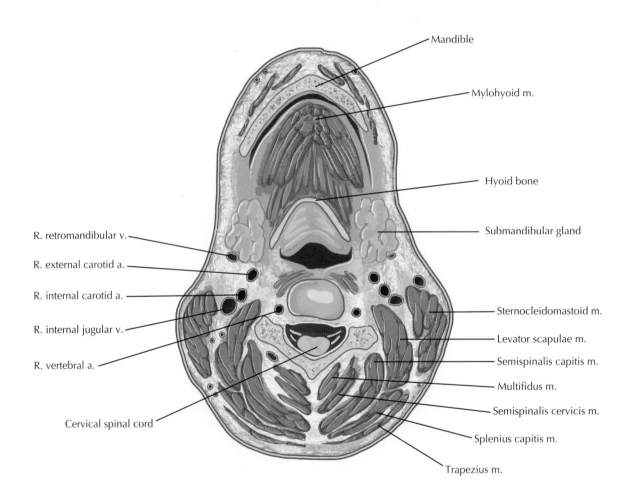

Mandible

Mylohyoid m.

Hyoid bone

Submandibular gland

R. retromandibular v.

R. external carotid a.

R. internal carotid a.

R. internal jugular v.

R. vertebral a.

Cervical spinal cord

Sternocleidomastoid m.

Levator scapulae m.

Semispinalis capitis m.

Multifidus m.

Semispinalis cervicis m.

Splenius capitis m.

Trapezius m.

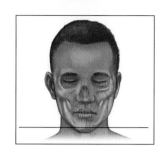

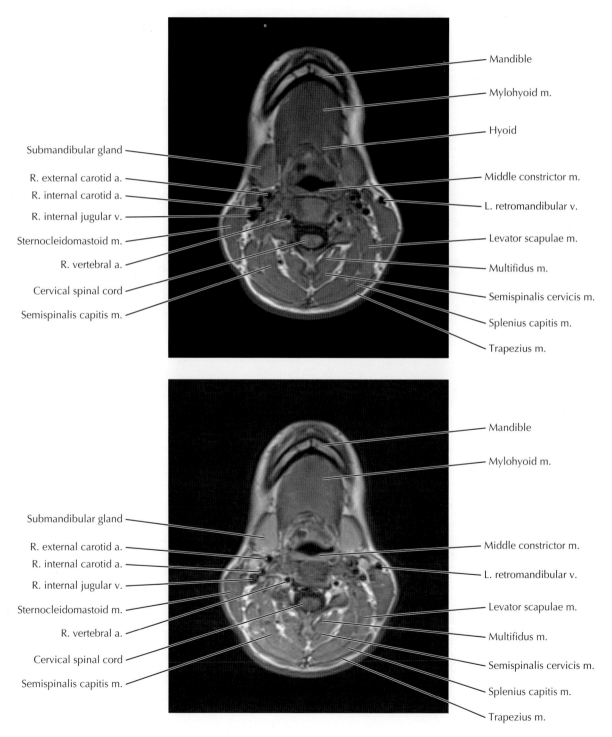

Mandible

Mylohyoid m.

Hyoid

Submandibular gland

R. external carotid a.

R. internal carotid a.

R. internal jugular v.

Sternocleidomastoid m.

R. vertebral a.

Cervical spinal cord

Semispinalis capitis m.

Middle constrictor m.

L. retromandibular v.

Levator scapulae m.

Multifidus m.

Semispinalis cervicis m.

Splenius capitis m.

Trapezius m.

Mandible

Mylohyoid m.

Submandibular gland

R. external carotid a.

R. internal carotid a.

R. internal jugular v.

Sternocleidomastoid m.

R. vertebral a.

Cervical spinal cord

Semispinalis capitis m.

Middle constrictor m.

L. retromandibular v.

Levator scapulae m.

Multifidus m.

Semispinalis cervicis m.

Splenius capitis m.

Trapezius m.

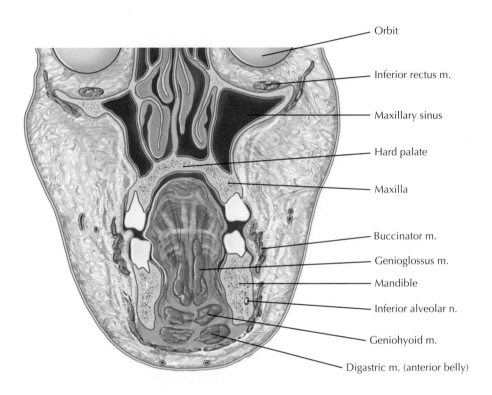

Orbit

Inferior rectus m.

Maxillary sinus

Hard palate

Maxilla

Buccinator m.

Genioglossus m.

Mandible

Inferior alveolar n.

Geniohyoid m.

Digastric m. (anterior belly)

IMAGING TECHNIQUE CONSIDERATION

Note the conspicuous contrast enhancement of the mucosal surfaces of the nasal passages on the lower postcontrast T1- weighted MR image in Coronal 1.

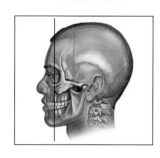

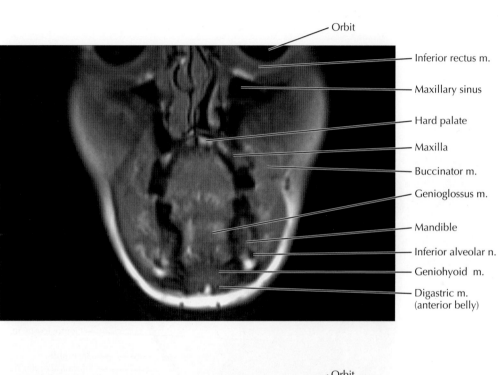

Orbit

Inferior rectus m.

Maxillary sinus

Hard palate

Maxilla

Buccinator m.

Genioglossus m.

Mandible

Inferior alveolar n.

Geniohyoid m.

Digastric m.
(anterior belly)

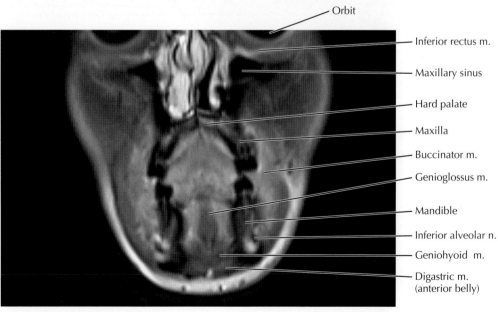

Orbit

Inferior rectus m.

Maxillary sinus

Hard palate

Maxilla

Buccinator m.

Genioglossus m.

Mandible

Inferior alveolar n.

Geniohyoid m.

Digastric m.
(anterior belly)

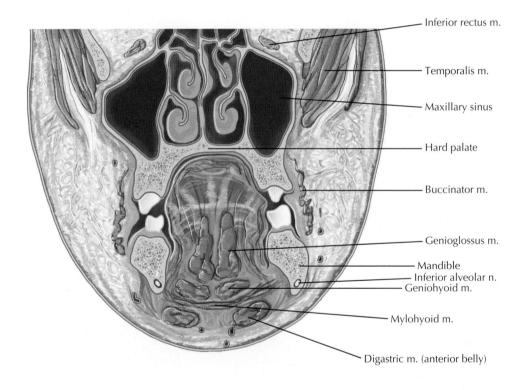

Inferior rectus m.

Temporalis m.

Maxillary sinus

Hard palate

Buccinator m.

Genioglossus m.

Mandible

Inferior alveolar n.

Geniohyoid m.

Mylohyoid m.

Digastric m. (anterior belly)

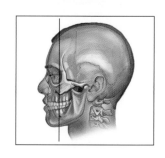

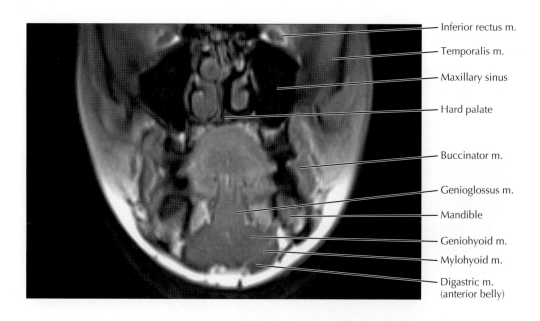

- Inferior rectus m.
- Temporalis m.
- Maxillary sinus
- Hard palate
- Buccinator m.
- Genioglossus m.
- Mandible
- Geniohyoid m.
- Mylohyoid m.
- Digastric m. (anterior belly)

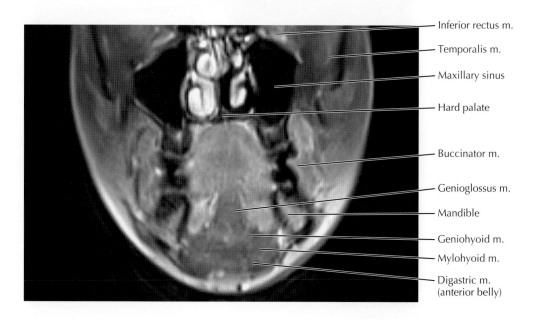

- Inferior rectus m.
- Temporalis m.
- Maxillary sinus
- Hard palate
- Buccinator m.
- Genioglossus m.
- Mandible
- Geniohyoid m.
- Mylohyoid m.
- Digastric m. (anterior belly)

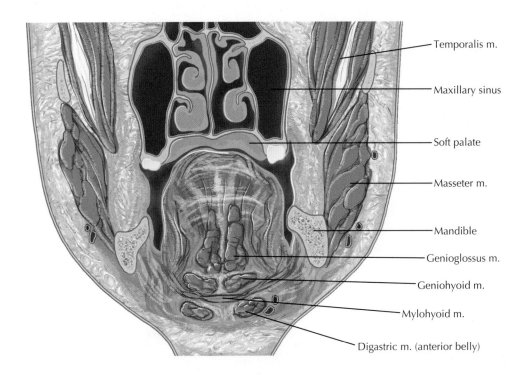

Temporalis m.

Maxillary sinus

Soft palate

Masseter m.

Mandible

Genioglossus m.

Geniohyoid m.

Mylohyoid m.

Digastric m. (anterior belly)

DIAGNOSTIC CONSIDERATION

Coronal imaging is often the best plane on MRI to assess a tongue lesion extending into the floor of mouth. The floor of the mouth is supported by the mylohyoid muscle (Greek *mylai*, "molar teeth"), which courses from the mandible to the hyoid bone.

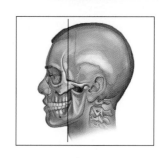

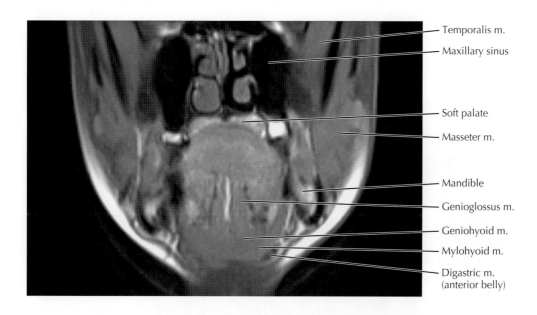

Temporalis m.
Maxillary sinus

Soft palate
Masseter m.

Mandible
Genioglossus m.
Geniohyoid m.
Mylohyoid m.
Digastric m. (anterior belly)

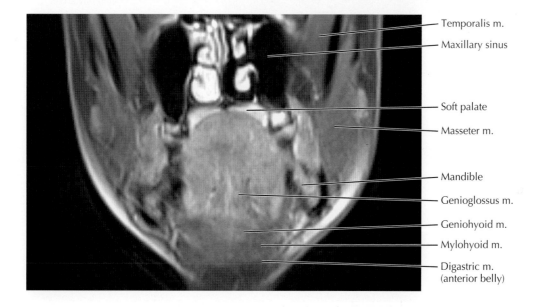

Temporalis m.
Maxillary sinus

Soft palate
Masseter m.

Mandible
Genioglossus m.
Geniohyoid m.
Mylohyoid m.
Digastric m. (anterior belly)

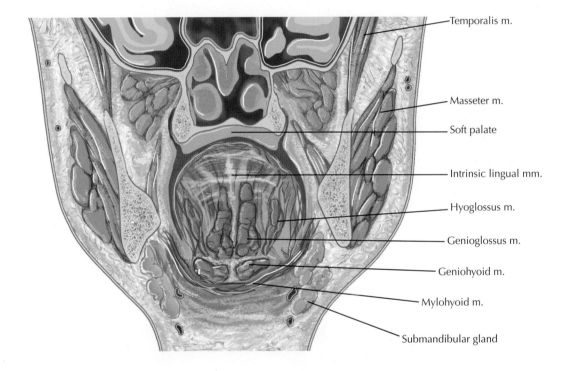

Temporalis m.

Masseter m.

Soft palate

Intrinsic lingual mm.

Hyoglossus m.

Genioglossus m.

Geniohyoid m.

Mylohyoid m.

Submandibular gland

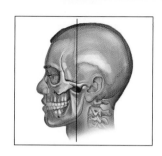

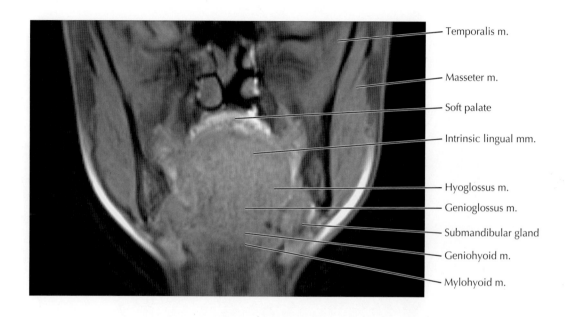

- Temporalis m.
- Masseter m.
- Soft palate
- Intrinsic lingual mm.
- Hyoglossus m.
- Genioglossus m.
- Submandibular gland
- Geniohyoid m.
- Mylohyoid m.

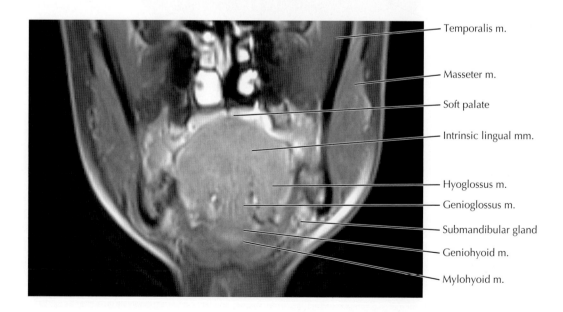

- Temporalis m.
- Masseter m.
- Soft palate
- Intrinsic lingual mm.
- Hyoglossus m.
- Genioglossus m.
- Submandibular gland
- Geniohyoid m.
- Mylohyoid m.

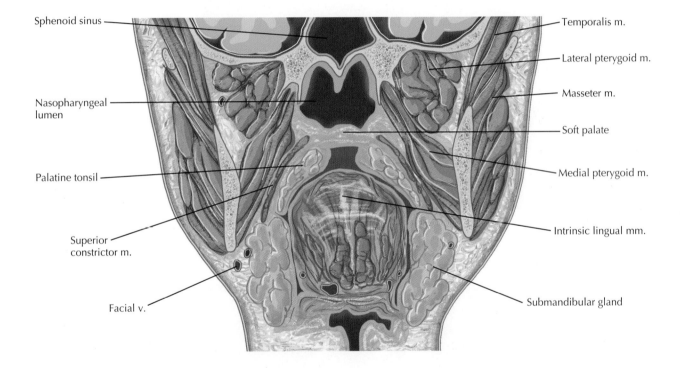

Sphenoid sinus

Nasopharyngeal lumen

Palatine tonsil

Superior constrictor m.

Facial v.

Temporalis m.

Lateral pterygoid m.

Masseter m.

Soft palate

Medial pterygoid m.

Intrinsic lingual mm.

Submandibular gland

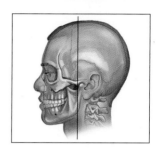

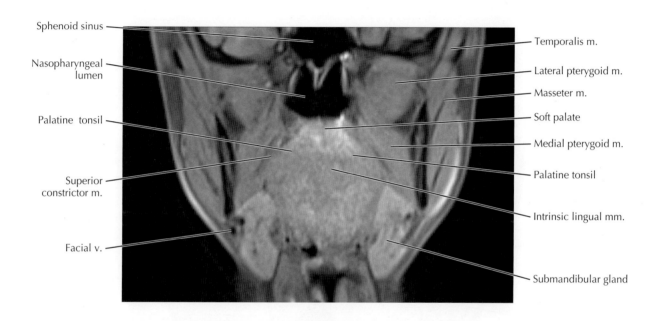

Sphenoid sinus

Nasopharyngeal lumen

Palatine tonsil

Superior constrictor m.

Facial v.

Temporalis m.

Lateral pterygoid m.

Masseter m.

Soft palate

Medial pterygoid m.

Palatine tonsil

Intrinsic lingual mm.

Submandibular gland

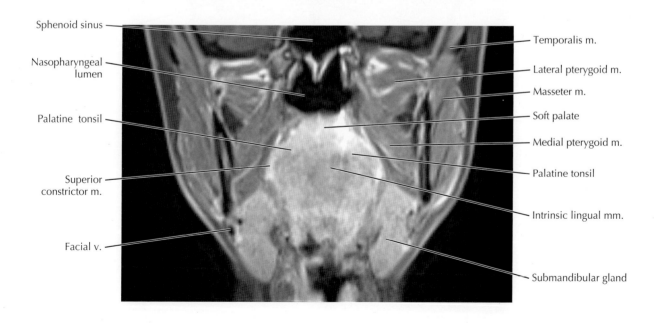

Sphenoid sinus

Nasopharyngeal lumen

Palatine tonsil

Superior constrictor m.

Facial v.

Temporalis m.

Lateral pterygoid m.

Masseter m.

Soft palate

Medial pterygoid m.

Palatine tonsil

Intrinsic lingual mm.

Submandibular gland

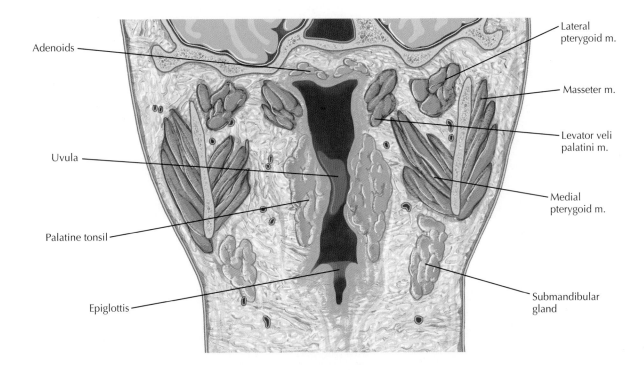

Adenoids

Lateral pterygoid m.

Masseter m.

Levator veli palatini m.

Uvula

Medial pterygoid m.

Palatine tonsil

Epiglottis

Submandibular gland

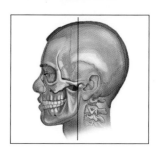

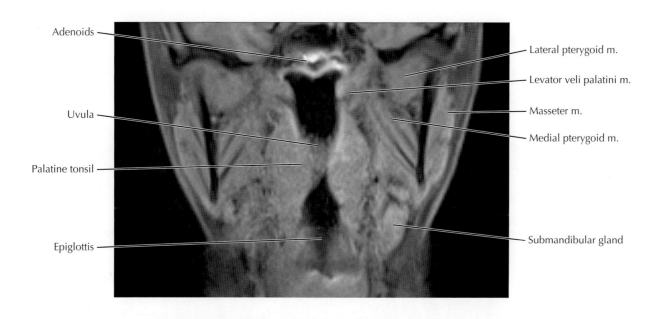

Adenoids

Uvula

Palatine tonsil

Epiglottis

Lateral pterygoid m.

Levator veli palatini m.

Masseter m.

Medial pterygoid m.

Submandibular gland

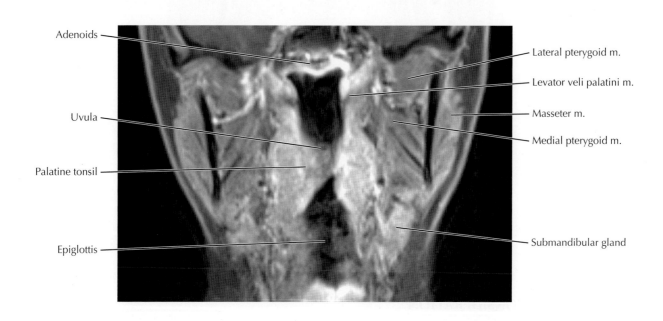

Adenoids

Uvula

Palatine tonsil

Epiglottis

Lateral pterygoid m.

Levator veli palatini m.

Masseter m.

Medial pterygoid m.

Submandibular gland

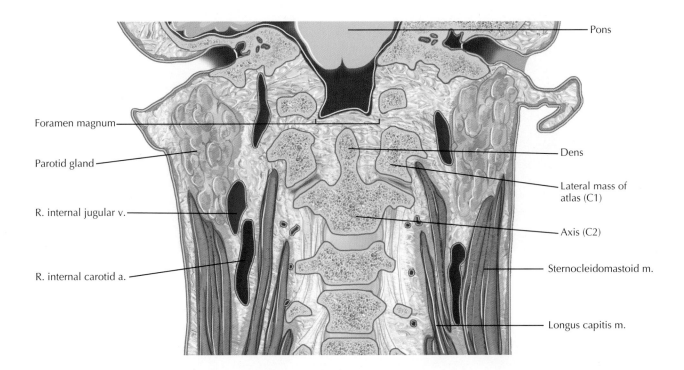

Pons

Foramen magnum

Parotid gland

R. internal jugular v.

R. internal carotid a.

Dens

Lateral mass of atlas (C1)

Axis (C2)

Sternocleidomastoid m.

Longus capitis m.

DIAGNOSTIC CONSIDERATION

Although axial imaging is the plane conventionally used for measuring the long axis of neck lymph nodes, the coronal plane is often useful for visualizing the entire craniocaudal length of the jugular and spinal accessory lymph node chains.

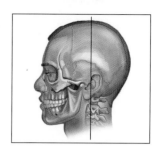

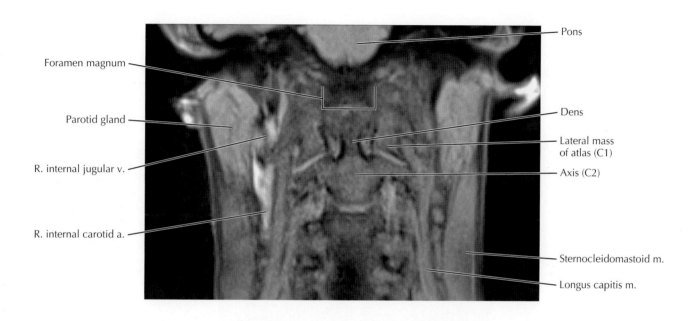

Foramen magnum

Parotid gland

R. internal jugular v.

R. internal carotid a.

Pons

Dens

Lateral mass of atlas (C1)

Axis (C2)

Sternocleidomastoid m.

Longus capitis m.

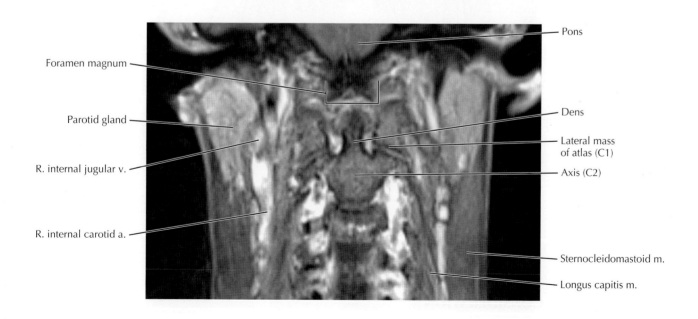

Foramen magnum

Parotid gland

R. internal jugular v.

R. internal carotid a.

Pons

Dens

Lateral mass of atlas (C1)

Axis (C2)

Sternocleidomastoid m.

Longus capitis m.

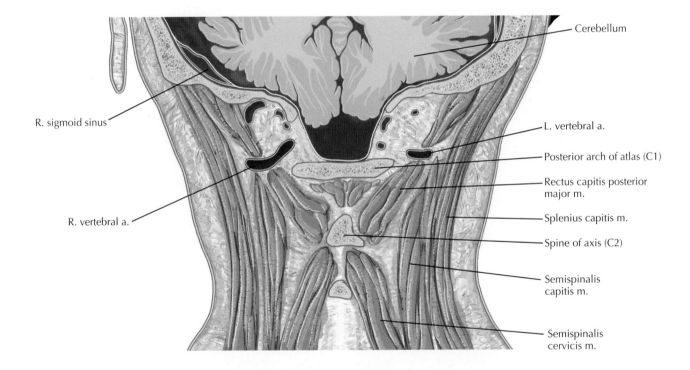

R. sigmoid sinus

R. vertebral a.

Cerebellum

L. vertebral a.

Posterior arch of atlas (C1)

Rectus capitis posterior major m.

Splenius capitis m.

Spine of axis (C2)

Semispinalis capitis m.

Semispinalis cervicis m.

DIAGNOSTIC CONSIDERATION

Tumors may arise from muscle, such as leiomyosarcoma, but are relatively rare. Muscles are often a source of pain, but this is usually benign. Bone, however, particularly vertebral body marrow, is a common target for metastases.

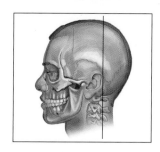

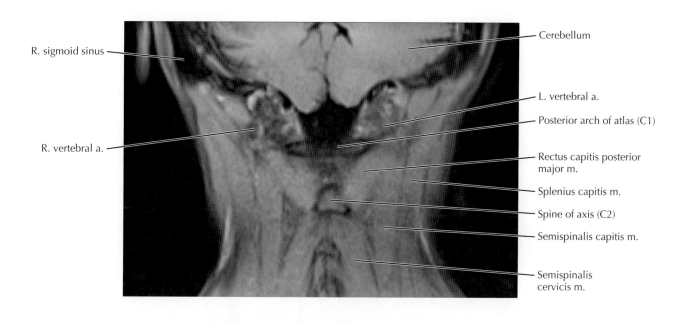

R. sigmoid sinus

R. vertebral a.

Cerebellum

L. vertebral a.

Posterior arch of atlas (C1)

Rectus capitis posterior major m.

Splenius capitis m.

Spine of axis (C2)

Semispinalis capitis m.

Semispinalis cervicis m.

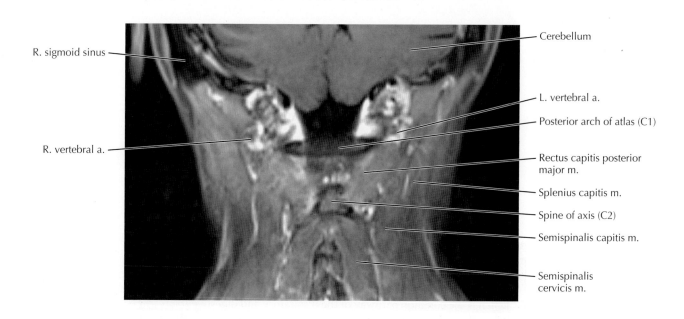

R. sigmoid sinus

R. vertebral a.

Cerebellum

L. vertebral a.

Posterior arch of atlas (C1)

Rectus capitis posterior major m.

Splenius capitis m.

Spine of axis (C2)

Semispinalis capitis m.

Semispinalis cervicis m.

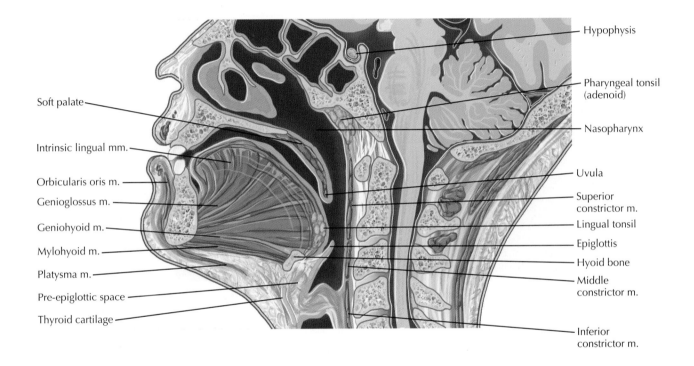

Soft palate

Intrinsic lingual mm.

Orbicularis oris m.

Genioglossus m.

Geniohyoid m.

Mylohyoid m.

Platysma m.

Pre-epiglottic space

Thyroid cartilage

Hypophysis

Pharyngeal tonsil (adenoid)

Nasopharynx

Uvula

Superior constrictor m.

Lingual tonsil

Epiglottis

Hyoid bone

Middle constrictor m.

Inferior constrictor m.

NORMAL ANATOMY

Note that the midline MR image in Sagittal 1 is aligned on the pharynx, which consists of the oropharynx, nasopharynx, and hypopharynx (nose is slightly off midline). The pharyngeal lumen is the common pathway of the respiratory and digestive tracts. Air enters the nose, passes inferiorly and anteriorly to the trachea, crossing over the path of food entering the mouth, which then passes inferiorly and posteriorly to the esophagus. The anterior location of the trachea allows for safe percutaneous access through the cricothyroid membrane in patients with upper airway obstruction at or above the level of the vocal cords.

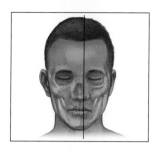

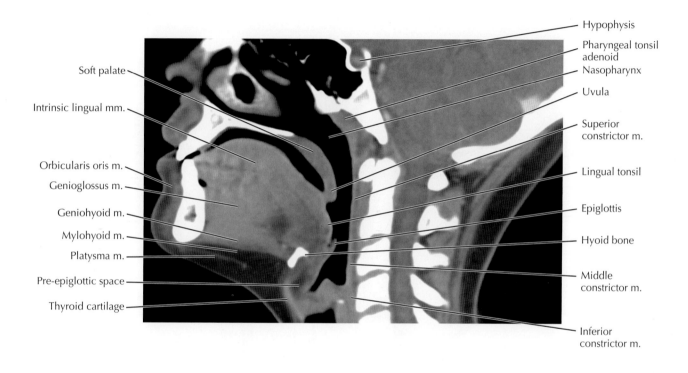

Soft palate

Intrinsic lingual mm.

Orbicularis oris m.

Genioglossus m.

Geniohyoid m.

Mylohyoid m.

Platysma m.

Pre-epiglottic space

Thyroid cartilage

Hypophysis

Pharyngeal tonsil adenoid

Nasopharynx

Uvula

Superior constrictor m.

Lingual tonsil

Epiglottis

Hyoid bone

Middle constrictor m.

Inferior constrictor m.

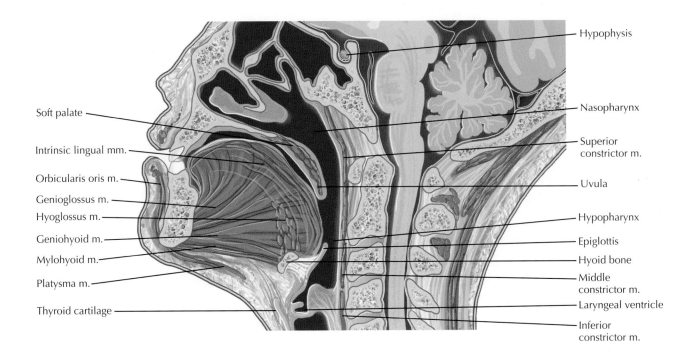

Soft palate

Intrinsic lingual mm.

Orbicularis oris m.

Genioglossus m.

Hyoglossus m.

Geniohyoid m.

Mylohyoid m.

Platysma m.

Thyroid cartilage

Hypophysis

Nasopharynx

Superior constrictor m.

Uvula

Hypopharynx

Epiglottis

Hyoid bone

Middle constrictor m.

Laryngeal ventricle

Inferior constrictor m.

DIAGNOSTIC CONSIDERATION

Sagittal imaging may be the best plane for assessing invasion by nasopharyngeal carcinoma into the clivus or incidental metastasis of vertebral bodies.

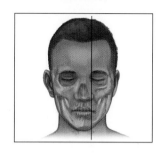

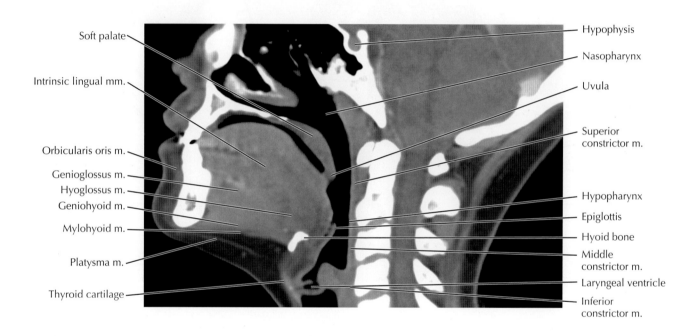

Soft palate

Intrinsic lingual mm.

Orbicularis oris m.

Genioglossus m.

Hyoglossus m.

Geniohyoid m.

Mylohyoid m.

Platysma m.

Thyroid cartilage

Hypophysis

Nasopharynx

Uvula

Superior constrictor m.

Hypopharynx

Epiglottis

Hyoid bone

Middle constrictor m.

Laryngeal ventricle

Inferior constrictor m.

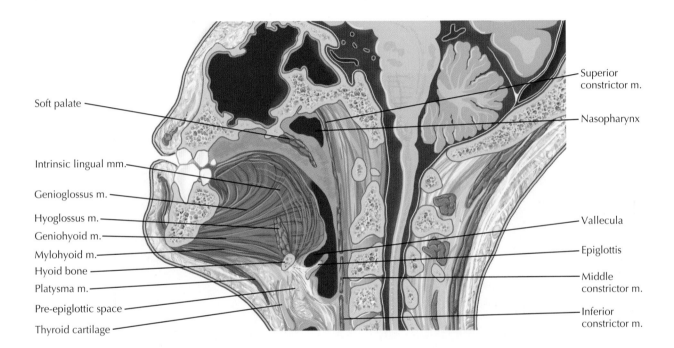

Soft palate

Intrinsic lingual mm.

Genioglossus m.

Hyoglossus m.

Geniohyoid m.

Mylohyoid m.

Hyoid bone

Platysma m.

Pre-epiglottic space

Thyroid cartilage

Superior constrictor m.

Nasopharynx

Vallecula

Epiglottis

Middle constrictor m.

Inferior constrictor m.

PATHOLOGIC PROCESS

Note the thinness of the epiglottis. Marked thickening of the epiglottis may result from viral infection (supraglottitis, epiglottitis) in children. The "thumbprint" sign on lateral radiographs identifies epiglottic thickening, which can lead to life-threatening airway obstruction. With the advent of *Haemophilus influenzae* type B vaccine, the incidence of supraglottitis has decreased greatly. Currently, the most common reason for epiglottic thickening is post–radiation therapy changes in adult patients.

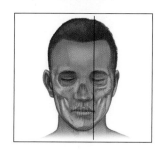

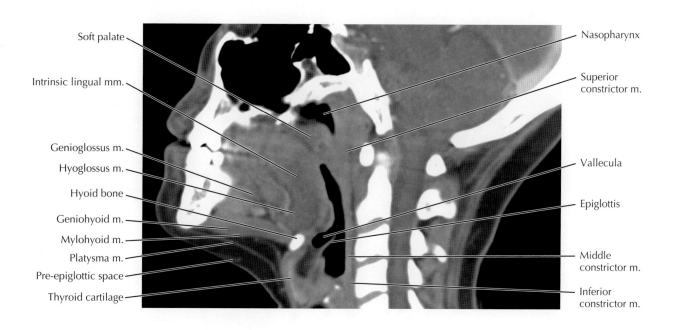

Soft palate

Intrinsic lingual mm.

Genioglossus m.

Hyoglossus m.

Hyoid bone

Geniohyoid m.

Mylohyoid m.

Platysma m.

Pre-epiglottic space

Thyroid cartilage

Nasopharynx

Superior constrictor m.

Vallecula

Epiglottis

Middle constrictor m.

Inferior constrictor m.

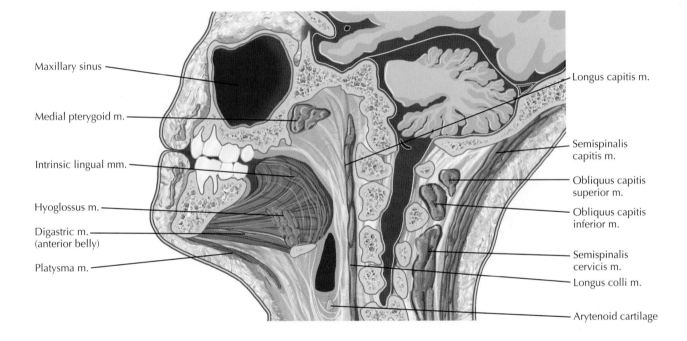

Maxillary sinus

Medial pterygoid m.

Intrinsic lingual mm.

Hyoglossus m.

Digastric m.
(anterior belly)

Platysma m.

Longus capitis m.

Semispinalis
capitis m.

Obliquus capitis
superior m.

Obliquus capitis
inferior m.

Semispinalis
cervicis m.

Longus colli m.

Arytenoid cartilage

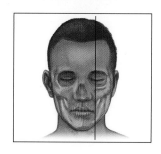

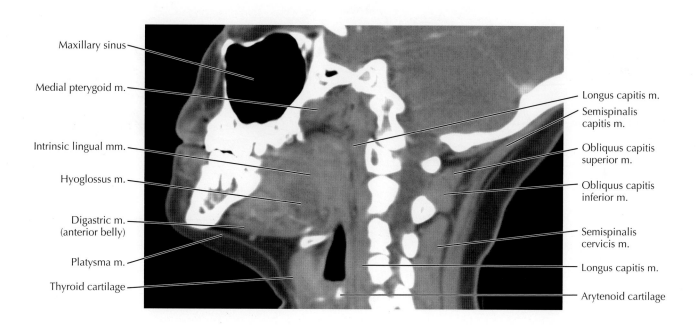

Maxillary sinus

Medial pterygoid m.

Intrinsic lingual mm.

Hyoglossus m.

Digastric m. (anterior belly)

Platysma m.

Thyroid cartilage

Longus capitis m.

Semispinalis capitis m.

Obliquus capitis superior m.

Obliquus capitis inferior m.

Semispinalis cervicis m.

Longus capitis m.

Arytenoid cartilage

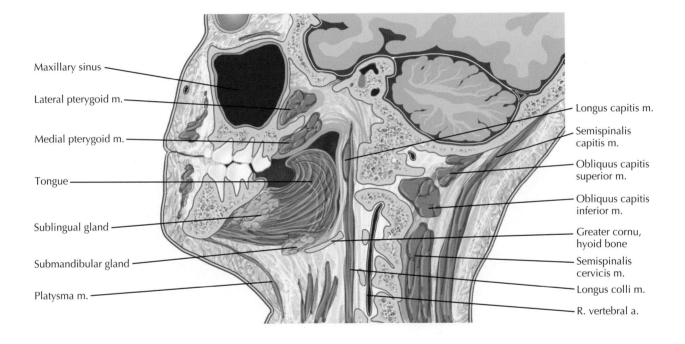

Maxillary sinus

Lateral pterygoid m.

Medial pterygoid m.

Tongue

Sublingual gland

Submandibular gland

Platysma m.

Longus capitis m.

Semispinalis capitis m.

Obliquus capitis superior m.

Obliquus capitis inferior m.

Greater cornu, hyoid bone

Semispinalis cervicis m.

Longus colli m.

R. vertebral a.

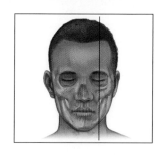

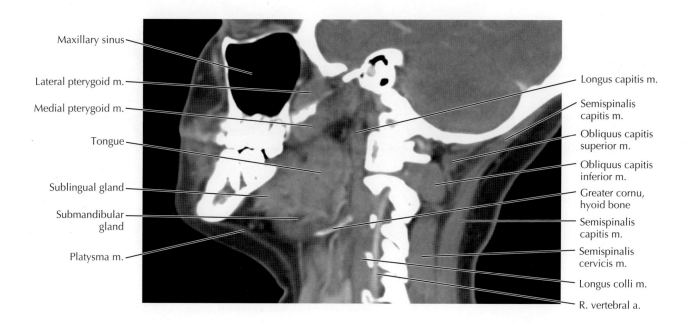

Maxillary sinus

Lateral pterygoid m.

Medial pterygoid m.

Tongue

Sublingual gland

Submandibular gland

Platysma m.

Longus capitis m.

Semispinalis capitis m.

Obliquus capitis superior m.

Obliquus capitis inferior m.

Greater cornu, hyoid bone

Semispinalis capitis m.

Semispinalis cervicis m.

Longus colli m.

R. vertebral a.

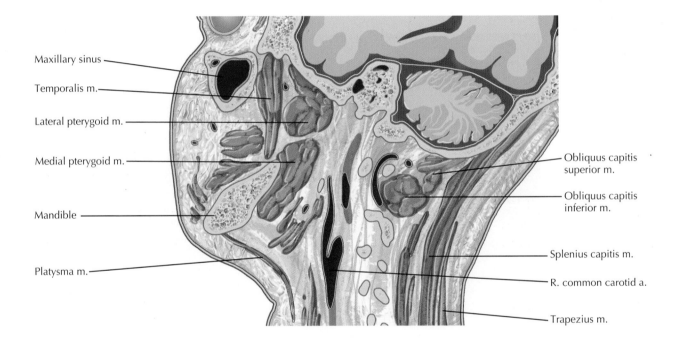

Maxillary sinus

Temporalis m.

Lateral pterygoid m.

Medial pterygoid m.

Mandible

Platysma m.

Obliquus capitis superior m.

Obliquus capitis inferior m.

Splenius capitis m.

R. common carotid a.

Trapezius m.

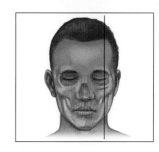

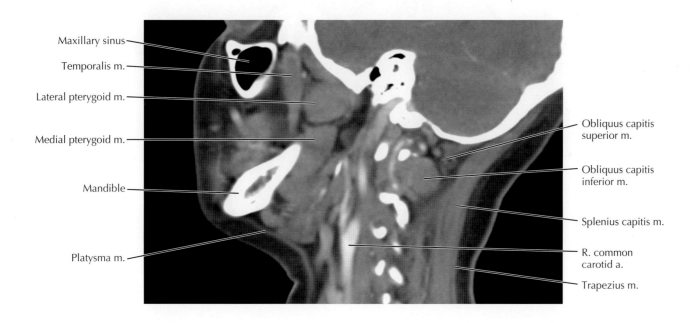

Maxillary sinus

Temporalis m.

Lateral pterygoid m.

Medial pterygoid m.

Mandible

Platysma m.

Obliquus capitis superior m.

Obliquus capitis inferior m.

Splenius capitis m.

R. common carotid a.

Trapezius m.

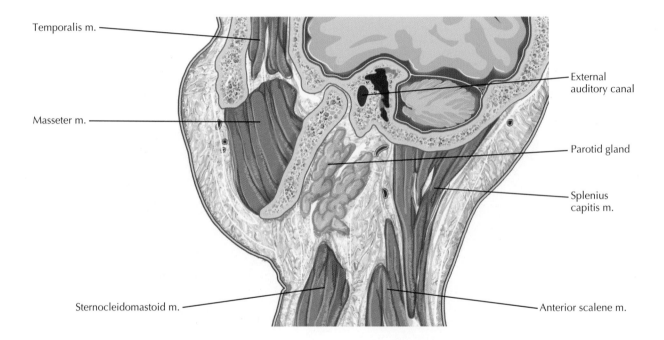

Temporalis m.

Masseter m.

External auditory canal

Parotid gland

Splenius capitis m.

Sternocleidomastoid m.

Anterior scalene m.

DIAGNOSTIC CONSIDERATION

The off-midline sagittal CT images are typically of limited diagnostic utility given the lack of symmetry as on axial images. Certain structures, however, such as the occipitocervical junction and facet joints, can be better assessed on the sagittal plane.

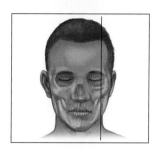

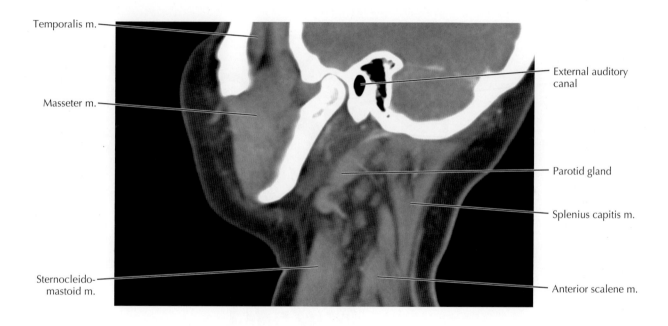

Temporalis m.

Masseter m.

Sternocleido-
mastoid m.

External auditory
canal

Parotid gland

Splenius capitis m.

Anterior scalene m.

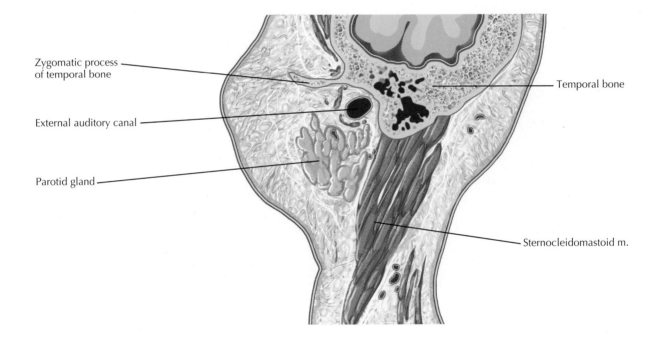

Zygomatic process
of temporal bone

Temporal bone

External auditory canal

Parotid gland

Sternocleidomastoid m.

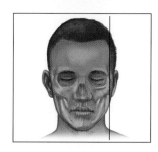

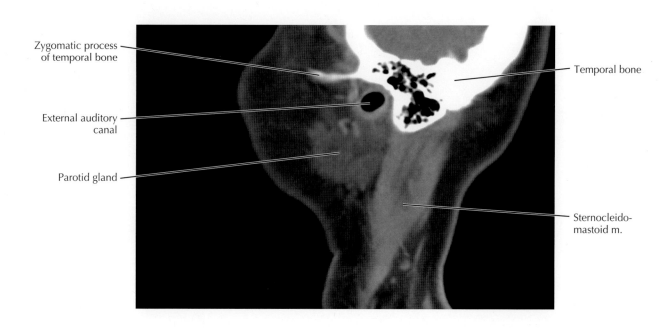

Zygomatic process
of temporal bone

Temporal bone

External auditory
canal

Parotid gland

Sternocleido-
mastoid m.

Chapter 14 HYPOPHARYNX, LARYNX, AND INFRAHYOID NECK

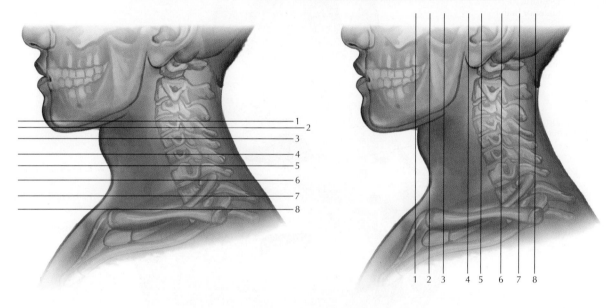

AXIAL   472

CORONAL   488

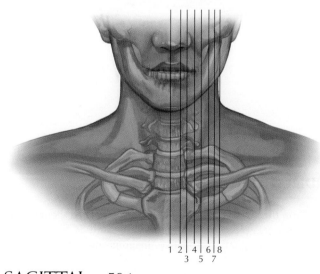

SAGITTAL   504

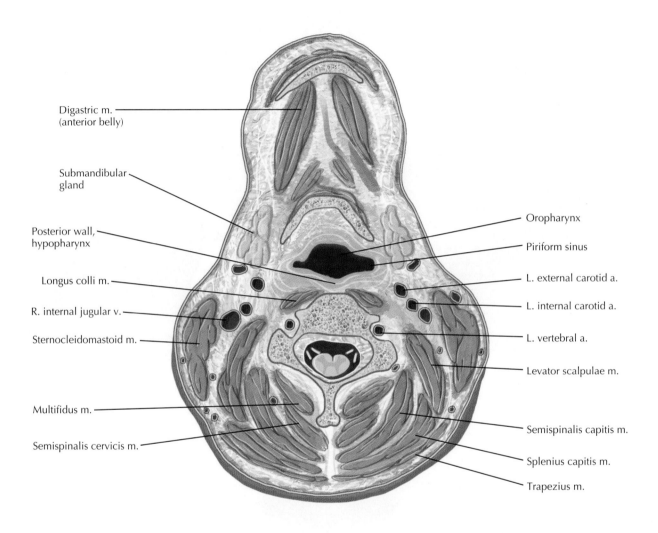

Digastric m.
(anterior belly)

Submandibular
gland

Posterior wall,
hypopharynx

Longus colli m.

R. internal jugular v.

Sternocleidomastoid m.

Multifidus m.

Semispinalis cervicis m.

Oropharynx

Piriform sinus

L. external carotid a.

L. internal carotid a.

L. vertebral a.

Levator scalpulae m.

Semispinalis capitis m.

Splenius capitis m.

Trapezius m.

DIAGNOSTIC CONSIDERATION

Axial 1 on the next page shows both a T2-weighted sequence (upper image) and a T1-weighted image (lower). Note that cerebrospinal fluid (CSF) around the spinal cord is bright on T2-weighted magnetic resonance imaging and dark gray on T1-weighted MRI. Usually the brightest structure on T1-weighted imaging is fat. Note that the fat is somewhat bright on T2-weighted imaging because most T2 MRIs are now performed with fast spin-echo or "turbo" spin-echo techniques that use multiple radiofrequency (RF) pulses per echo time and make fat signal appear more like water signal.

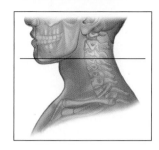

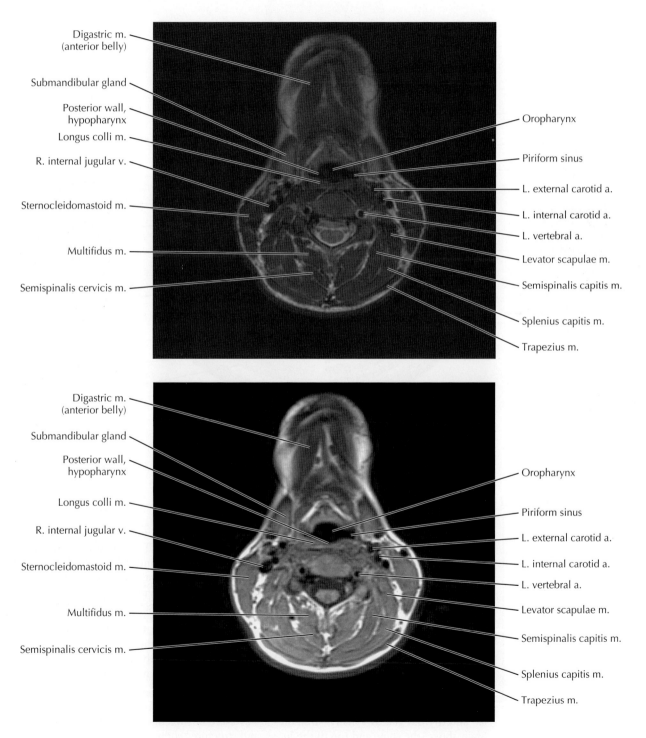

Digastric m. (anterior belly)

Submandibular gland

Posterior wall, hypopharynx

Longus colli m.

R. internal jugular v.

Sternocleidomastoid m.

Multifidus m.

Semispinalis cervicis m.

Oropharynx

Piriform sinus

L. external carotid a.

L. internal carotid a.

L. vertebral a.

Levator scapulae m.

Semispinalis capitis m.

Splenius capitis m.

Trapezius m.

Digastric m. (anterior belly)

Submandibular gland

Posterior wall, hypopharynx

Longus colli m.

R. internal jugular v.

Sternocleidomastoid m.

Multifidus m.

Semispinalis cervicis m.

Oropharynx

Piriform sinus

L. external carotid a.

L. internal carotid a.

L. vertebral a.

Levator scapulae m.

Semispinalis capitis m.

Splenius capitis m.

Trapezius m.

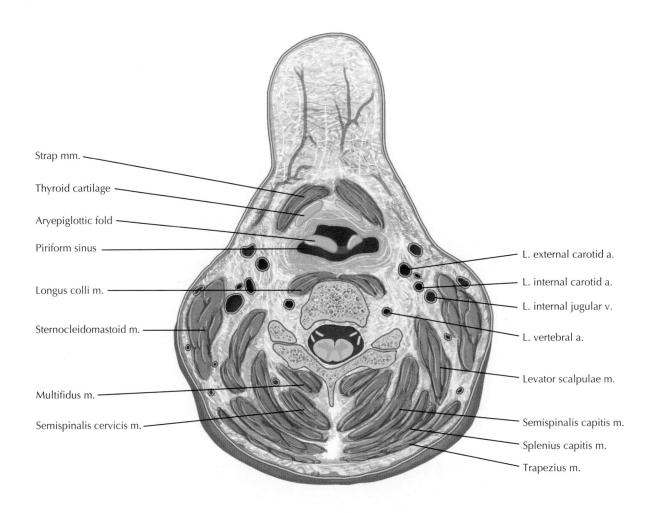

Strap mm.

Thyroid cartilage

Aryepiglottic fold

Piriform sinus

Longus colli m.

Sternocleidomastoid m.

Multifidus m.

Semispinalis cervicis m.

L. external carotid a.

L. internal carotid a.

L. internal jugular v.

L. vertebral a.

Levator scalpulae m.

Semispinalis capitis m.

Splenius capitis m.

Trapezius m.

DIAGNOSTIC CONSIDERATION

Imaging of the neck can be difficult because many critical structures are compressed within a relatively small space. One diagnostic approach to MRI and CT of the neck is to assess the structures from central to peripheral, starting with the *airway*. Impending airway obstruction should be recognized early in evaluation of the neck. The airway is often the first structure to be exposed to carcinogenic agents and viruses. A primary hypopharyngeal squamous cell carcinoma may first appear as a slight asymmetry in the mucosal surfaces of the hypopharynx.

The next structure to assess is the usual site of malignancy spread, the *lymph nodes*, which generally follow the venous structures. The largest venous structure in the neck is the internal jugular vein, and thus the jugular lymph node chain typically contains the largest lymph nodes. The largest node is at the top of this chain, the jugulodigastric lymph node, which serves as a common point of lymphatic drainage for the head.

Next, specialized glands of the head and neck can be assessed, including parotid, submandibular, and thyroid glands. Finally, structures are assessed at the edge of a neck study, such as the brain above, the spine and top of the lungs, and structures common to many parts of the body (e.g., vessels, bones, muscles, subcutaneous tissue, skin contours).

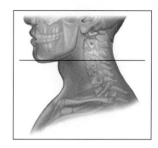

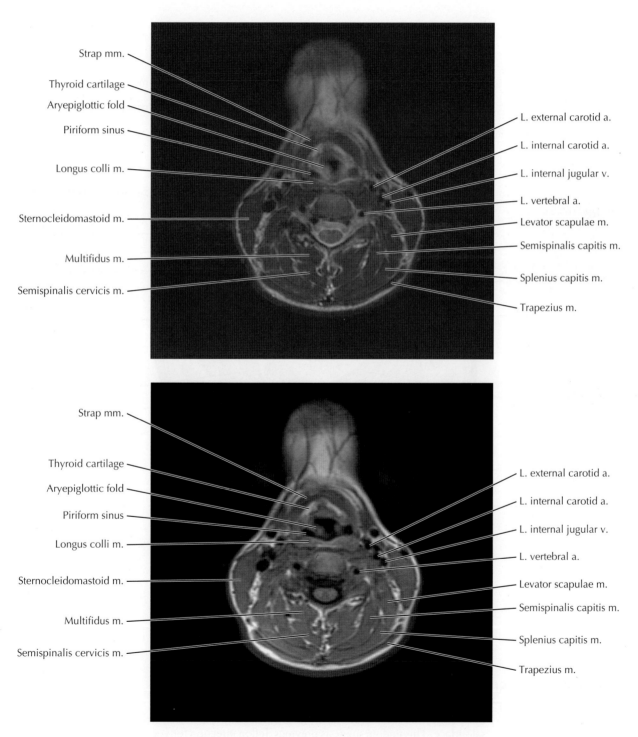

Strap mm.

Thyroid cartilage

Aryepiglottic fold

Piriform sinus

Longus colli m.

Sternocleidomastoid m.

Multifidus m.

Semispinalis cervicis m.

L. external carotid a.

L. internal carotid a.

L. internal jugular v.

L. vertebral a.

Levator scapulae m.

Semispinalis capitis m.

Splenius capitis m.

Trapezius m.

Strap mm.

Thyroid cartilage

Aryepiglottic fold

Piriform sinus

Longus colli m.

Sternocleidomastoid m.

Multifidus m.

Semispinalis cervicis m.

L. external carotid a.

L. internal carotid a.

L. internal jugular v.

L. vertebral a.

Levator scapulae m.

Semispinalis capitis m.

Splenius capitis m.

Trapezius m.

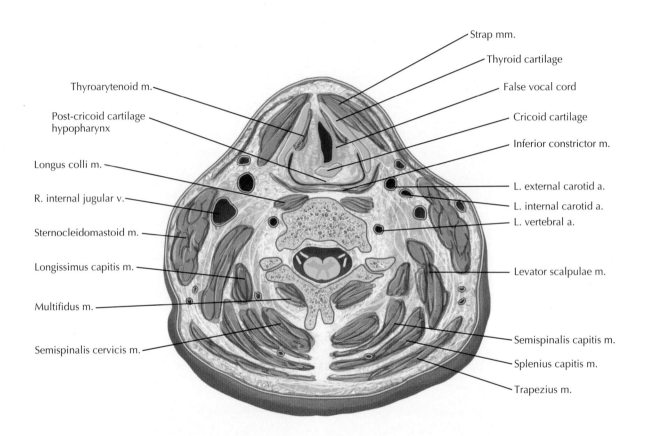

Strap mm.

Thyroid cartilage

False vocal cord

Cricoid cartilage

Inferior constrictor m.

L. external carotid a.

L. internal carotid a.

L. vertebral a.

Levator scalpulae m.

Semispinalis capitis m.

Splenius capitis m.

Trapezius m.

Thyroarytenoid m.

Post-cricoid cartilage hypopharynx

Longus colli m.

R. internal jugular v.

Sternocleidomastoid m.

Longissimus capitis m.

Multifidus m.

Semispinalis cervicis m.

PATHOLOGIC CONSIDERATION

Note the medial deviation of the right vocal cord with a focus of dark signal deep to the mucosal surface. This finding suggests previous Teflon injection for vocal cord paralysis, to help bring one cord in contact with the normal-moving cord.

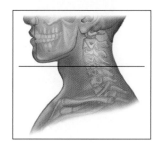

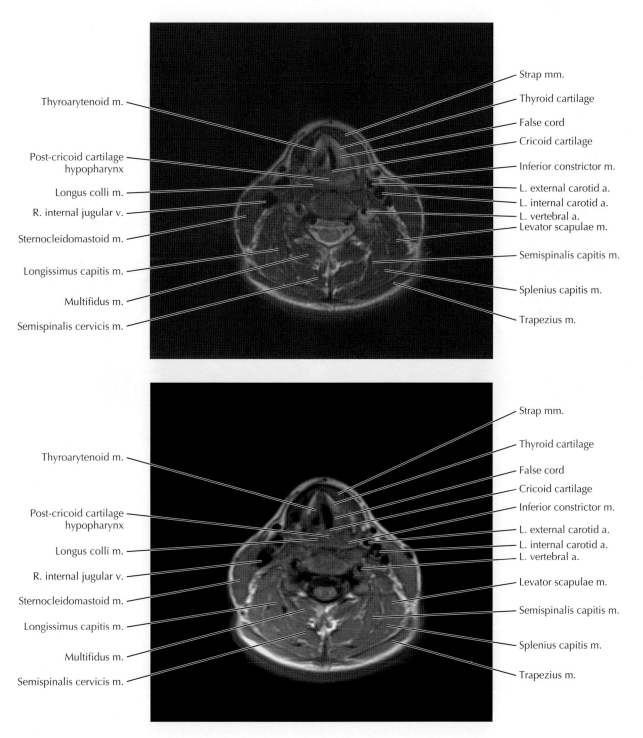

Thyroarytenoid m.

Post-cricoid cartilage hypopharynx

Longus colli m.

R. internal jugular v.

Sternocleidomastoid m.

Longissimus capitis m.

Multifidus m.

Semispinalis cervicis m.

Strap mm.

Thyroid cartilage

False cord

Cricoid cartilage

Inferior constrictor m.

L. external carotid a.

L. internal carotid a.

L. vertebral a.

Levator scapulae m.

Semispinalis capitis m.

Splenius capitis m.

Trapezius m.

Thyroarytenoid m.

Post-cricoid cartilage hypopharynx

Longus colli m.

R. internal jugular v.

Sternocleidomastoid m.

Longissimus capitis m.

Multifidus m.

Semispinalis cervicis m.

Strap mm.

Thyroid cartilage

False cord

Cricoid cartilage

Inferior constrictor m.

L. external carotid a.

L. internal carotid a.

L. vertebral a.

Levator scapulae m.

Semispinalis capitis m.

Splenius capitis m.

Trapezius m.

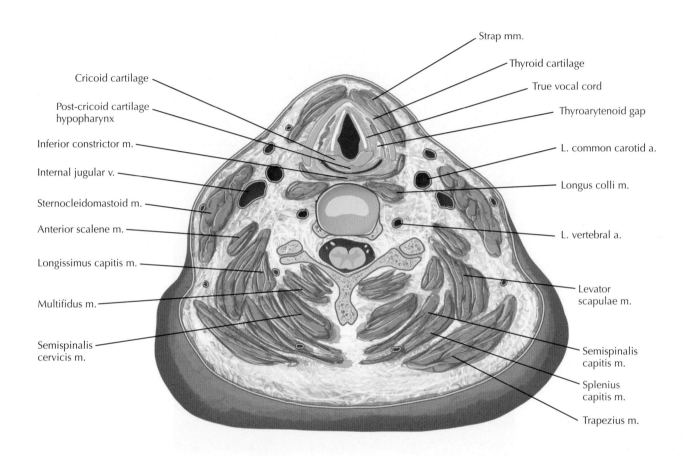

Strap mm.

Thyroid cartilage

True vocal cord

Thyroarytenoid gap

L. common carotid a.

Longus colli m.

L. vertebral a.

Levator scapulae m.

Semispinalis capitis m.

Splenius capitis m.

Trapezius m.

Cricoid cartilage

Post-cricoid cartilage hypopharynx

Inferior constrictor m.

Internal jugular v.

Sternocleidomastoid m.

Anterior scalene m.

Longissimus capitis m.

Multifidus m.

Semispinalis cervicis m.

IMAGING TECHNIQUE CONSIDERATION

The vocal cords should be symmetric. Medial deviation of one of the vocal cords suggests palsy, and the neuroradiologist should look carefully for a lesion or enlarged lymph node along the course of the recurrent laryngeal nerves.

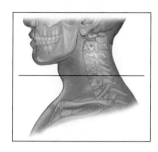

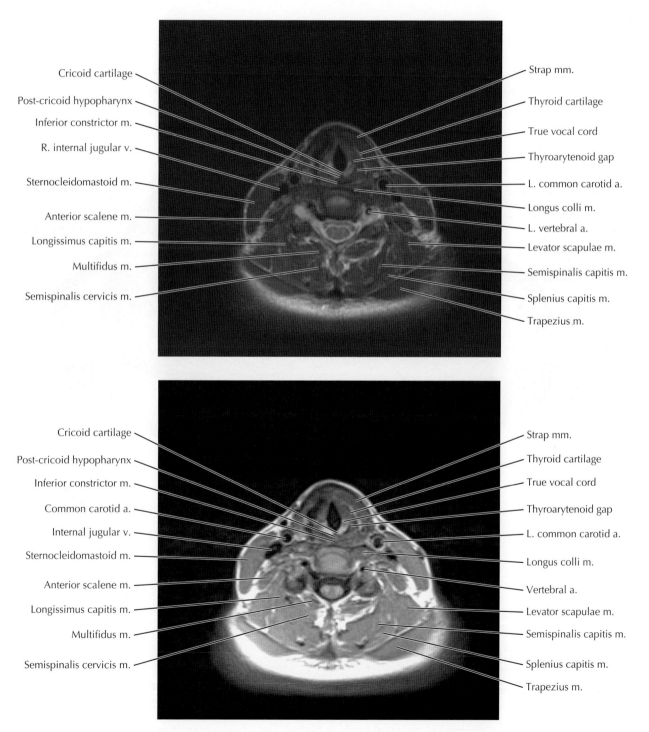

Cricoid cartilage

Post-cricoid hypopharynx

Inferior constrictor m.

R. internal jugular v.

Sternocleidomastoid m.

Anterior scalene m.

Longissimus capitis m.

Multifidus m.

Semispinalis cervicis m.

Strap mm.

Thyroid cartilage

True vocal cord

Thyroarytenoid gap

L. common carotid a.

Longus colli m.

L. vertebral a.

Levator scapulae m.

Semispinalis capitis m.

Splenius capitis m.

Trapezius m.

Cricoid cartilage

Post-cricoid hypopharynx

Inferior constrictor m.

Common carotid a.

Internal jugular v.

Sternocleidomastoid m.

Anterior scalene m.

Longissimus capitis m.

Multifidus m.

Semispinalis cervicis m.

Strap mm.

Thyroid cartilage

True vocal cord

Thyroarytenoid gap

L. common carotid a.

Longus colli m.

Vertebral a.

Levator scapulae m.

Semispinalis capitis m.

Splenius capitis m.

Trapezius m.

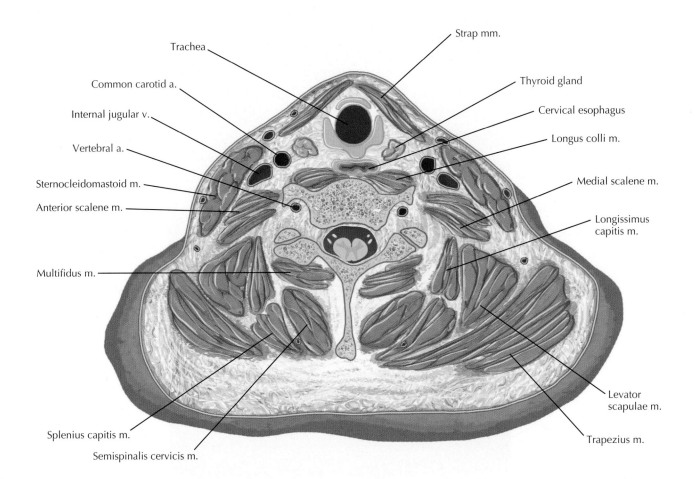

Trachea

Common carotid a.

Internal jugular v.

Vertebral a.

Sternocleidomastoid m.

Anterior scalene m.

Multifidus m.

Splenius capitis m.

Semispinalis cervicis m.

Strap mm.

Thyroid gland

Cervical esophagus

Longus colli m.

Medial scalene m.

Longissimus capitis m.

Levator scapulae m.

Trapezius m.

PATHOLOGIC PROCESS

The membranous space in the midline between the thyroid cartilage caudally and the cricoid ring caudally is the site for emergency cricothyrotomy (cricoid tracheotomy). Puncture of the cricothyroid membrane with an angiocatheter allows airway access in cases of obstruction at the level of the vocal cords or higher. The subcutaneous spaces in the midline are relatively avascular.

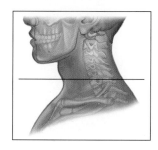

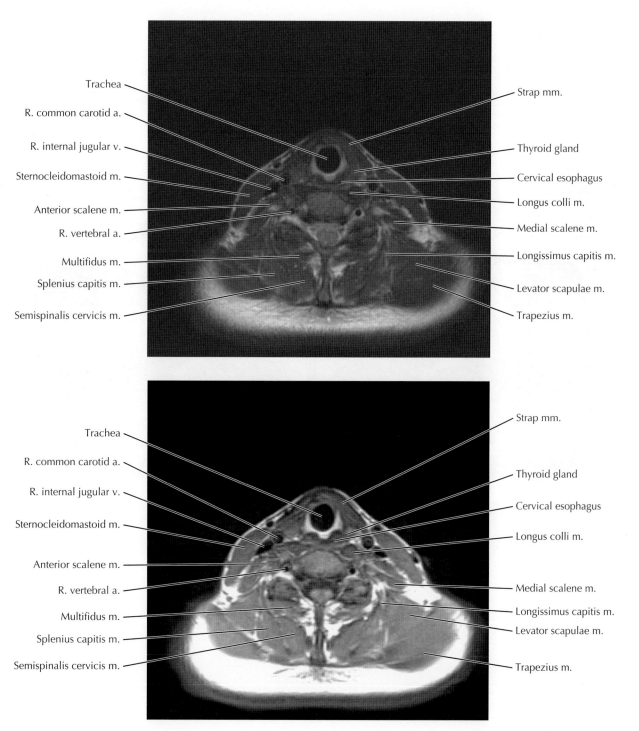

Trachea

R. common carotid a.

R. internal jugular v.

Sternocleidomastoid m.

Anterior scalene m.

R. vertebral a.

Multifidus m.

Splenius capitis m.

Semispinalis cervicis m.

Strap mm.

Thyroid gland

Cervical esophagus

Longus colli m.

Medial scalene m.

Longissimus capitis m.

Levator scapulae m.

Trapezius m.

Trachea

R. common carotid a.

R. internal jugular v.

Sternocleidomastoid m.

Anterior scalene m.

R. vertebral a.

Multifidus m.

Splenius capitis m.

Semispinalis cervicis m.

Strap mm.

Thyroid gland

Cervical esophagus

Longus colli m.

Medial scalene m.

Longissimus capitis m.

Levator scapulae m.

Trapezius m.

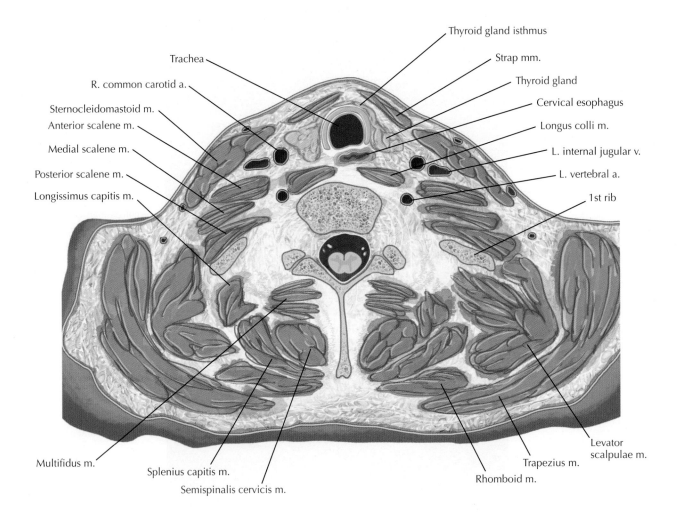

Thyroid gland isthmus

Trachea

Strap mm.

R. common carotid a.

Thyroid gland

Sternocleidomastoid m.

Cervical esophagus

Anterior scalene m.

Longus colli m.

Medial scalene m.

L. internal jugular v.

Posterior scalene m.

L. vertebral a.

Longissimus capitis m.

1st rib

Multifidus m.

Levator scalpulae m.

Splenius capitis m.

Trapezius m.

Semispinalis cervicis m.

Rhomboid m.

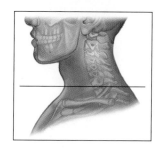

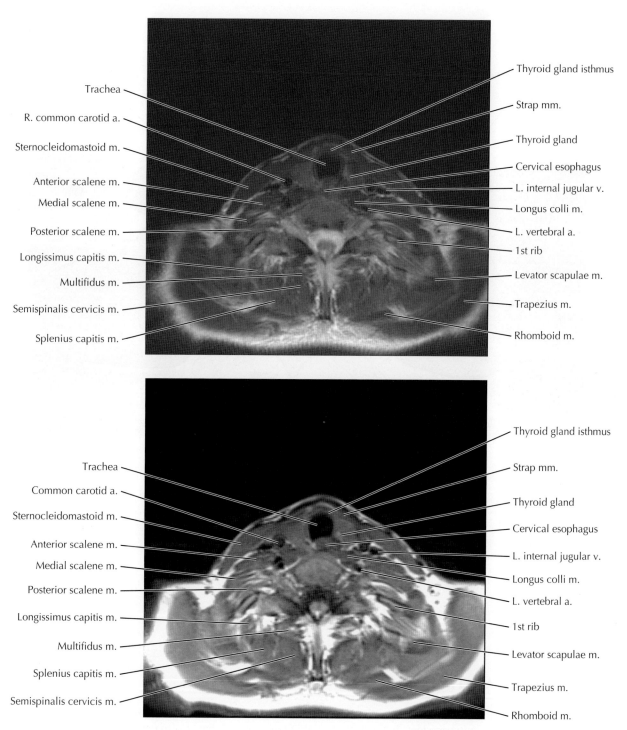

Trachea

R. common carotid a.

Sternocleidomastoid m.

Anterior scalene m.

Medial scalene m.

Posterior scalene m.

Longissimus capitis m.

Multifidus m.

Semispinalis cervicis m.

Splenius capitis m.

Thyroid gland isthmus

Strap mm.

Thyroid gland

Cervical esophagus

L. internal jugular v.

Longus colli m.

L. vertebral a.

1st rib

Levator scapulae m.

Trapezius m.

Rhomboid m.

Trachea

Common carotid a.

Sternocleidomastoid m.

Anterior scalene m.

Medial scalene m.

Posterior scalene m.

Longissimus capitis m.

Multifidus m.

Splenius capitis m.

Semispinalis cervicis m.

Thyroid gland isthmus

Strap mm.

Thyroid gland

Cervical esophagus

L. internal jugular v.

Longus colli m.

L. vertebral a.

1st rib

Levator scapulae m.

Trapezius m.

Rhomboid m.

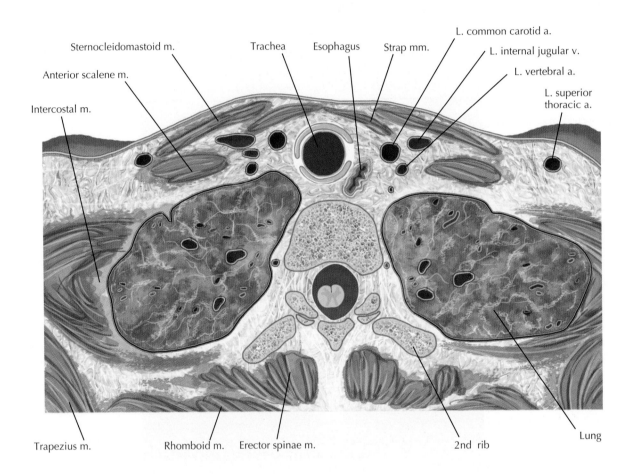

Sternocleidomastoid m.

Anterior scalene m.

Intercostal m.

Trachea

Esophagus

Strap mm.

L. common carotid a.

L. internal jugular v.

L. vertebral a.

L. superior thoracic a.

Trapezius m.

Rhomboid m.

Erector spinae m.

2nd rib

Lung

NORMAL ANATOMY

The trachea below the bony cricoid ring has firm, cartilaginous material along the lateral and anterior sides, but a softer, membranous portion that is often straight (or concave) along the posterior wall.

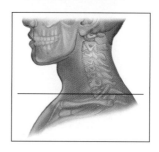

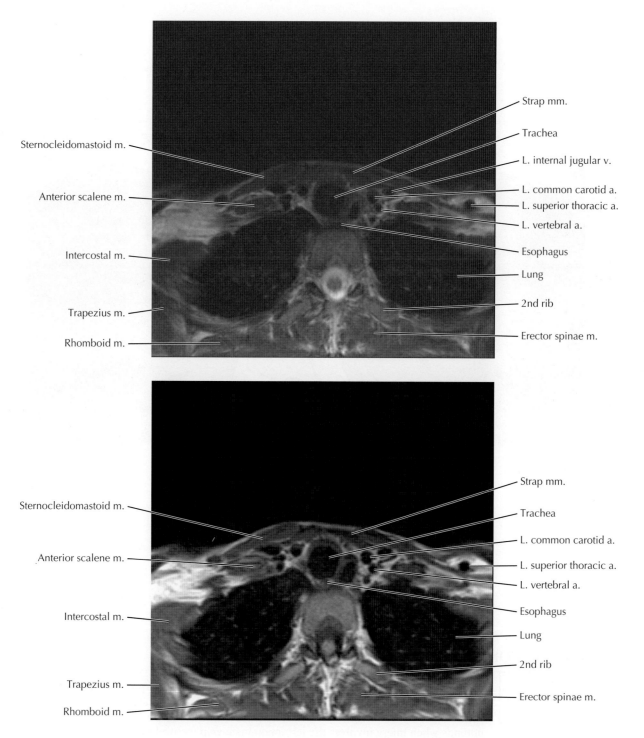

Strap mm.

Trachea

L. internal jugular v.

L. common carotid a.

L. superior thoracic a.

L. vertebral a.

Esophagus

Lung

2nd rib

Erector spinae m.

Sternocleidomastoid m.

Anterior scalene m.

Intercostal m.

Trapezius m.

Rhomboid m.

Strap mm.

Trachea

L. common carotid a.

L. superior thoracic a.

L. vertebral a.

Esophagus

Lung

2nd rib

Erector spinae m.

Sternocleidomastoid m.

Anterior scalene m.

Intercostal m.

Trapezius m.

Rhomboid m.

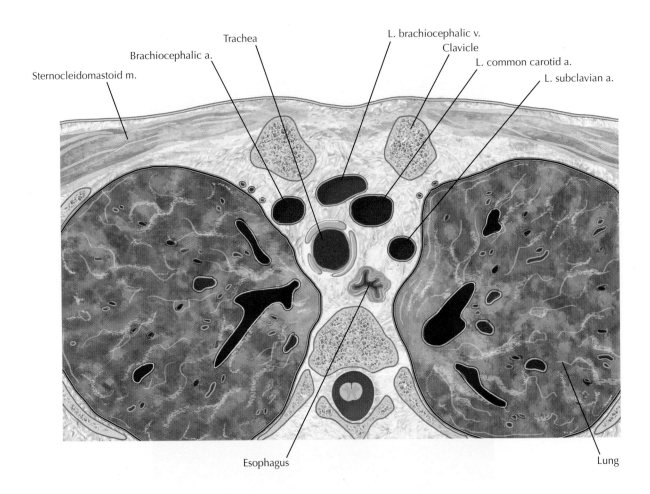

Sternocleidomastoid m.

Brachiocephalic a.

Trachea

L. brachiocephalic v.

Clavicle

L. common carotid a.

L. subclavian a.

Esophagus

Lung

SURGICAL CONSIDERATION

The left innominate (brachiocephalic) vein passes immediately posterior to the suprasternal notch. It drains venous blood from the left internal jugular vein and left subclavian vein, crosses the midline, and joins right innominate vein to form the superior vena cava. In midline sternotomy, when injury involves the left innominate vein, control can be obtained by hooking a finger deep to the suprasternal notch and pulling upward.

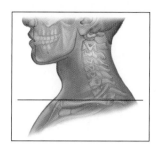

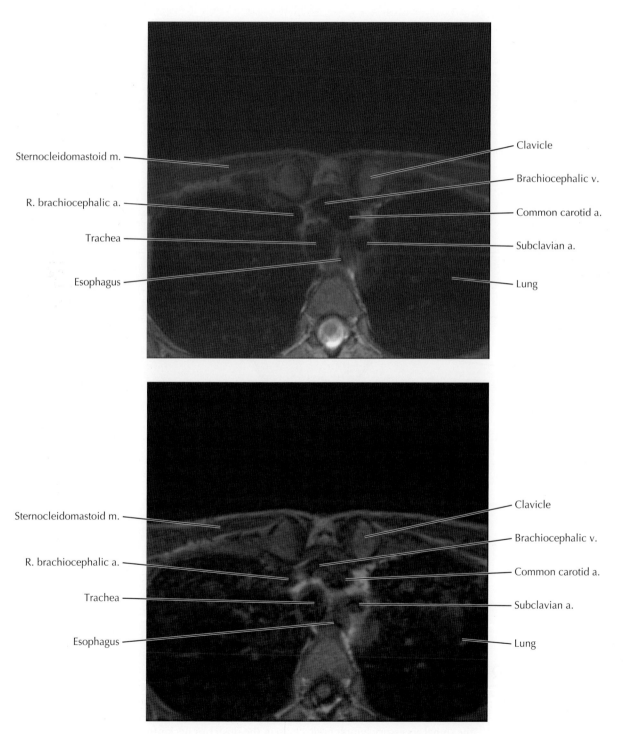

Sternocleidomastoid m.

R. brachiocephalic a.

Trachea

Esophagus

Clavicle

Brachiocephalic v.

Common carotid a.

Subclavian a.

Lung

Sternocleidomastoid m.

R. brachiocephalic a.

Trachea

Esophagus

Clavicle

Brachiocephalic v.

Common carotid a.

Subclavian a.

Lung

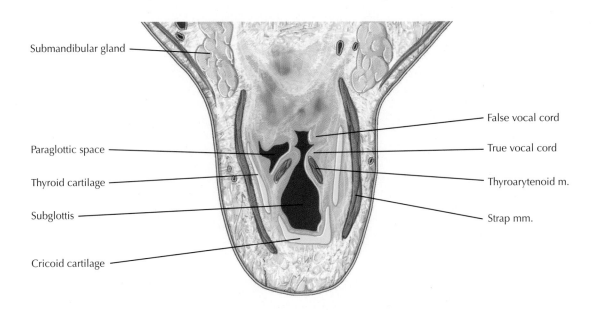

Submandibular gland

Paraglottic space

Thyroid cartilage

Subglottis

Cricoid cartilage

False vocal cord

True vocal cord

Thyroarytenoid m.

Strap mm.

IMAGING TECHNIQUE CONSIDERATION

Coronal imaging is used less often than axial imaging when assessing the neck. However, the ability to see the craniocaudal extent of the jugular lymph node chain in the anterior neck and the spinal accessory lymph node chain in the posterior neck often makes enlarged lymph nodes more conspicuous on coronal MR images.

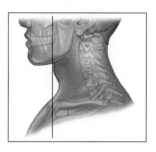

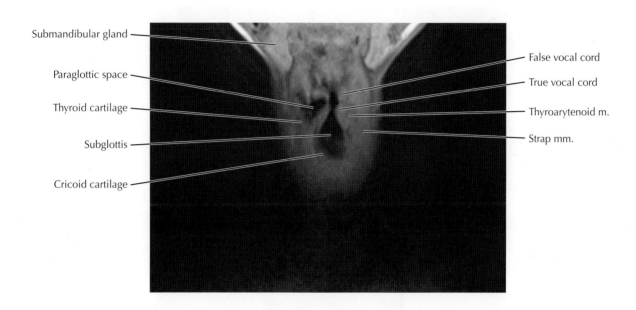

Submandibular gland

Paraglottic space

Thyroid cartilage

Subglottis

Cricoid cartilage

False vocal cord

True vocal cord

Thyroarytenoid m.

Strap mm.

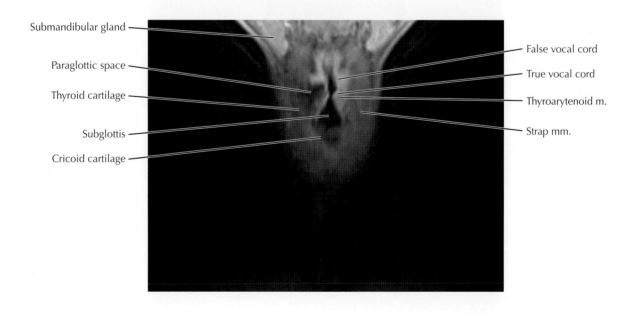

Submandibular gland

Paraglottic space

Thyroid cartilage

Subglottis

Cricoid cartilage

False vocal cord

True vocal cord

Thyroarytenoid m.

Strap mm.

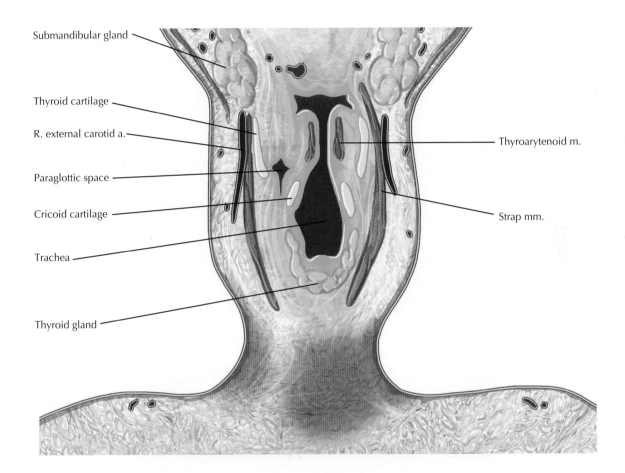

Submandibular gland

Thyroid cartilage

R. external carotid a.

Paraglottic space

Cricoid cartilage

Trachea

Thyroid gland

Thyroarytenoid m.

Strap mm.

PATHOLOGIC PROCESS

Note the asymmetric dark focus associated with the right vocal cord, suggestive of previous Teflon injection for vocal cord palsy.

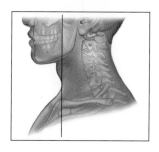

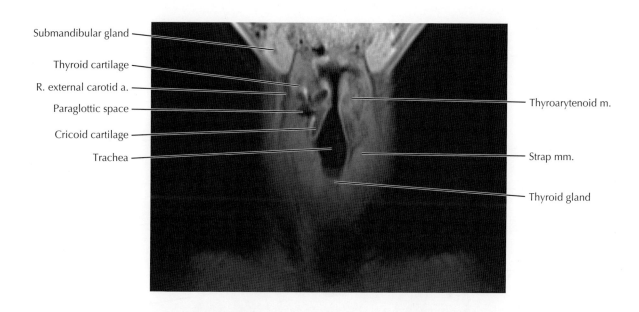

Submandibular gland

Thyroid cartilage

R. external carotid a.

Paraglottic space

Cricoid cartilage

Trachea

Thyroarytenoid m.

Strap mm.

Thyroid gland

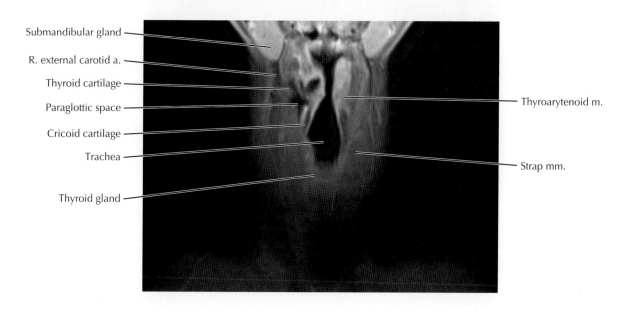

Submandibular gland

R. external carotid a.

Thyroid cartilage

Paraglottic space

Cricoid cartilage

Trachea

Thyroid gland

Thyroarytenoid m.

Strap mm.

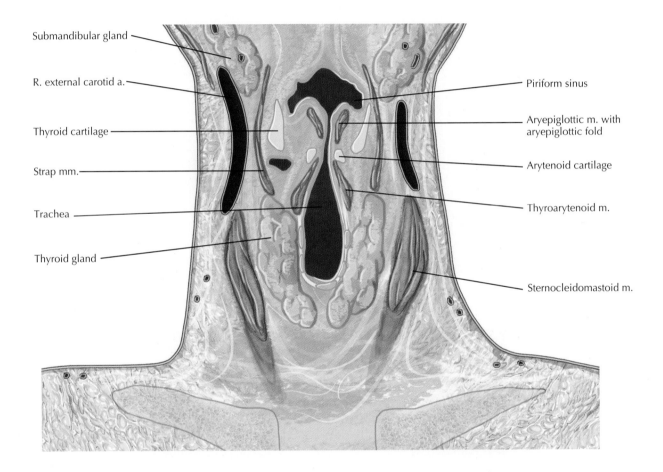

Submandibular gland

R. external carotid a.

Thyroid cartilage

Strap mm.

Trachea

Thyroid gland

Piriform sinus

Aryepiglottic m. with
aryepiglottic fold

Arytenoid cartilage

Thyroarytenoid m.

Sternocleidomastoid m.

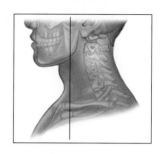

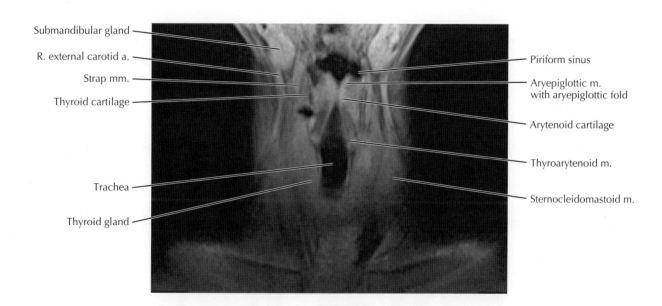

Submandibular gland

R. external carotid a.

Strap mm.

Thyroid cartilage

Trachea

Thyroid gland

Piriform sinus

Aryepiglottic m. with aryepiglottic fold

Arytenoid cartilage

Thyroarytenoid m.

Sternocleidomastoid m.

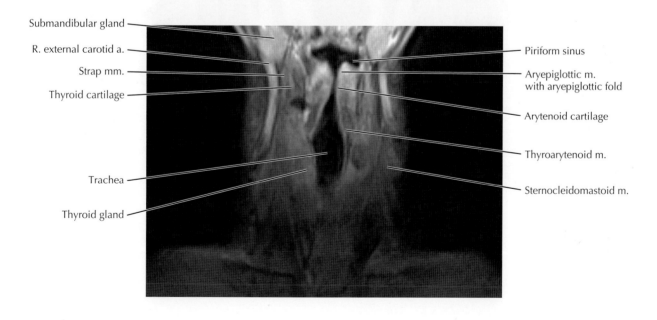

Submandibular gland

R. external carotid a.

Strap mm.

Thyroid cartilage

Trachea

Thyroid gland

Piriform sinus

Aryepiglottic m. with aryepiglottic fold

Arytenoid cartilage

Thyroarytenoid m.

Sternocleidomastoid m.

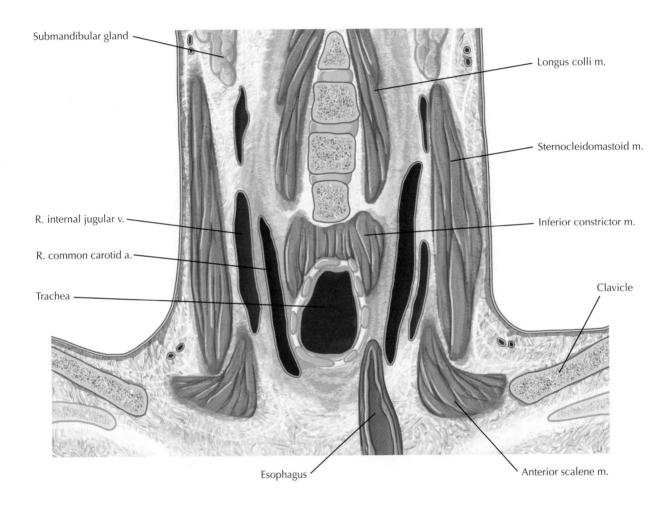

Submandibular gland

Longus colli m.

Sternocleidomastoid m.

R. internal jugular v.

Inferior constrictor m.

R. common carotid a.

Clavicle

Trachea

Esophagus

Anterior scalene m.

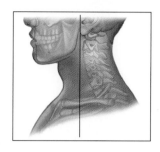

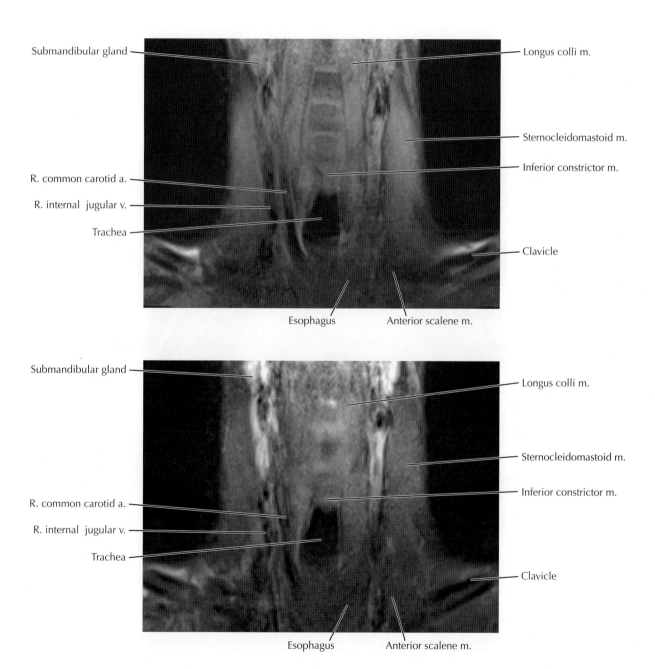

Submandibular gland — Longus colli m.

Sternocleidomastoid m.

Inferior constrictor m.

R. common carotid a.

R. internal jugular v.

Trachea

Clavicle

Esophagus   Anterior scalene m.

Submandibular gland — Longus colli m.

Sternocleidomastoid m.

Inferior constrictor m.

R. common carotid a.

R. internal jugular v.

Trachea

Clavicle

Esophagus   Anterior scalene m.

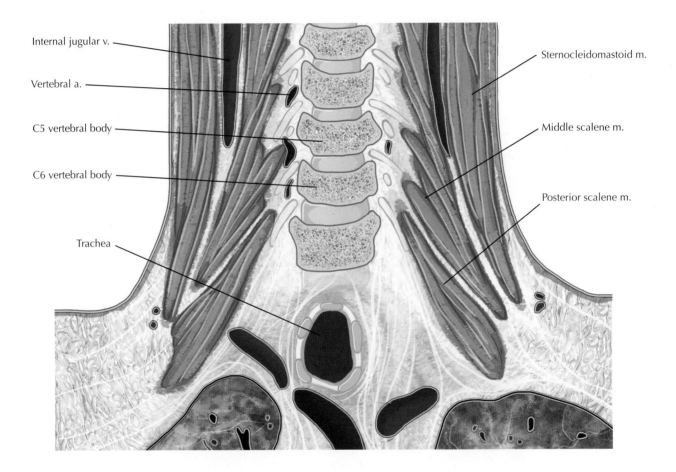

Internal jugular v.

Vertebral a.

C5 vertebral body

C6 vertebral body

Trachea

Sternocleidomastoid m.

Middle scalene m.

Posterior scalene m.

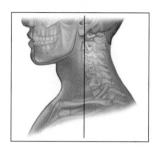

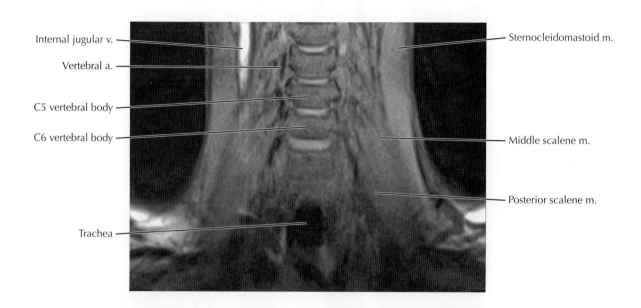

Internal jugular v.

Vertebral a.

C5 vertebral body

C6 vertebral body

Trachea

Sternocleidomastoid m.

Middle scalene m.

Posterior scalene m.

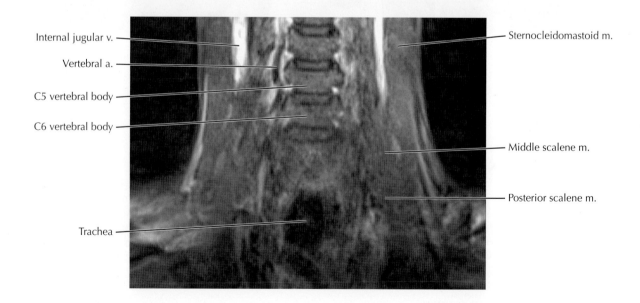

Internal jugular v.

Vertebral a.

C5 vertebral body

C6 vertebral body

Trachea

Sternocleidomastoid m.

Middle scalene m.

Posterior scalene m.

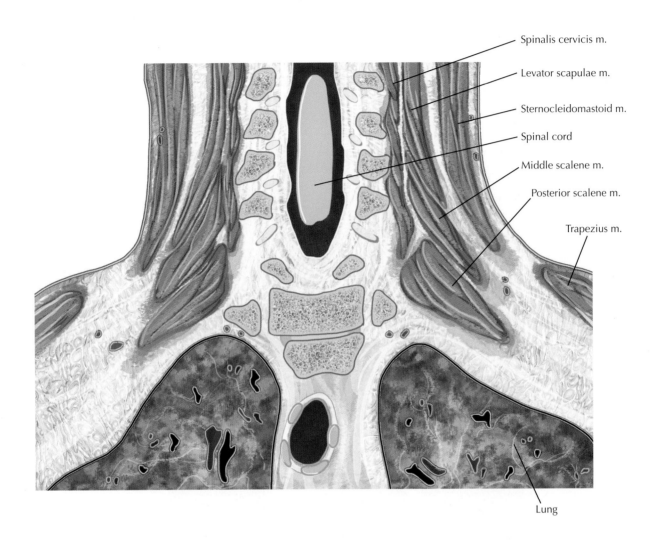

Spinalis cervicis m.

Levator scapulae m.

Sternocleidomastoid m.

Spinal cord

Middle scalene m.

Posterior scalene m.

Trapezius m.

Lung

NORMAL ANATOMY

On the Coronal 6 image, cervical nerve roots are seen exiting the foramina to form the brachial plexus. This plexus is formed at cervical vertebrae C5, C6, C7, and C8 and the first thoracic vertebra (T1). Note that C8 is the only nerve without a corresponding vertebra; thus it exits through the C7-T1 foramen. Nerves above this level exit above the corresponding vertebra (e.g., C7 exits spinal canal through C6-C7 foramen), and nerves below this level exit below the corresponding vertebra (e.g., T1 exits through T1-T2 foramen).

PATHOLOGIC PROCESS

Metastatic lymph nodes in the neck typically are anterior to the spinal column and do not invade the brachial plexus, except in florid disease. More often, a tumor in the top of the lungs may involve the brachial plexus, known as a *Pancoast tumor* (pulmonary sulcus tumor).

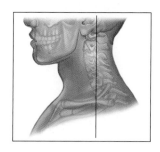

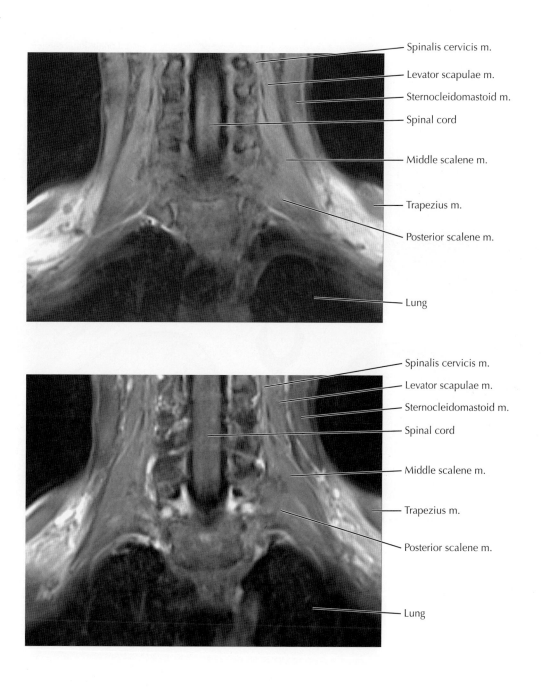

Spinalis cervicis m.

Levator scapulae m.

Sternocleidomastoid m.

Spinal cord

Middle scalene m.

Trapezius m.

Posterior scalene m.

Lung

Spinalis cervicis m.

Levator scapulae m.

Sternocleidomastoid m.

Spinal cord

Middle scalene m.

Trapezius m.

Posterior scalene m.

Lung

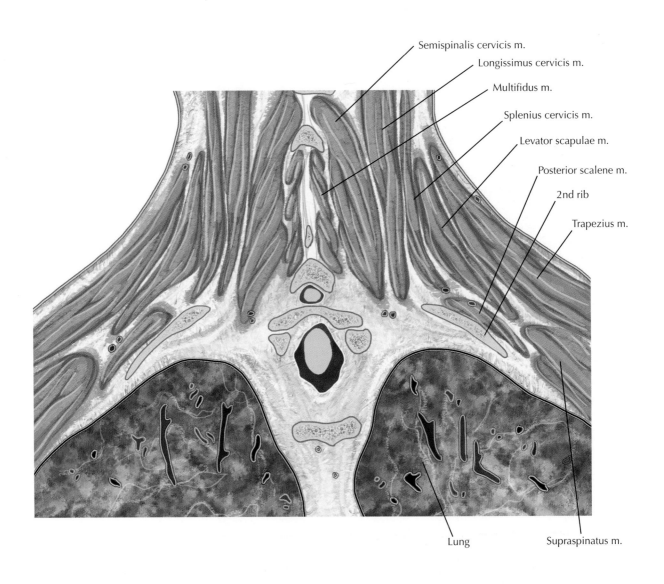

Semispinalis cervicis m.

Longissimus cervicis m.

Multifidus m.

Splenius cervicis m.

Levator scapulae m.

Posterior scalene m.

2nd rib

Trapezius m.

Lung

Supraspinatus m.

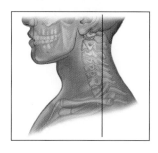

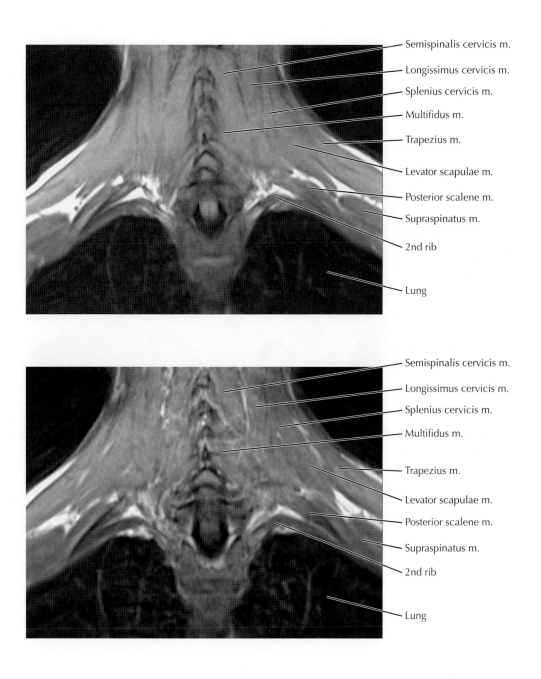

Semispinalis cervicis m.

Longissimus cervicis m.

Splenius cervicis m.

Multifidus m.

Trapezius m.

Levator scapulae m.

Posterior scalene m.

Supraspinatus m.

2nd rib

Lung

Semispinalis cervicis m.

Longissimus cervicis m.

Splenius cervicis m.

Multifidus m.

Trapezius m.

Levator scapulae m.

Posterior scalene m.

Supraspinatus m.

2nd rib

Lung

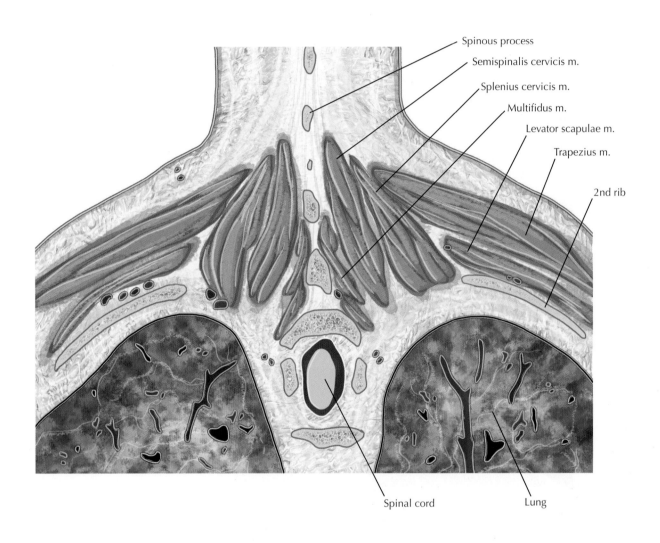

Spinous process

Semispinalis cervicis m.

Splenius cervicis m.

Multifidus m.

Levator scapulae m.

Trapezius m.

2nd rib

Spinal cord

Lung

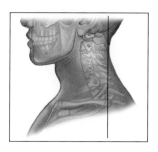

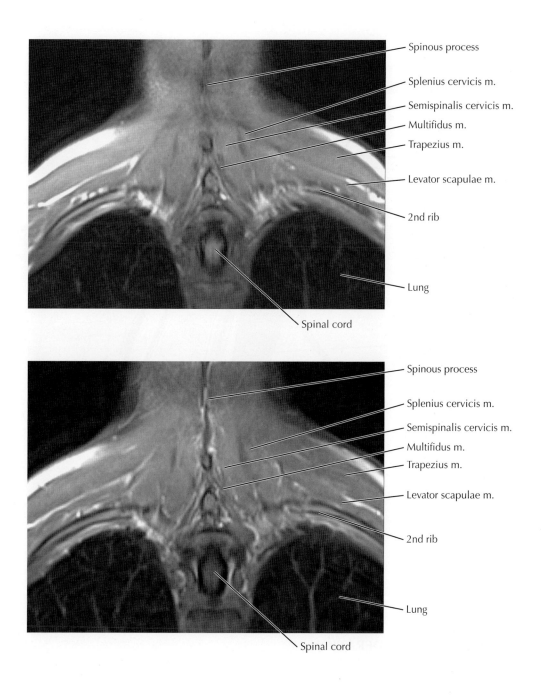

Spinous process

Splenius cervicis m.

Semispinalis cervicis m.

Multifidus m.

Trapezius m.

Levator scapulae m.

2nd rib

Lung

Spinal cord

Spinous process

Splenius cervicis m.

Semispinalis cervicis m.

Multifidus m.

Trapezius m.

Levator scapulae m.

2nd rib

Lung

Spinal cord

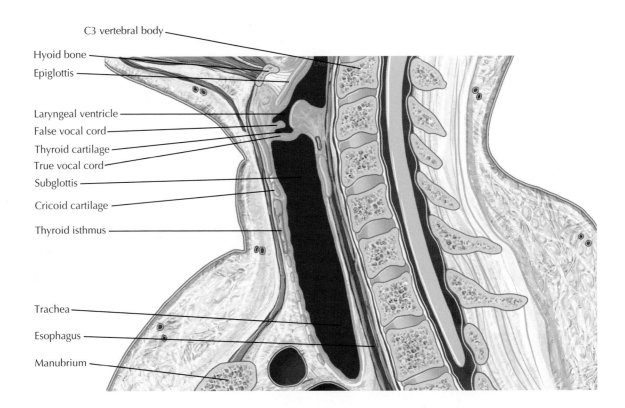

C3 vertebral body

Hyoid bone

Epiglottis

Laryngeal ventricle

False vocal cord

Thyroid cartilage

True vocal cord

Subglottis

Cricoid cartilage

Thyroid isthmus

Trachea

Esophagus

Manubrium

IMAGING TECHNIQUE CONSIDERATION

Although the Sagittal 1 plane is ideally a midline image, most patients will show a slight curvature caused by positioning or scoliosis. This sagittal image is fairly well centered on the hypopharynx and upper trachea, although the lower trachea is seen curving off the plane of image, as are the lower cervical and upper thoracic spinous processes.

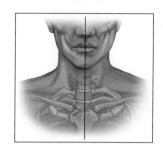

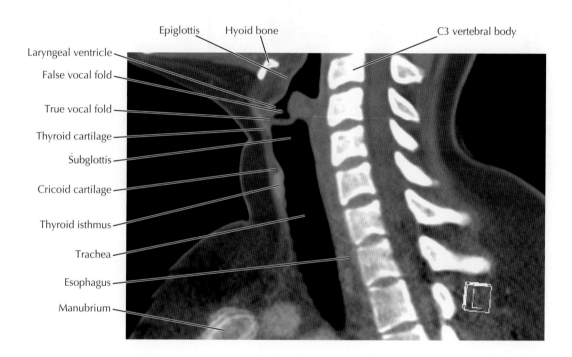

Epiglottis   Hyoid bone   C3 vertebral body

Laryngeal ventricle

False vocal fold

True vocal fold

Thyroid cartilage

Subglottis

Cricoid cartilage

Thyroid isthmus

Trachea

Esophagus

Manubrium

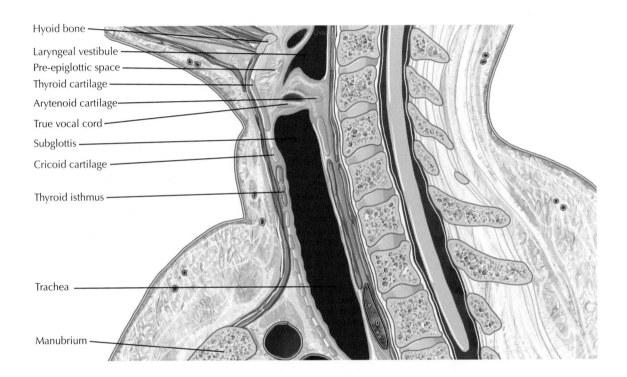

Hyoid bone
Laryngeal vestibule
Pre-epiglottic space
Thyroid cartilage
Arytenoid cartilage
True vocal cord
Subglottis
Cricoid cartilage
Thyroid isthmus
Trachea
Manubrium

NORMAL ANATOMY

Usually the vertebra with the most palpable spinous process is C7. This patient has subcutaneous tissue that does not allow for palpation of the C7 spinous process tip. However, note how much farther posteriorly the C7 process extends than the tip of C3, C4, C5, or C6. The most accurate way of labeling spine levels is to count from C1. The hyoid bone is anterior to C3.

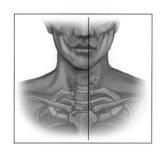

Hyoid bone

Pre-epiglottic space

Thyroid cartilage

True vocal fold

Arytenoid cartilage

Subglottis

Cricoid cartilage

Thyroid isthmus

Trachea

Manubrium

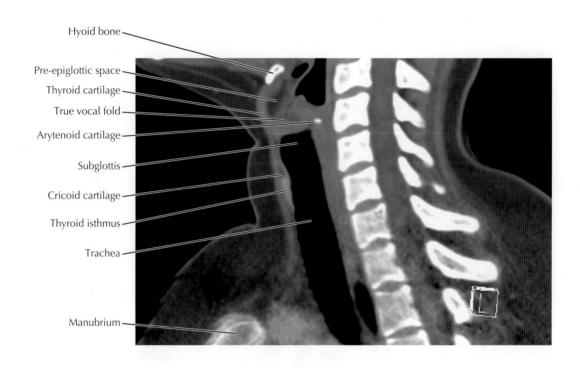

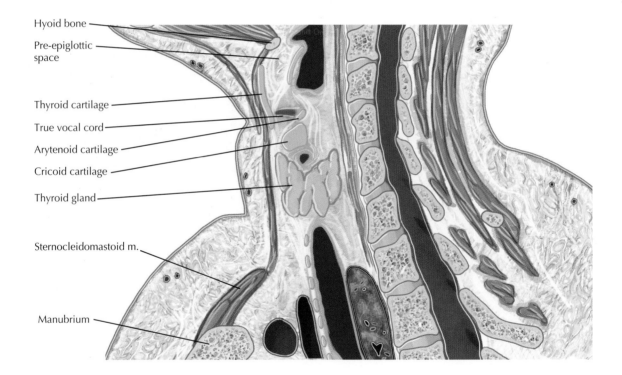

Hyoid bone

Pre-epiglottic space

Thyroid cartilage

True vocal cord

Arytenoid cartilage

Cricoid cartilage

Thyroid gland

Sternocleidomastoid m.

Manubrium

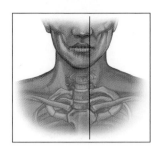

Hyoid bone

Pre-epiglottic space

Thyroid cartilage

True vocal fold

Arytenoid cartilage

Cricoid cartilage

Thyroid gland

Sternocleido-
mastoid m.

Manubrium

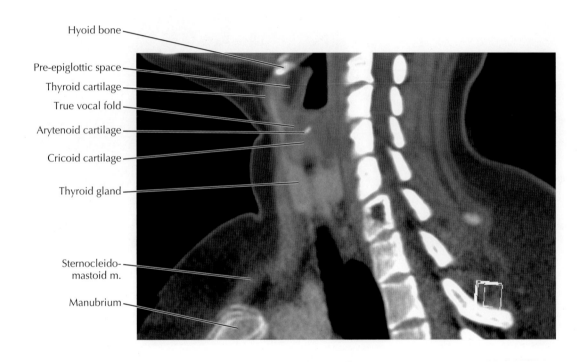

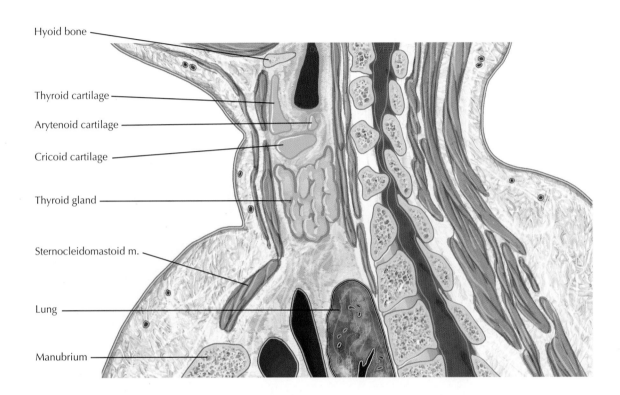

Hyoid bone

Thyroid cartilage

Arytenoid cartilage

Cricoid cartilage

Thyroid gland

Sternocleidomastoid m.

Lung

Manubrium

NORMAL ANATOMY

The cervical neural foramina rarely line up on a single plane as in lumbar imaging, where the anatomic structures such as the foramina and pedicles are much larger. In the Sagittal 4 CT image, the upper neural foramina can be seen, but not the lower foramina because of curvature of the cervical spine from positioning or scoliosis. Thus, assessment of cervical foraminal stenosis is often best done on axial images, where there is symmetry for comparison.

DIAGNOSTIC CONSIDERATION

Although measurement of cervical lymph nodes is performed on axial imaging by convention, the sagittal plane can often increase the conspicuity of an enlarged lymph node, because the internal jugular and spinal accessory lymph node chains can be seen along their entire length.

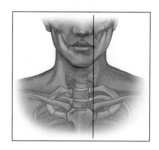

Hyoid bone

Thyroid cartilage

Arytenoid cartilage

Cricoid cartilage

Thyroid gland

Sternocleido-
mastoid m.

Manubrium

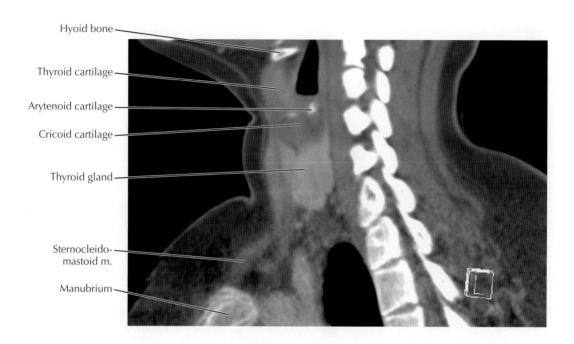

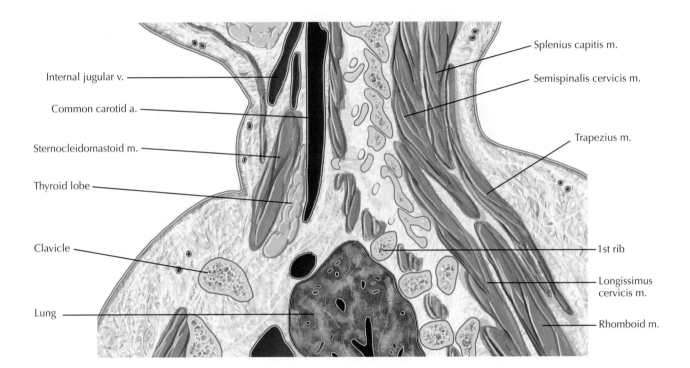

Internal jugular v.

Common carotid a.

Sternocleidomastoid m.

Thyroid lobe

Clavicle

Lung

Splenius capitis m.

Semispinalis cervicis m.

Trapezius m.

1st rib

Longissimus cervicis m.

Rhomboid m.

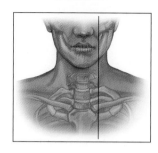

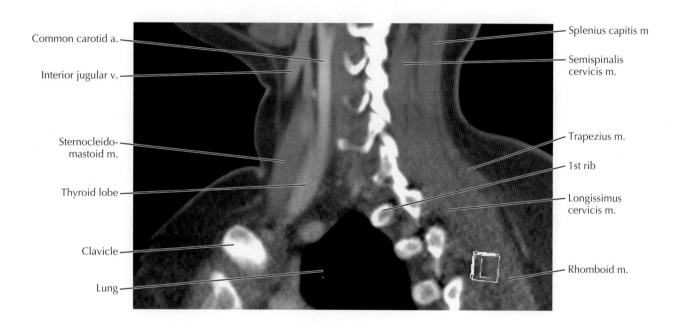

Common carotid a.

Interior jugular v.

Sternocleido-mastoid m.

Thyroid lobe

Clavicle

Lung

Splenius capitis m

Semispinalis cervicis m.

Trapezius m.

1st rib

Longissimus cervicis m.

Rhomboid m.

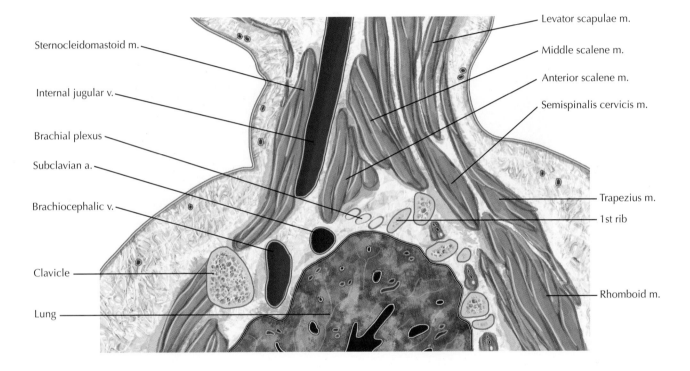

Sternocleidomastoid m.

Internal jugular v.

Brachial plexus

Subclavian a.

Brachiocephalic v.

Clavicle

Lung

Levator scapulae m.

Middle scalene m.

Anterior scalene m.

Semispinalis cervicis m.

Trapezius m.

1st rib

Rhomboid m.

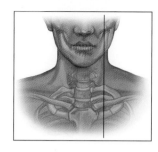

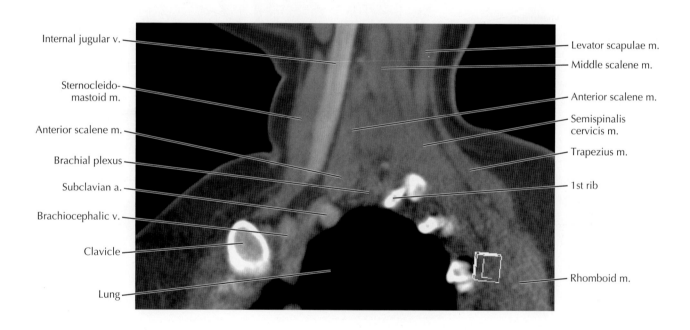

Internal jugular v.

Sternocleido-
mastoid m.

Anterior scalene m.

Brachial plexus

Subclavian a.

Brachiocephalic v.

Clavicle

Lung

Levator scapulae m.

Middle scalene m.

Anterior scalene m.

Semispinalis
cervicis m.

Trapezius m.

1st rib

Rhomboid m.

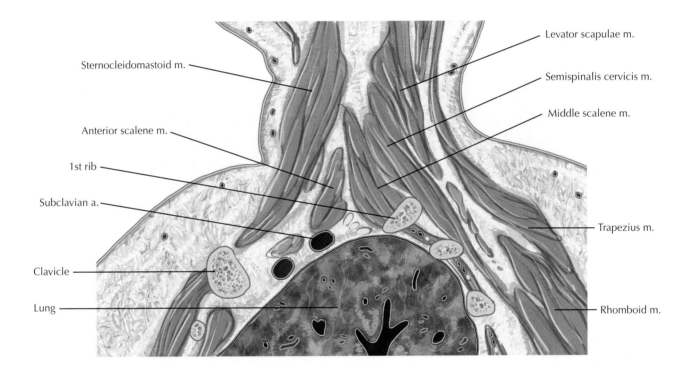

Sternocleidomastoid m.

Anterior scalene m.

1st rib

Subclavian a.

Clavicle

Lung

Levator scapulae m.

Semispinalis cervicis m.

Middle scalene m.

Trapezius m.

Rhomboid m.

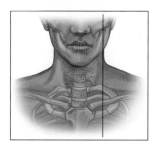

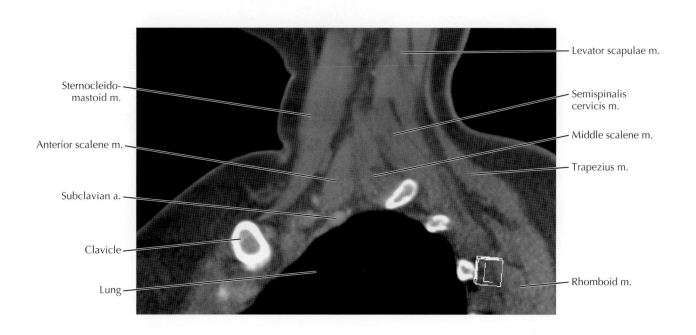

Sternocleido-
mastoid m.

Anterior scalene m.

Subclavian a.

Clavicle

Lung

Levator scapulae m.

Semispinalis
cervicis m.

Middle scalene m.

Trapezius m.

Rhomboid m.

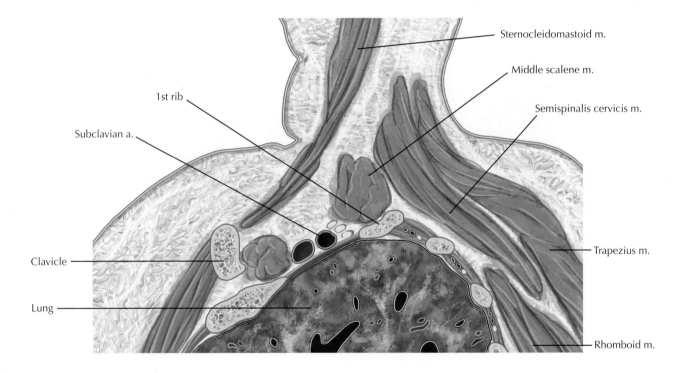

1st rib

Subclavian a.

Clavicle

Lung

Sternocleidomastoid m.

Middle scalene m.

Semispinalis cervicis m.

Trapezius m.

Rhomboid m.

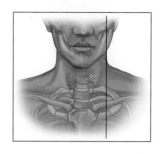

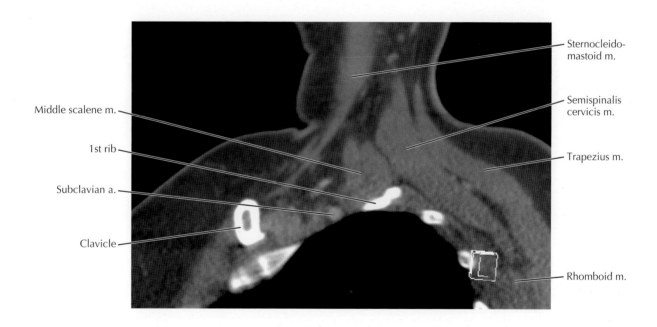

Sternocleido-
mastoid m.

Semispinalis
cervicis m.

Trapezius m.

Middle scalene m.

1st rib

Subclavian a.

Clavicle

Rhomboid m.

PART 3 SPINE

Chapter 15 OVERVIEW OF SPINE

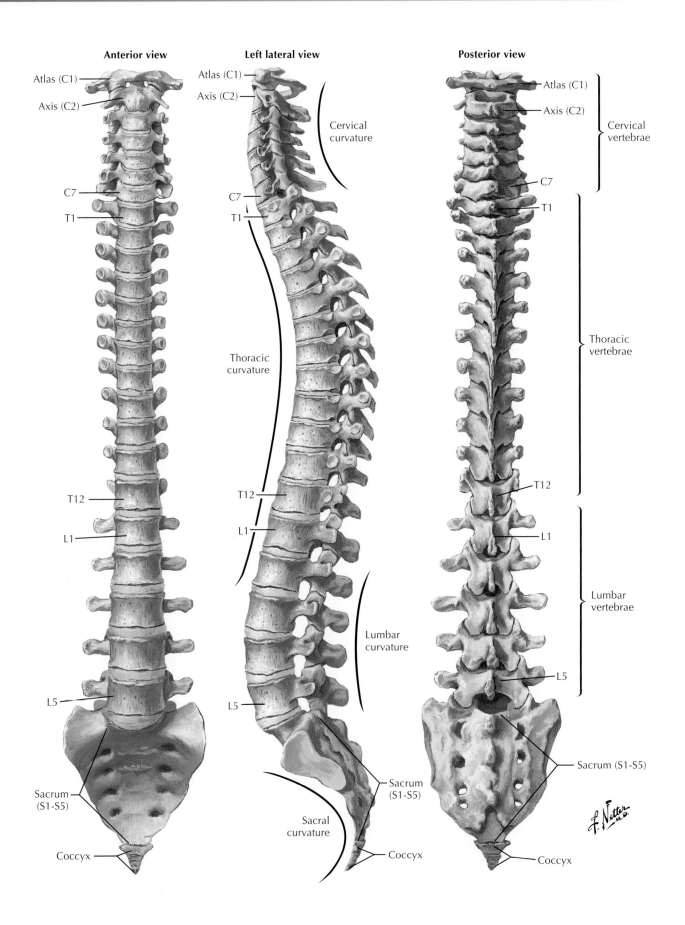

Anterior view

Atlas (C1)
Axis (C2)
C7
T1
T12
L1
L5
Sacrum (S1-S5)
Coccyx

Left lateral view

Atlas (C1)
Axis (C2)
Cervical curvature
C7
T1
Thoracic curvature
T12
L1
Lumbar curvature
L5
Sacrum (S1-S5)
Sacral curvature
Coccyx

Posterior view

Atlas (C1)
Axis (C2)
Cervical vertebrae
C7
T1
Thoracic vertebrae
T12
L1
Lumbar vertebrae
L5
Sacrum (S1-S5)
Coccyx

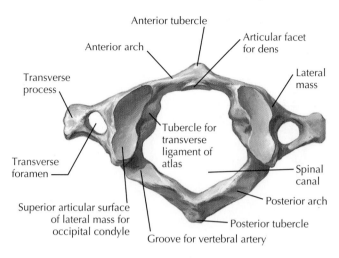

Atlas (C1): superior view

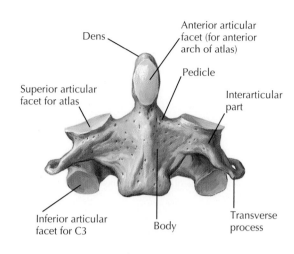

Axis (C2): anterior view

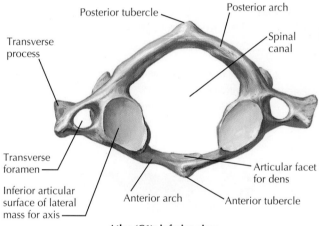

Atlas (C1): inferior view

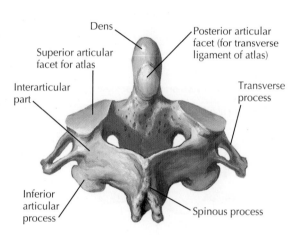

Axis (C2): posterosuperior view

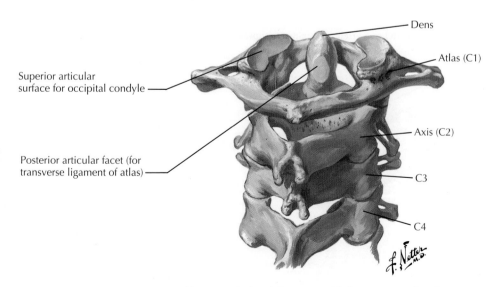

Upper cervical vertebrae, assembled: posterosuperior view

Inferior aspect of C3 and superior aspect of C4 showing the sites of the facet and uncovertebral articulations

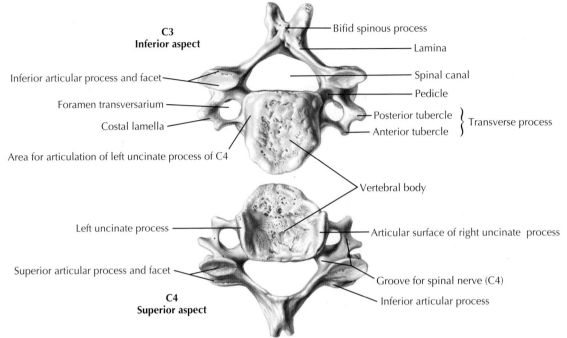

C3
Inferior aspect

Bifid spinous process
Lamina
Inferior articular process and facet
Spinal canal
Pedicle
Foramen transversarium
Posterior tubercle
Transverse process
Costal lamella
Anterior tubercle
Area for articulation of left uncinate process of C4
Vertebral body
Left uncinate process
Articular surface of right uncinate process
Superior articular process and facet
Groove for spinal nerve (C4)
Inferior articular process

C4
Superior aspect

4th cervical vertebra: anterior view

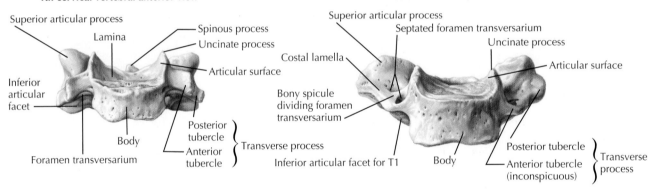

Superior articular process
Lamina
Spinous process
Uncinate process
Articular surface
Inferior articular facet
Posterior tubercle
Anterior tubercle
Transverse process
Body
Foramen transversarium

7th cervical vertebra: anterior view

Superior articular process
Septated foramen transversarium
Uncinate process
Costal lamella
Articular surface
Bony spicule dividing foramen transversarium
Posterior tubercle
Inferior articular facet for T1
Body
Anterior tubercle (inconspicuous)
Transverse process

7th cervical vertebra (vertebra prominens): superior view

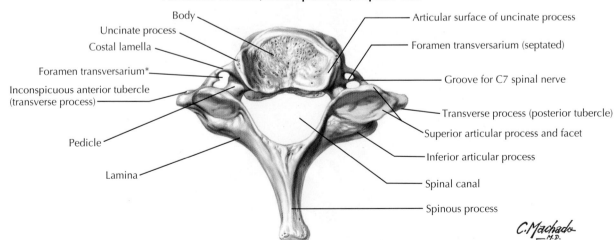

Body
Uncinate process
Costal lamella
Foramen transversarium*
Inconspicuous anterior tubercle (transverse process)
Pedicle
Lamina
Articular surface of uncinate process
Foramen transversarium (septated)
Groove for C7 spinal nerve
Transverse process (posterior tubercle)
Superior articular process and facet
Inferior articular process
Spinal canal
Spinous process

C. Machado
M.D.

The foramina transversaria of C7 transmit vertebral veins, but usually not the vertebral artery, and are asymmetric in this specimen.

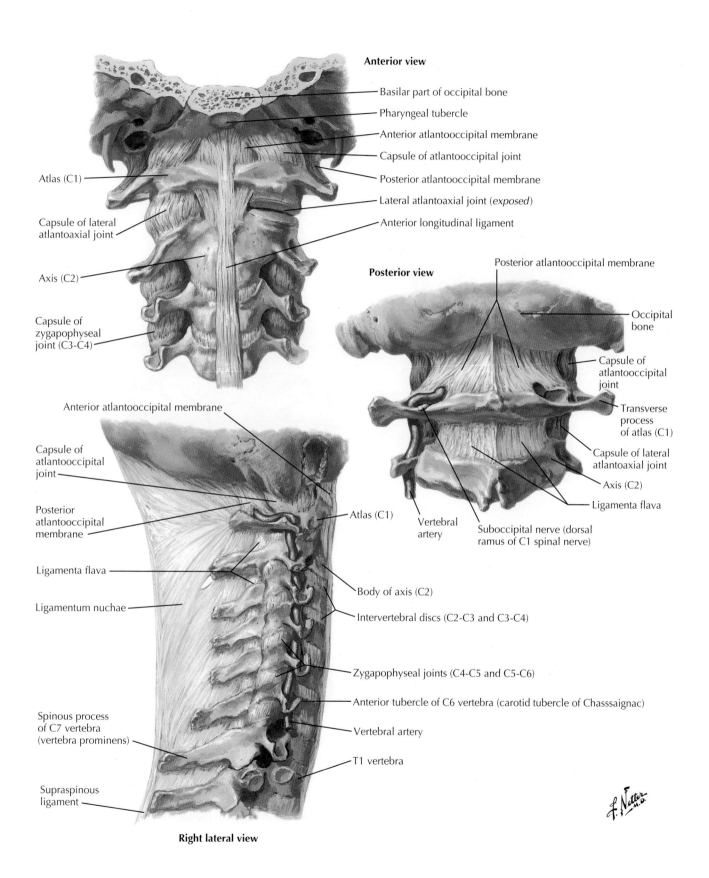

Anterior view

Basilar part of occipital bone

Pharyngeal tubercle

Anterior atlantooccipital membrane

Capsule of atlantooccipital joint

Posterior atlantooccipital membrane

Lateral atlantoaxial joint (*exposed*)

Anterior longitudinal ligament

Atlas (C1)

Capsule of lateral atlantoaxial joint

Axis (C2)

Capsule of zygapophyseal joint (C3-C4)

Posterior view

Posterior atlantooccipital membrane

Occipital bone

Capsule of atlantooccipital joint

Transverse process of atlas (C1)

Capsule of lateral atlantoaxial joint

Axis (C2)

Ligamenta flava

Vertebral artery

Suboccipital nerve (dorsal ramus of C1 spinal nerve)

Anterior atlantooccipital membrane

Capsule of atlantooccipital joint

Posterior atlantooccipital membrane

Ligamenta flava

Ligamentum nuchae

Atlas (C1)

Body of axis (C2)

Intervertebral discs (C2-C3 and C3-C4)

Zygapophyseal joints (C4-C5 and C5-C6)

Anterior tubercle of C6 vertebra (carotid tubercle of Chasssaignac)

Vertebral artery

Spinous process of C7 vertebra (vertebra prominens)

T1 vertebra

Supraspinous ligament

Right lateral view

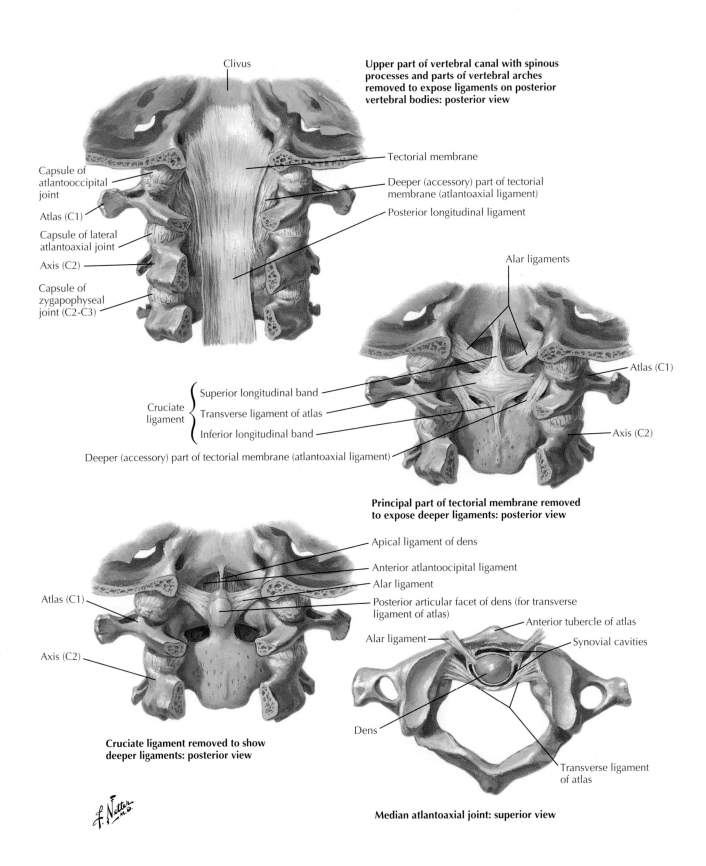

Clivus

Upper part of vertebral canal with spinous processes and parts of vertebral arches removed to expose ligaments on posterior vertebral bodies: posterior view

Tectorial membrane

Capsule of atlantooccipital joint

Deeper (accessory) part of tectorial membrane (atlantoaxial ligament)

Atlas (C1)

Posterior longitudinal ligament

Capsule of lateral atlantoaxial joint

Axis (C2)

Capsule of zygapophyseal joint (C2-C3)

Alar ligaments

Atlas (C1)

Cruciate ligament { Superior longitudinal band

Transverse ligament of atlas

Inferior longitudinal band

Axis (C2)

Deeper (accessory) part of tectorial membrane (atlantoaxial ligament)

Principal part of tectorial membrane removed to expose deeper ligaments: posterior view

Apical ligament of dens

Anterior atlantoocipital ligament

Alar ligament

Atlas (C1)

Posterior articular facet of dens (for transverse ligament of atlas)

Axis (C2)

Anterior tubercle of atlas

Alar ligament

Synovial cavities

Dens

Transverse ligament of atlas

Cruciate ligament removed to show deeper ligaments: posterior view

Median atlantoaxial joint: superior view

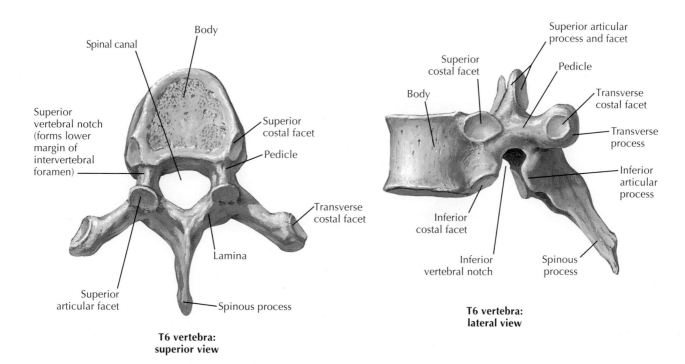

Spinal canal

Body

Superior vertebral notch (forms lower margin of intervertebral foramen)

Superior costal facet

Pedicle

Transverse costal facet

Lamina

Superior articular facet

Spinous process

T6 vertebra: superior view

Superior costal facet

Body

Superior articular process and facet

Pedicle

Transverse costal facet

Transverse process

Inferior articular process

Inferior costal facet

Inferior vertebral notch

Spinous process

T6 vertebra: lateral view

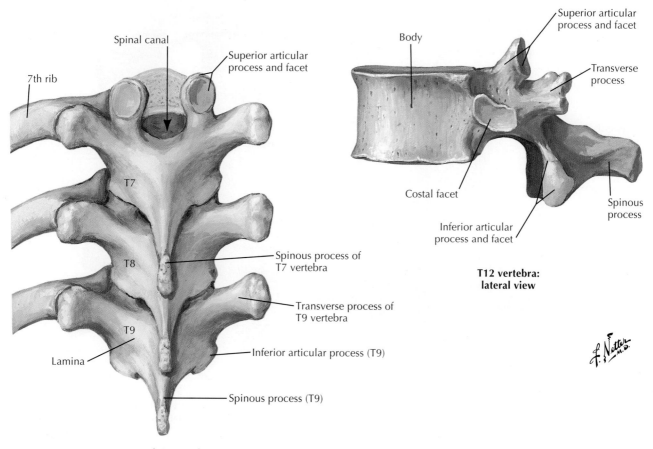

Spinal canal

Superior articular process and facet

7th rib

T7

T8

T9

Lamina

Spinous process of T7 vertebra

Transverse process of T9 vertebra

Inferior articular process (T9)

Spinous process (T9)

T7, T8, and T9 vertebrae: posterior view

Body

Superior articular process and facet

Transverse process

Costal facet

Inferior articular process and facet

Spinous process

T12 vertebra: lateral view

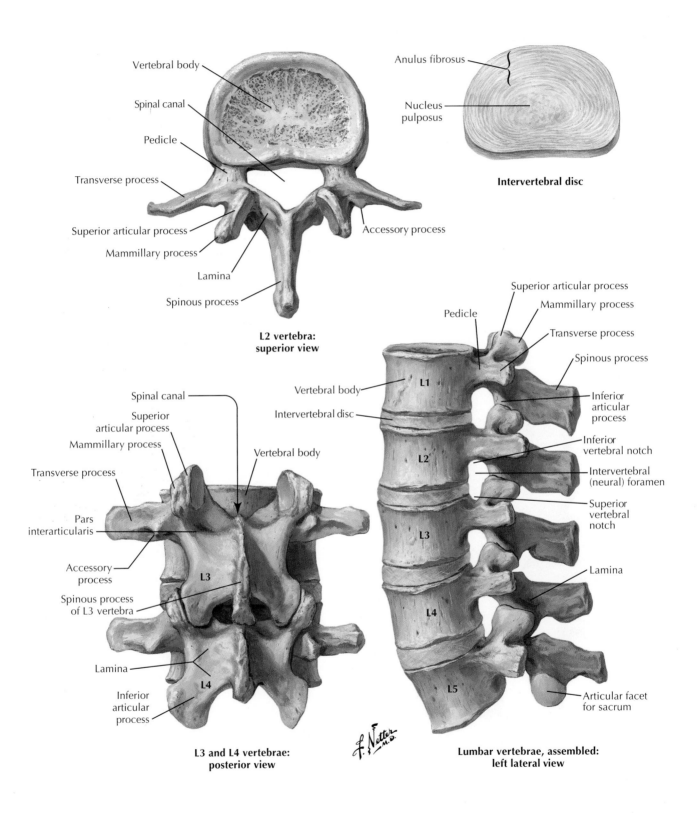

Vertebral body

Spinal canal

Pedicle

Transverse process

Superior articular process

Mammillary process

Lamina

Spinous process

L2 vertebra: superior view

Anulus fibrosus

Nucleus pulposus

Intervertebral disc

Spinal canal

Superior articular process

Mammillary process

Transverse process

Pars interarticularis

Accessory process

Spinous process of L3 vertebra

Lamina

Inferior articular process

Vertebral body

L3

L4

L3 and L4 vertebrae: posterior view

Pedicle

Superior articular process

Mammillary process

Transverse process

Spinous process

Inferior articular process

Inferior vertebral notch

Intervertebral (neural) foramen

Superior vertebral notch

Lamina

Articular facet for sacrum

Vertebral body

Intervertebral disc

L1

L2

L3

L4

L5

Lumbar vertebrae, assembled: left lateral view

Accessory process

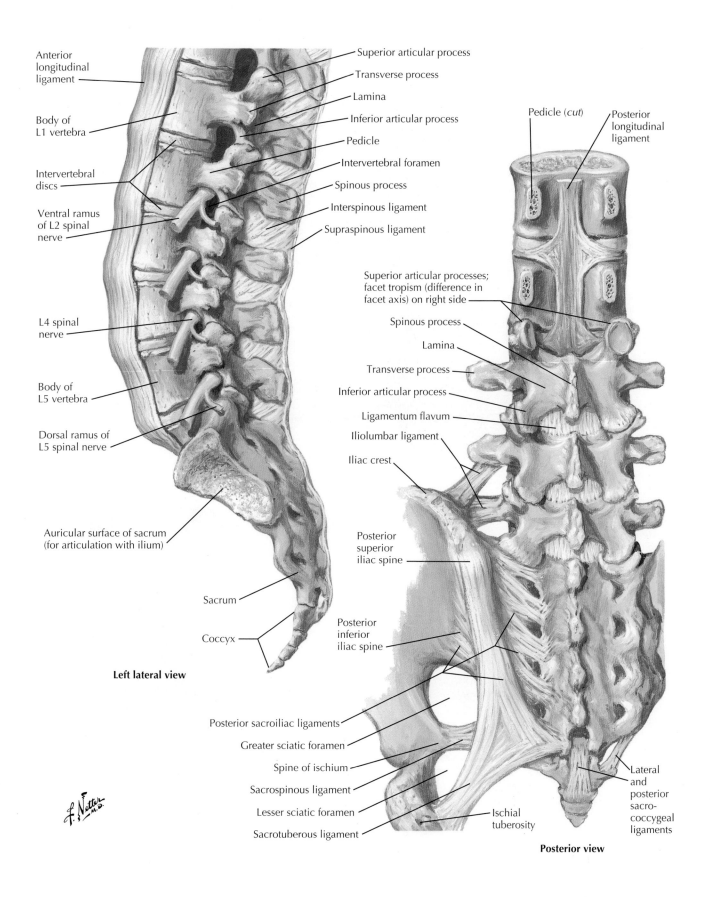

Anterior longitudinal ligament

Body of L1 vertebra

Intervertebral discs

Ventral ramus of L2 spinal nerve

L4 spinal nerve

Body of L5 vertebra

Dorsal ramus of L5 spinal nerve

Auricular surface of sacrum (for articulation with ilium)

Sacrum

Coccyx

Left lateral view

Superior articular process

Transverse process

Lamina

Inferior articular process

Pedicle

Intervertebral foramen

Spinous process

Interspinous ligament

Supraspinous ligament

Pedicle (*cut*)

Posterior longitudinal ligament

Superior articular processes; facet tropism (difference in facet axis) on right side

Spinous process

Lamina

Transverse process

Inferior articular process

Ligamentum flavum

Iliolumbar ligament

Iliac crest

Posterior superior iliac spine

Posterior inferior iliac spine

Posterior sacroiliac ligaments

Greater sciatic foramen

Spine of ischium

Sacrospinous ligament

Lesser sciatic foramen

Sacrotuberous ligament

Ischial tuberosity

Lateral and posterior sacro-coccygeal ligaments

Posterior view

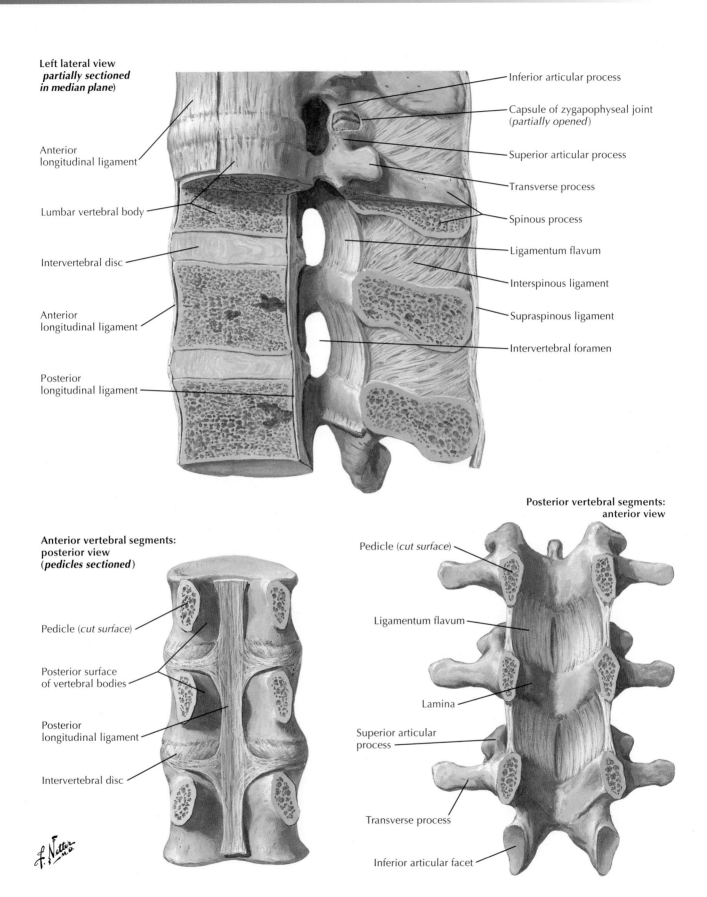

Left lateral view
partially sectioned in median plane)

Anterior longitudinal ligament

Lumbar vertebral body

Intervertebral disc

Anterior longitudinal ligament

Posterior longitudinal ligament

Inferior articular process

Capsule of zygapophyseal joint (*partially opened*)

Superior articular process

Transverse process

Spinous process

Ligamentum flavum

Interspinous ligament

Supraspinous ligament

Intervertebral foramen

Anterior vertebral segments: posterior view (*pedicles sectioned*)

Pedicle (*cut surface*)

Posterior surface of vertebral bodies

Posterior longitudinal ligament

Intervertebral disc

Posterior vertebral segments: anterior view

Pedicle (*cut surface*)

Ligamentum flavum

Lamina

Superior articular process

Transverse process

Inferior articular facet

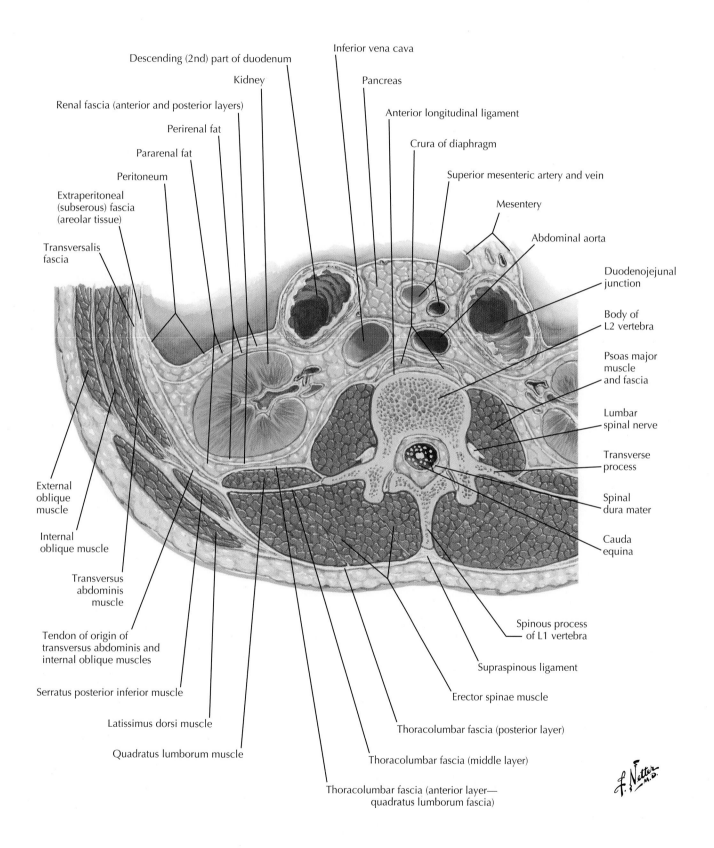

Descending (2nd) part of duodenum

Inferior vena cava

Kidney

Pancreas

Renal fascia (anterior and posterior layers)

Anterior longitudinal ligament

Perirenal fat

Crura of diaphragm

Pararenal fat

Superior mesenteric artery and vein

Peritoneum

Mesentery

Extraperitoneal (subserous) fascia (areolar tissue)

Abdominal aorta

Transversalis fascia

Duodenojejunal junction

Body of L2 vertebra

Psoas major muscle and fascia

Lumbar spinal nerve

Transverse process

External oblique muscle

Spinal dura mater

Internal oblique muscle

Cauda equina

Transversus abdominis muscle

Tendon of origin of transversus abdominis and internal oblique muscles

Serratus posterior inferior muscle

Spinous process of L1 vertebra

Supraspinous ligament

Latissimus dorsi muscle

Erector spinae muscle

Quadratus lumborum muscle

Thoracolumbar fascia (posterior layer)

Thoracolumbar fascia (middle layer)

Thoracolumbar fascia (anterior layer— quadratus lumborum fascia)

Chapter 16 SPINE

CERVICAL SPINE

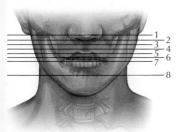

AXIAL   536

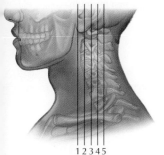

CORONAL   552

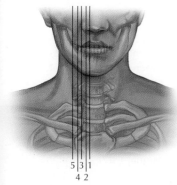

SAGITTAL   562

THORACIC SPINE

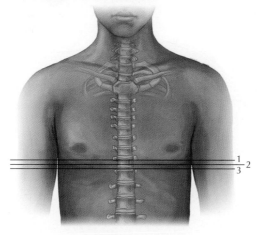

AXIAL   572

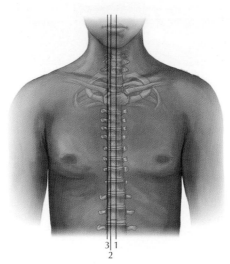

SAGITTAL   578

LUMBOSACRAL SPINE

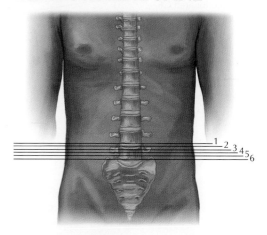

AXIAL   584

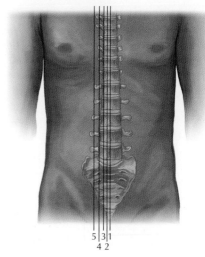

SAGITTAL   596

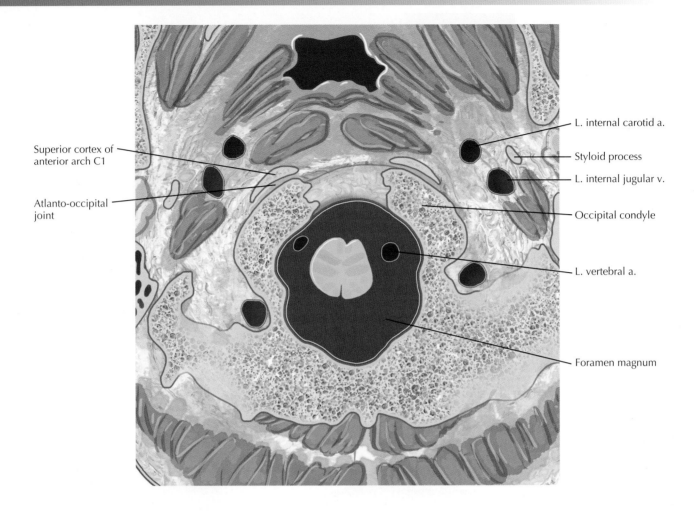

Superior cortex of
anterior arch C1

Atlanto-occipital
joint

L. internal carotid a.

Styloid process

L. internal jugular v.

Occipital condyle

L. vertebral a.

Foramen magnum

PATHOLOGIC PROCESS

Note on these images that the nasopharynx is often seen on cervical spine imaging. The neuroradiologist should always check for symmetry of the Eustachian tube opening and fossa of Rosenmüller just anterior to the longus capitis muscle to ensure that no nasopharyngeal lesion is present (see Chapter 13).

IMAGING TECHNIQUE CONSIDERATION

Spinal imaging can be daunting at first due to the complex three-dimensional (3D) anatomy of the vertebrae and the critical implications of damage to the spine. This is particularly true taking into account various signal characteristics on magnetic resonance imaging (MRI) and motion artifact from vessel pulsation and respiration. A good principle is that computed tomography (CT) and MRI are complementary. In general, CT better delineates the architecture of the dense bones, the cortex of which does not provide much MR signal, and MRI is better at providing contrast to the soft tissues, such as the spinal cord. Although CT (top image) would be better at showing a subtle fracture of the vertebral artery foramen, MRI (bottom image) would be better at delineating hematoma in the wall of the vertebral artery from dissection.

Another good principle for learning spinal anatomy is that the lower the level in the spine, the larger the vertebrae and the easier it is to understand the anatomy. Thus it is often best to start with the lumbar spine, learning both diagnostic principles and image-guided intervention, and to work up the spine as familiarity with spinal anatomy increases.

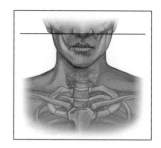

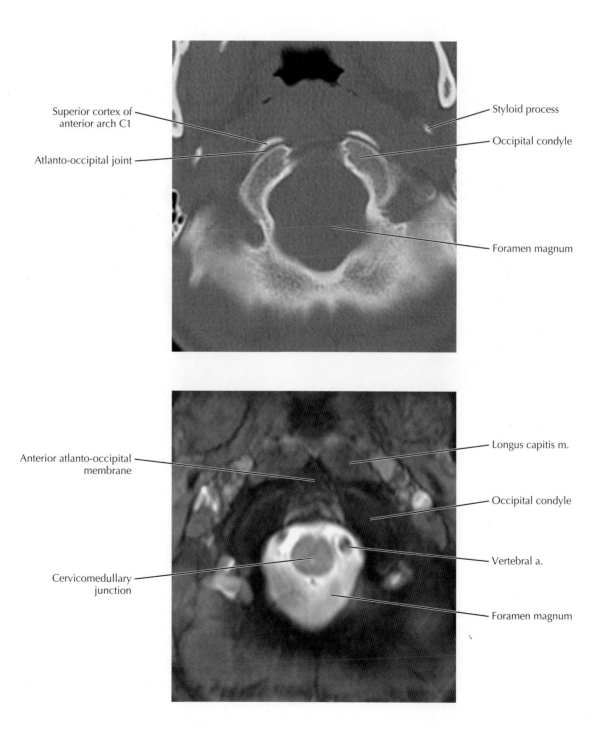

Superior cortex of anterior arch C1

Atlanto-occipital joint

Styloid process

Occipital condyle

Foramen magnum

Anterior atlanto-occipital membrane

Cervicomedullary junction

Longus capitis m.

Occipital condyle

Vertebral a.

Foramen magnum

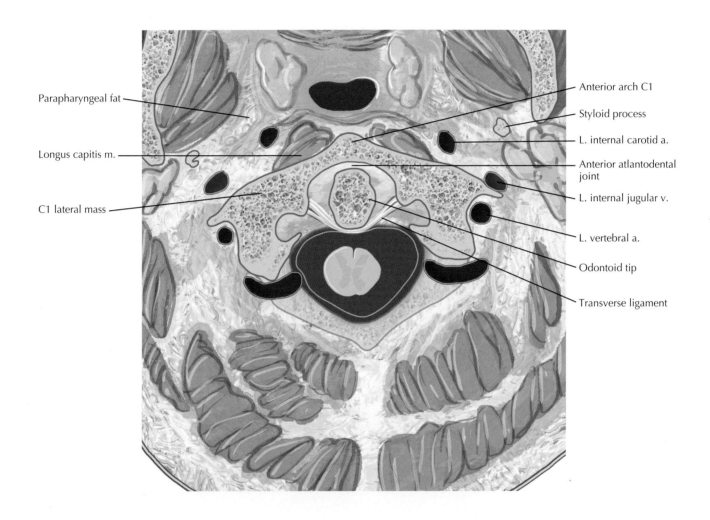

Parapharyngeal fat

Longus capitis m.

C1 lateral mass

Anterior arch C1

Styloid process

L. internal carotid a.

Anterior atlantodental joint

L. internal jugular v.

L. vertebral a.

Odontoid tip

Transverse ligament

DIAGNOSTIC CONSIDERATION

The *predental space*, or distance between the anterior aspect of the dens and the posterior border of the anterior arch of C1 (atlas), should measure 3 mm or less in the adult patient. Widening of this space or asymmetry of soft tissue lateral to the odontoid raises concern for cruciate ligament injury. The best imaging test is voluntary flexion and extension sequences on lateral cervical radiographs to check for change in the predental space measurement. However, in the patient who has pain limiting motion, or in the unconscious patient, CT or MRI can provide secondary signs such as fracture of C1 or C2 (axis), hemorrhage along the dura, and edema within the soft tissues.

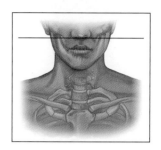

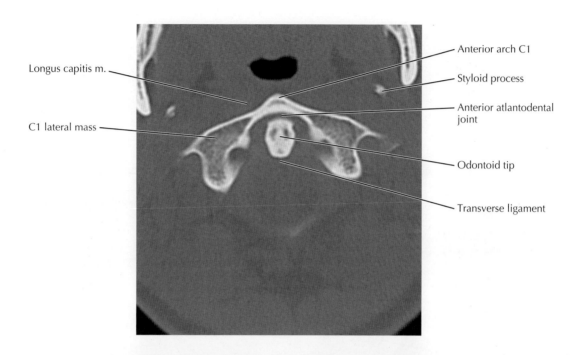

Longus capitis m.

C1 lateral mass

Anterior arch C1

Styloid process

Anterior atlantodental joint

Odontoid tip

Transverse ligament

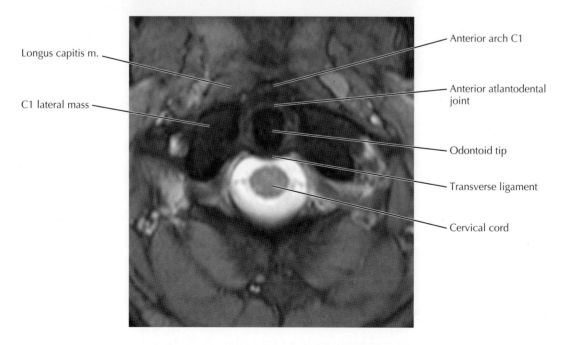

Longus capitis m.

C1 lateral mass

Anterior arch C1

Anterior atlantodental joint

Odontoid tip

Transverse ligament

Cervical cord

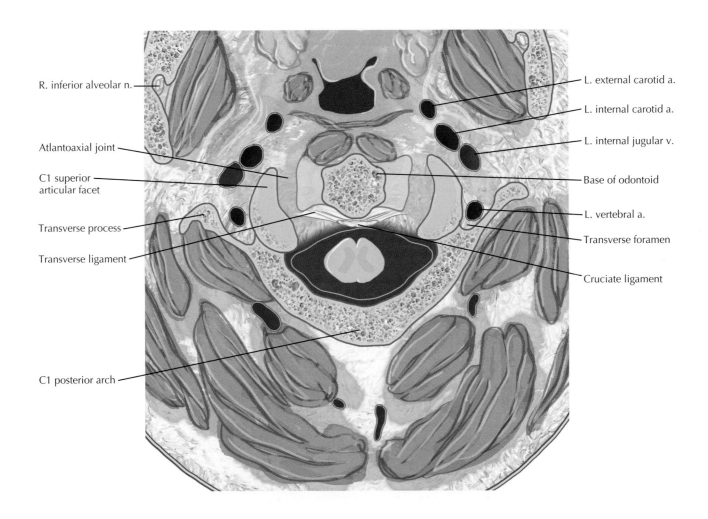

R. inferior alveolar n.

Atlantoaxial joint

C1 superior
articular facet

Transverse process

Transverse ligament

C1 posterior arch

L. external carotid a.

L. internal carotid a.

L. internal jugular v.

Base of odontoid

L. vertebral a.

Transverse foramen

Cruciate ligament

PATHOLOGIC PROCESS

Somewhat counterintuitively, a fracture through the larger base of the odontoid process is less serious than a fracture more superiorly near the tip. The better, more proximal blood supply at the odontoid base allows better healing and less chance of avascular necrosis.

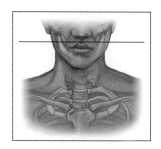

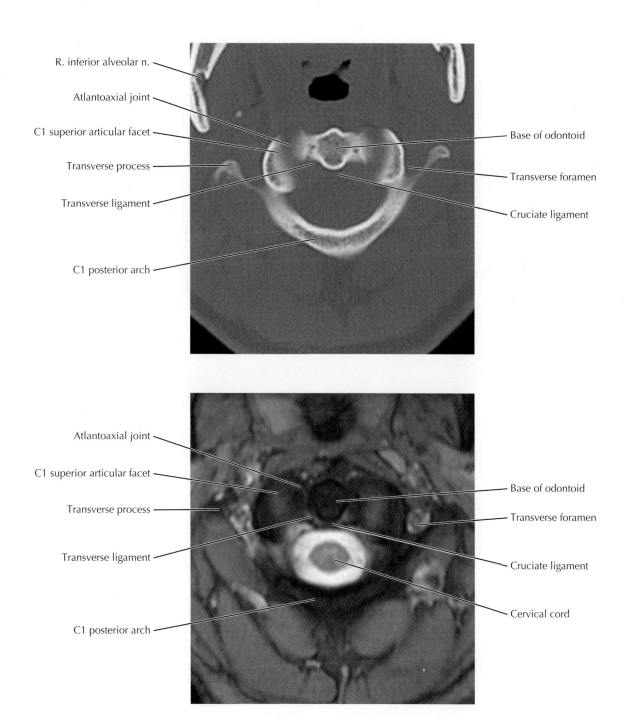

R. inferior alveolar n.

Atlantoaxial joint

C1 superior articular facet

Transverse process

Transverse ligament

C1 posterior arch

Base of odontoid

Transverse foramen

Cruciate ligament

Atlantoaxial joint

C1 superior articular facet

Transverse process

Transverse ligament

C1 posterior arch

Base of odontoid

Transverse foramen

Cruciate ligament

Cervical cord

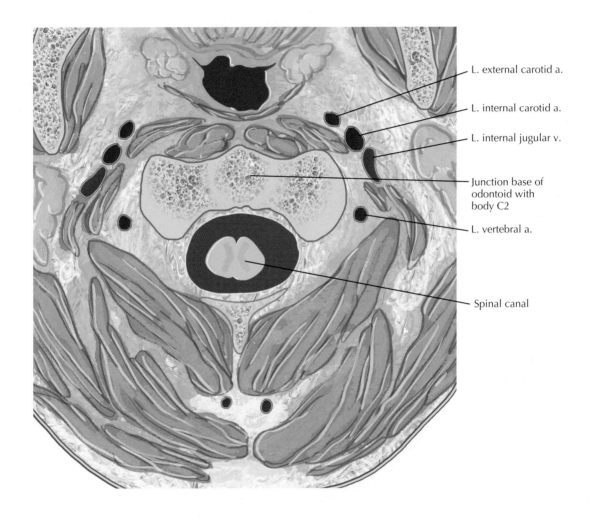

L. external carotid a.

L. internal carotid a.

L. internal jugular v.

Junction base of odontoid with body C2

L. vertebral a.

Spinal canal

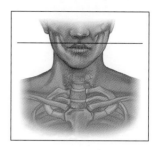

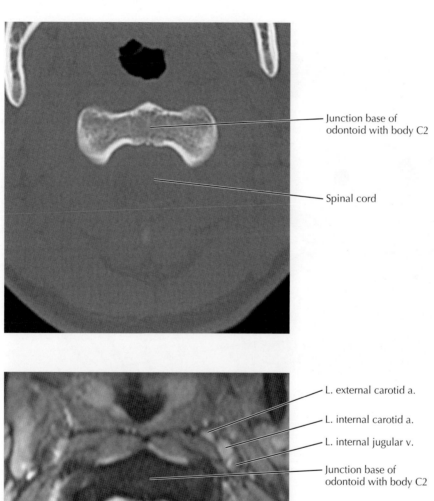

Junction base of
odontoid with body C2

Spinal cord

L. external carotid a.

L. internal carotid a.

L. internal jugular v.

Junction base of
odontoid with body C2

L. vertebral a.

Spinal cord

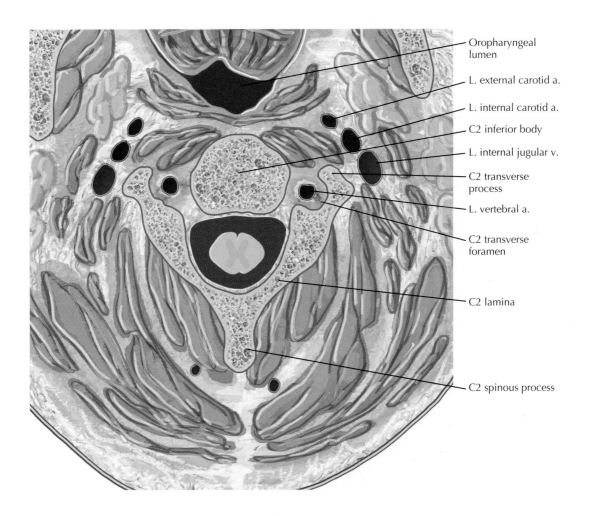

Oropharyngeal lumen

L. external carotid a.

L. internal carotid a.

C2 inferior body

L. internal jugular v.

C2 transverse process

L. vertebral a.

C2 transverse foramen

C2 lamina

C2 spinous process

IMAGING TECHNIQUE CONSIDERATION

The MR images (lower) are axial 3D T2* gradient images. The advantages over standard 2D spin-echo sequences are the higher spatial resolution and the ability to reformat in any plane. Motion, however, tends to cause all the images of the sequence to become blurred.

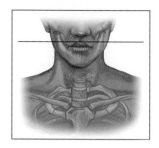

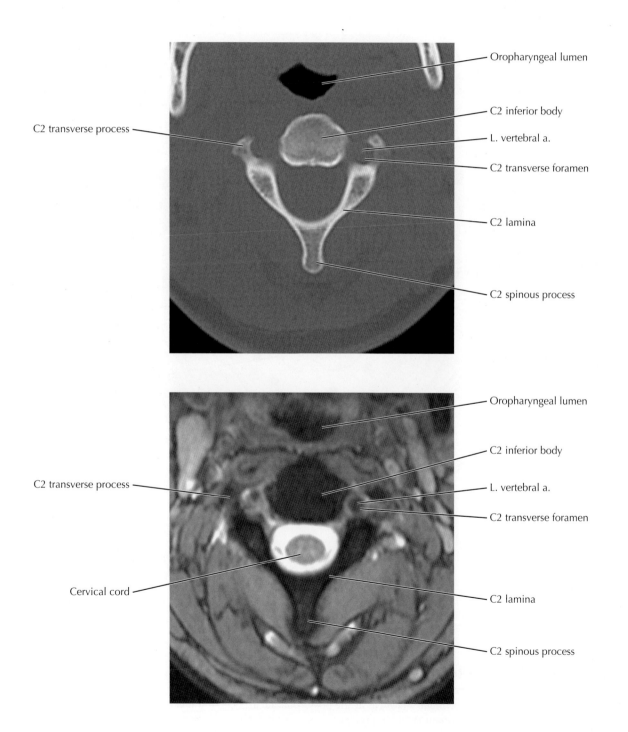

Oropharyngeal lumen

C2 inferior body

L. vertebral a.

C2 transverse foramen

C2 transverse process

C2 lamina

C2 spinous process

Oropharyngeal lumen

C2 inferior body

C2 transverse process

L. vertebral a.

C2 transverse foramen

Cervical cord

C2 lamina

C2 spinous process

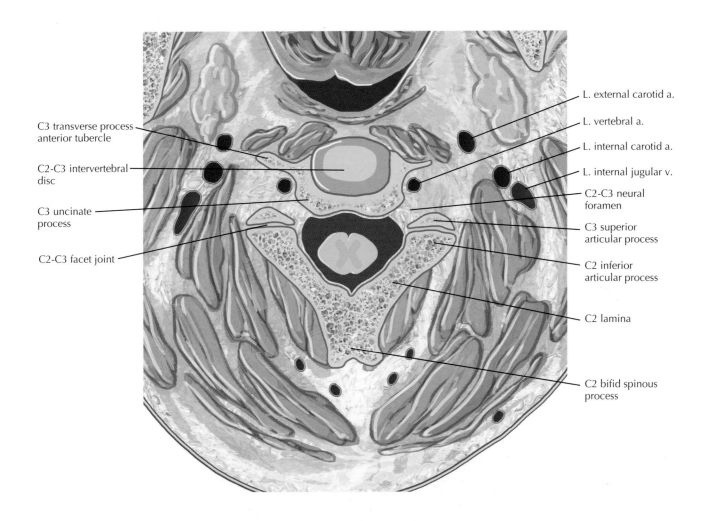

C3 transverse process anterior tubercle

C2-C3 intervertebral disc

C3 uncinate process

C2-C3 facet joint

L. external carotid a.

L. vertebral a.

L. internal carotid a.

L. internal jugular v.

C2-C3 neural foramen

C3 superior articular process

C2 inferior articular process

C2 lamina

C2 bifid spinous process

PATHOLOGIC PROCESS

Uncovertebral osteophytes at the posterolateral aspects of the vertebral body can cause narrowing of the foramina and impingement of exiting nerve roots. Some osteophytes may be confluent with a broad-based disc-osteophyte complex across the entire posterior aspect of the vertebral body that can chronically flatten the spinal cord.

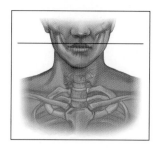

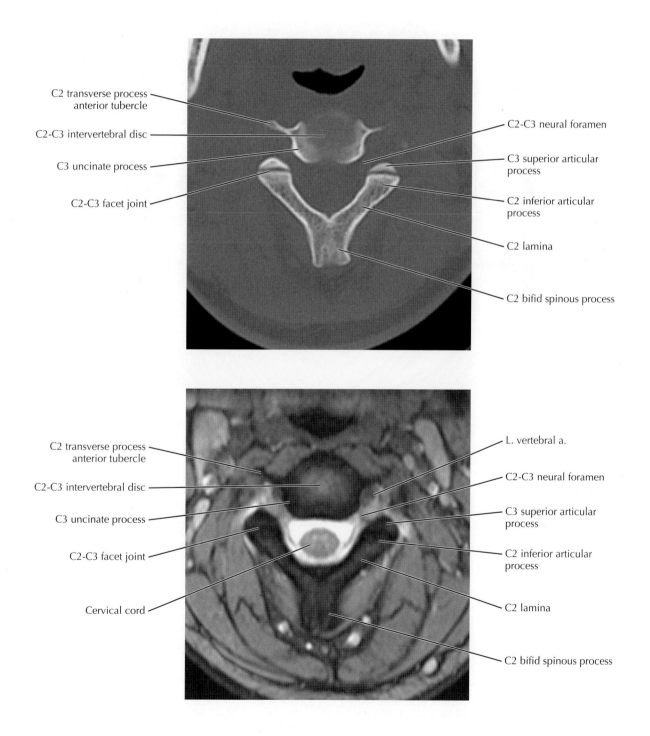

C2 transverse process anterior tubercle

C2-C3 intervertebral disc

C3 uncinate process

C2-C3 facet joint

C2-C3 neural foramen

C3 superior articular process

C2 inferior articular process

C2 lamina

C2 bifid spinous process

C2 transverse process anterior tubercle

C2-C3 intervertebral disc

C3 uncinate process

C2-C3 facet joint

Cervical cord

L. vertebral a.

C2-C3 neural foramen

C3 superior articular process

C2 inferior articular process

C2 lamina

C2 bifid spinous process

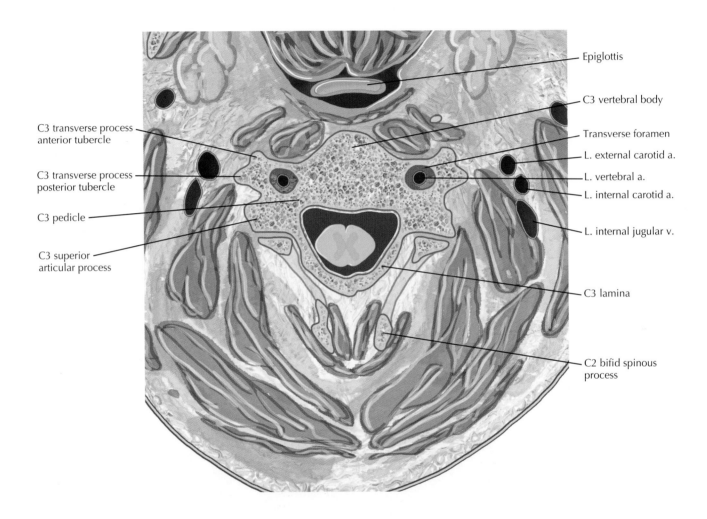

C3 transverse process anterior tubercle

C3 transverse process posterior tubercle

C3 pedicle

C3 superior articular process

Epiglottis

C3 vertebral body

Transverse foramen

L. external carotid a.

L. vertebral a.

L. internal carotid a.

L. internal jugular v.

C3 lamina

C2 bifid spinous process

DIAGNOSTIC CONSIDERATION

Note that the bony vertebral artery foramina, also called transverse foramina, are symmetric in this patient (Cervical Axial 7). A careful search for fracture lines across these foramina in the setting of trauma will help reveal vertebral artery dissection. Angiography (CTA or MRA) of the cervical arteries often shows some asymmetry in the lumina. If corresponding asymmetry exists in the bony foramina, the cause is likely a congenitally hypoplastic side rather than a dissection.

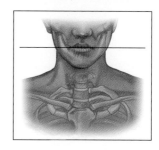

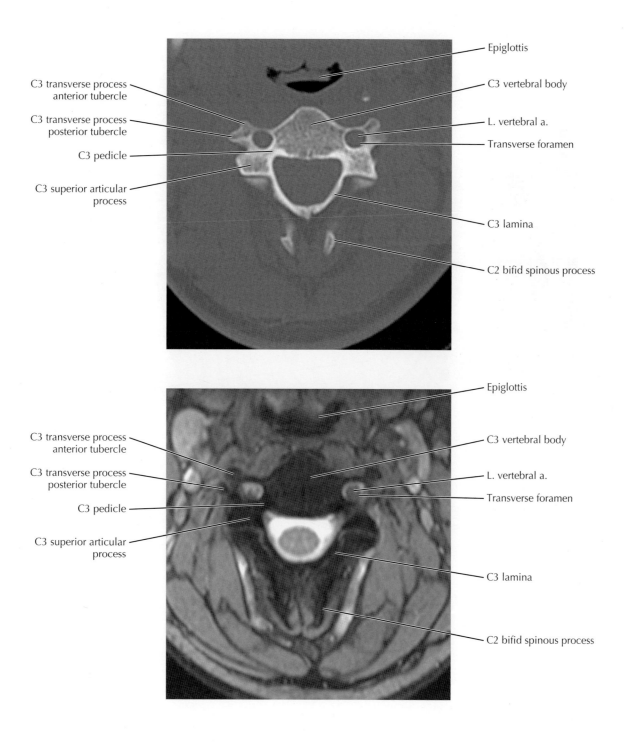

C3 transverse process anterior tubercle

C3 transverse process posterior tubercle

C3 pedicle

C3 superior articular process

Epiglottis

C3 vertebral body

L. vertebral a.

Transverse foramen

C3 lamina

C2 bifid spinous process

C3 transverse process anterior tubercle

C3 transverse process posterior tubercle

C3 pedicle

C3 superior articular process

Epiglottis

C3 vertebral body

L. vertebral a.

Transverse foramen

C3 lamina

C2 bifid spinous process

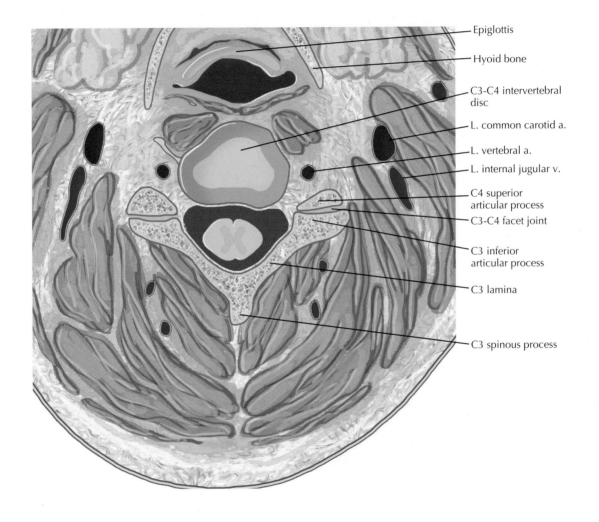

Epiglottis

Hyoid bone

C3-C4 intervertebral disc

L. common carotid a.

L. vertebral a.

L. internal jugular v.

C4 superior articular process

C3-C4 facet joint

C3 inferior articular process

C3 lamina

C3 spinous process

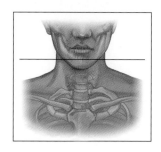

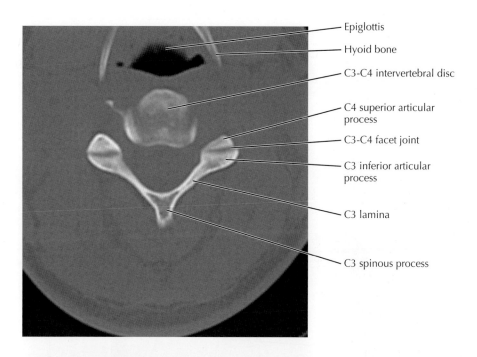

- Epiglottis
- Hyoid bone
- C3-C4 intervertebral disc
- C4 superior articular process
- C3-C4 facet joint
- C3 inferior articular process
- C3 lamina
- C3 spinous process

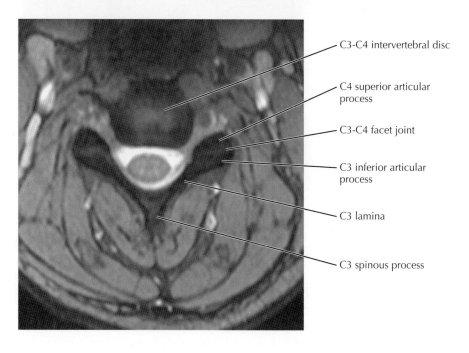

- C3-C4 intervertebral disc
- C4 superior articular process
- C3-C4 facet joint
- C3 inferior articular process
- C3 lamina
- C3 spinous process

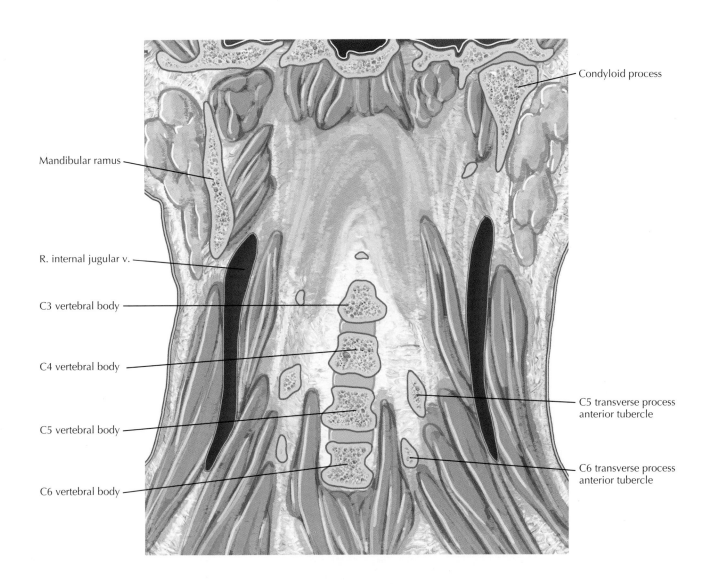

Condyloid process

Mandibular ramus

R. internal jugular v.

C3 vertebral body

C4 vertebral body

C5 transverse process anterior tubercle

C5 vertebral body

C6 transverse process anterior tubercle

C6 vertebral body

IMAGING TECHNIQUE CONSIDERATION

The temporomandibular joints (TMJs) can often be seen in coronal imaging of the cervical spine. In Cervical Spine Coronal 1, there is slight rotation of positioning such that the patient's left TMJ on the right side of the image is slightly more anterior and better seen than the right TMJ.

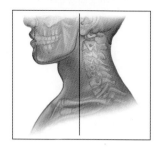

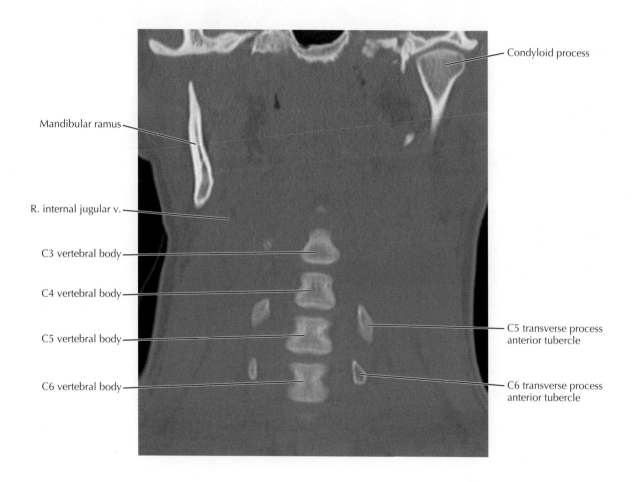

Condyloid process

Mandibular ramus

R. internal jugular v.

C3 vertebral body

C4 vertebral body

C5 vertebral body

C6 vertebral body

C5 transverse process anterior tubercle

C6 transverse process anterior tubercle

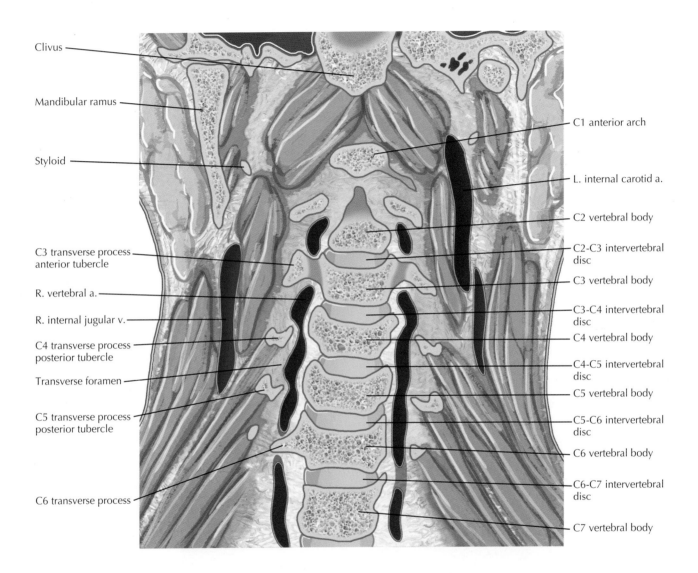

Clivus

Mandibular ramus

Styloid

C3 transverse process anterior tubercle

R. vertebral a.

R. internal jugular v.

C4 transverse process posterior tubercle

Transverse foramen

C5 transverse process posterior tubercle

C6 transverse process

C1 anterior arch

L. internal carotid a.

C2 vertebral body

C2-C3 intervertebral disc

C3 vertebral body

C3-C4 intervertebral disc

C4 vertebral body

C4-C5 intervertebral disc

C5 vertebral body

C5-C6 intervertebral disc

C6 vertebral body

C6-C7 intervertebral disc

C7 vertebral body

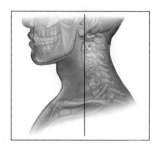

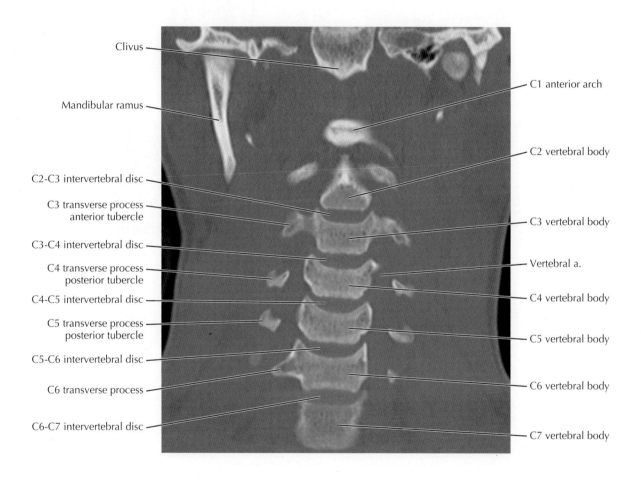

Clivus

C1 anterior arch

Mandibular ramus

C2 vertebral body

C2-C3 intervertebral disc

C3 transverse process anterior tubercle

C3 vertebral body

C3-C4 intervertebral disc

C4 transverse process posterior tubercle

Vertebral a.

C4-C5 intervertebral disc

C4 vertebral body

C5 transverse process posterior tubercle

C5 vertebral body

C5-C6 intervertebral disc

C6 transverse process

C6 vertebral body

C6-C7 intervertebral disc

C7 vertebral body

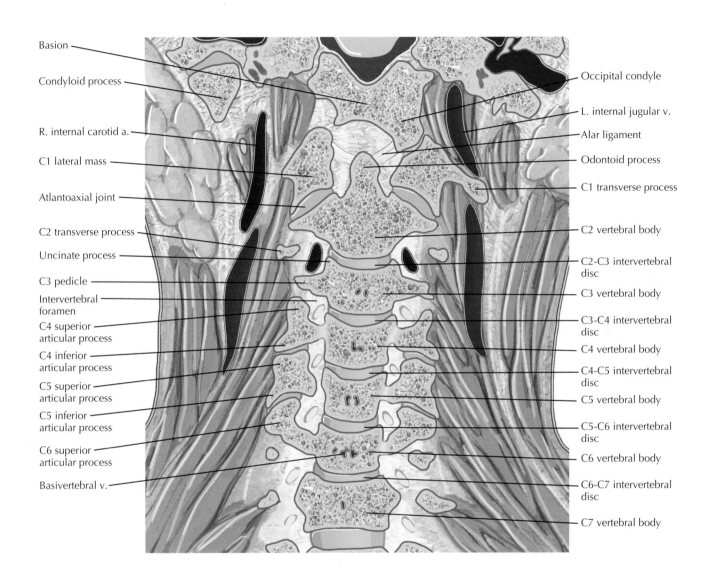

Basion
Condyloid process
R. internal carotid a.
C1 lateral mass
Atlantoaxial joint
C2 transverse process
Uncinate process
C3 pedicle
Intervertebral foramen
C4 superior articular process
C4 inferior articular process
C5 superior articular process
C5 inferior articular process
C6 superior articular process
Basivertebral v.

Occipital condyle
L. internal jugular v.
Alar ligament
Odontoid process
C1 transverse process
C2 vertebral body
C2-C3 intervertebral disc
C3 vertebral body
C3-C4 intervertebral disc
C4 vertebral body
C4-C5 intervertebral disc
C5 vertebral body
C5-C6 intervertebral disc
C6 vertebral body
C6-C7 intervertebral disc
C7 vertebral body

DIAGNOSTIC CONSIDERATION

The coronal image is a good plane on which to assess for asymmetric positioning of the odontoid process. Note that in Cervical Spine Coronal 3 there is slightly more space to the right side of the patient's odontoid (left side of the image), although this is likely caused by slight rotation of the patient's neck or perhaps slight normal variation rather than trauma in this patient. The edges of the atlantoaxial joints are shown to be well aligned.

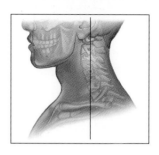

Basion

Condyloid process

C1 lateral mass

Atlantoaxial joint

C2 transverse process

Uncinate process

C3 pedicle

Intervertebral foramen

C4 superior articular process

C5 superior articular process

C5 inferior articular process

C6 inferior articular process

Basivertebral v.

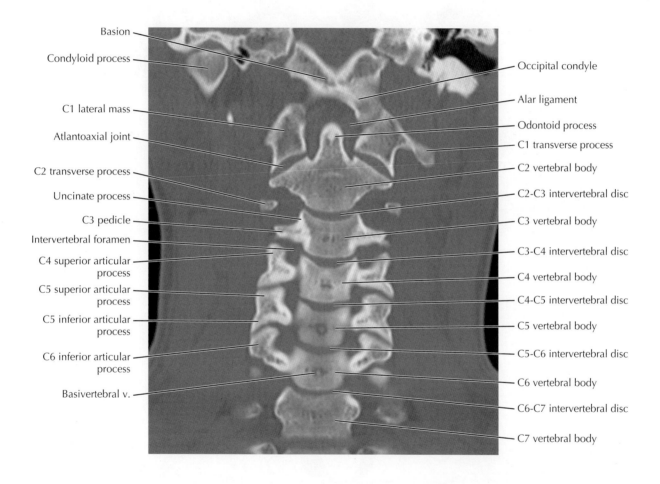

Occipital condyle

Alar ligament

Odontoid process

C1 transverse process

C2 vertebral body

C2-C3 intervertebral disc

C3 vertebral body

C3-C4 intervertebral disc

C4 vertebral body

C4-C5 intervertebral disc

C5 vertebral body

C5-C6 intervertebral disc

C6 vertebral body

C6-C7 intervertebral disc

C7 vertebral body

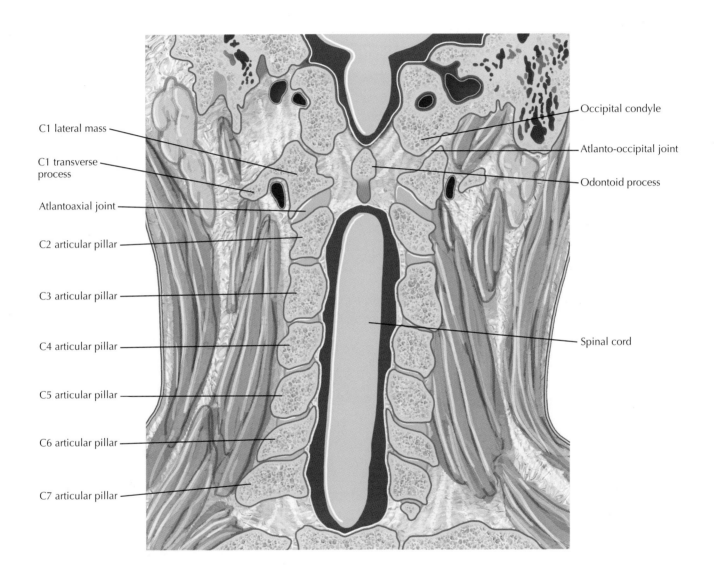

C1 lateral mass

C1 transverse process

Atlantoaxial joint

C2 articular pillar

C3 articular pillar

C4 articular pillar

C5 articular pillar

C6 articular pillar

C7 articular pillar

Occipital condyle

Atlanto-occipital joint

Odontoid process

Spinal cord

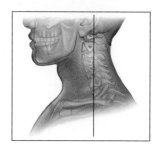

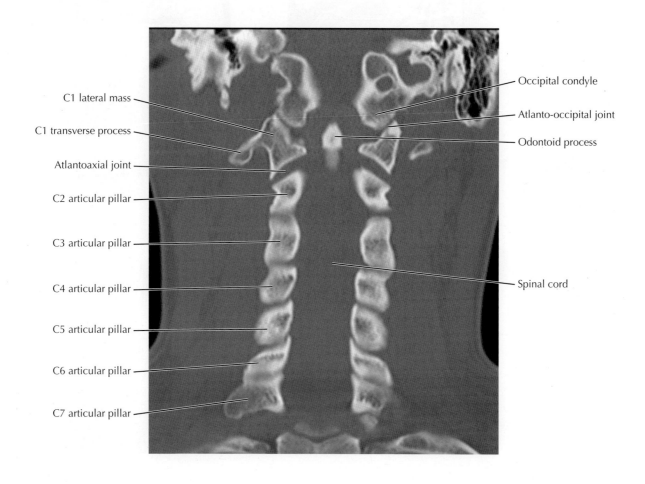

C1 lateral mass

C1 transverse process

Atlantoaxial joint

C2 articular pillar

C3 articular pillar

C4 articular pillar

C5 articular pillar

C6 articular pillar

C7 articular pillar

Occipital condyle

Atlanto-occipital joint

Odontoid process

Spinal cord

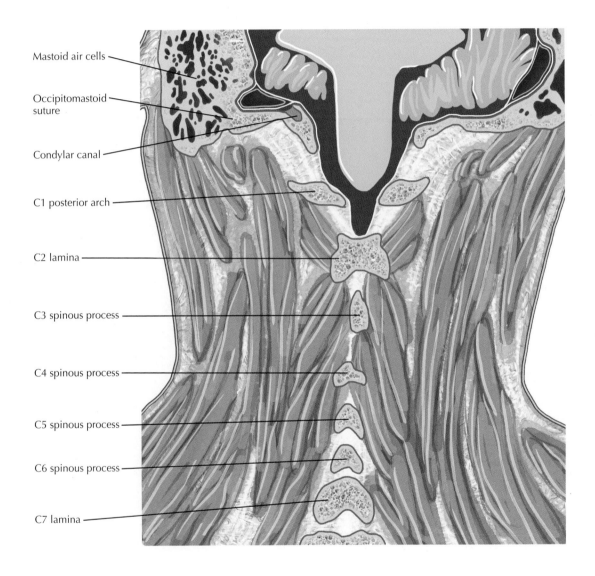

Mastoid air cells

Occipitomastoid suture

Condylar canal

C1 posterior arch

C2 lamina

C3 spinous process

C4 spinous process

C5 spinous process

C6 spinous process

C7 lamina

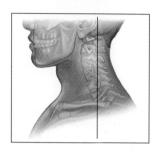

Mastoid air cells

Occipitomastoid suture

Condylar canal

C1 posterior arch

C2 lamina

C3 spinous process

C4 spinous process

C5 spinous process

C6 spinous process

C7 lamina

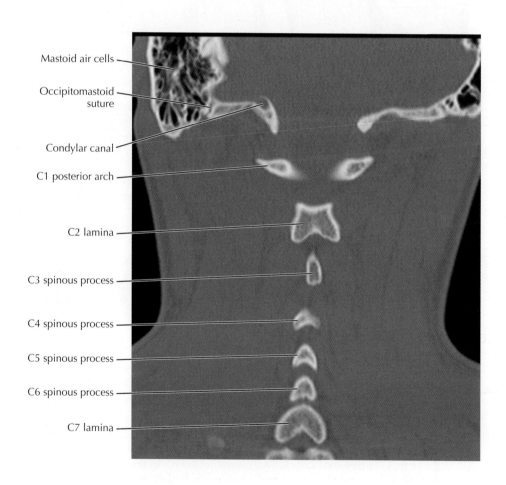

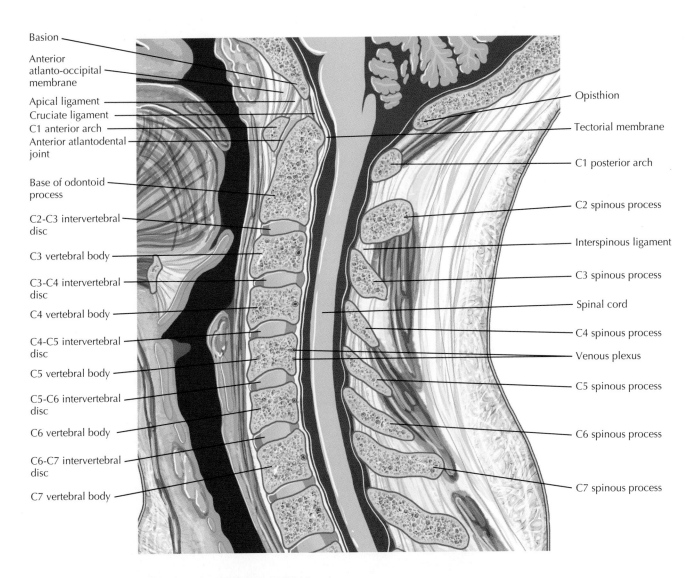

Basion
Anterior atlanto-occipital membrane
Apical ligament
Cruciate ligament
C1 anterior arch
Anterior atlantodental joint
Base of odontoid process
C2-C3 intervertebral disc
C3 vertebral body
C3-C4 intervertebral disc
C4 vertebral body
C4-C5 intervertebral disc
C5 vertebral body
C5-C6 intervertebral disc
C6 vertebral body
C6-C7 intervertebral disc
C7 vertebral body

Opisthion
Tectorial membrane
C1 posterior arch
C2 spinous process
Interspinous ligament
C3 spinous process
Spinal cord
C4 spinous process
Venous plexus
C5 spinous process
C6 spinous process
C7 spinous process

IMAGING TECHNIQUE CONSIDERATION

The midline sagittal cervical image is arguably the most important image in spinal imaging. Injury to the cord above C3 can lead to respiratory loss and death. The diaphragms are innervated by C3, C4, and C5 ("C3, 4, 5 keep the diaphragm alive"), and cord injury below this level can lead to quadriplegia.

The most palpable spinous process is usually that of C7. Recall that there are eight cervical nerves, so in the cervical region, a nerve root exits just above its corresponding vertebral body (e.g., C7 nerve root exits C6-C7 neural foramen). In the thoracic region, where there are typically 12 exiting nerve roots and 12 vertebral bodies, and in the lumbar region, where there are typically five lumbar vertebral bodies and five exiting nerve roots, the nerve root exits just below the corresponding vertebral body (e.g., L5 nerve root exits at L5-S1 neural foramen). Considerable variation exists, however, such as a lumbarized first sacral (S1) vertebral body or an accessory rib; thus, with any spinal imaging analysis, the examiner should declare the numbering of levels used. The best method is to count down from C1.

Note the clear view of the aerodigestive tract lumen, which should always be assessed. Narrowing of the lumen from prevertebral soft tissue swelling may indicate cervical spine injury. Above C4, the prevertebral soft tissue should be not more than one-third the distance of the anterior-to-posterior measurement of the vertebral body. The nasopharynx is somewhat bulky in this case because of normally prominent adenoidal tissue in this relatively young patient, with little cervical degenerative disc disease.

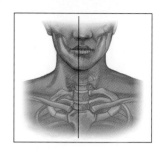

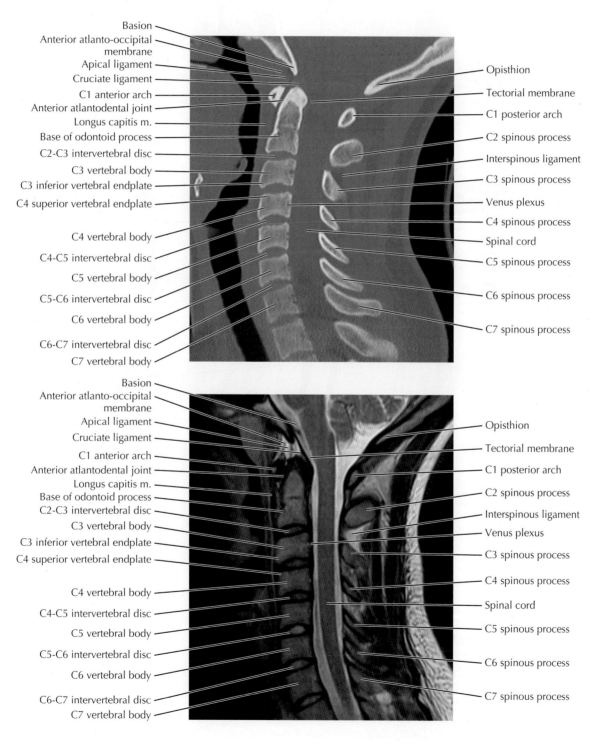

Basion
Anterior atlanto-occipital membrane
Apical ligament
Cruciate ligament
C1 anterior arch
Anterior atlantodental joint
Longus capitis m.
Base of odontoid process
C2-C3 intervertebral disc
C3 vertebral body
C3 inferior vertebral endplate
C4 superior vertebral endplate
C4 vertebral body
C4-C5 intervertebral disc
C5 vertebral body
C5-C6 intervertebral disc
C6 vertebral body
C6-C7 intervertebral disc
C7 vertebral body

Opisthion
Tectorial membrane
C1 posterior arch
C2 spinous process
Interspinous ligament
C3 spinous process
Venus plexus
C4 spinous process
Spinal cord
C5 spinous process
C6 spinous process
C7 spinous process

Basion
Anterior atlanto-occipital membrane
Apical ligament
Cruciate ligament
C1 anterior arch
Anterior atlantodental joint
Longus capitis m.
Base of odontoid process
C2-C3 intervertebral disc
C3 vertebral body
C3 inferior vertebral endplate
C4 superior vertebral endplate
C4 vertebral body
C4-C5 intervertebral disc
C5 vertebral body
C5-C6 intervertebral disc
C6 vertebral body
C6-C7 intervertebral disc
C7 vertebral body

Opisthion
Tectorial membrane
C1 posterior arch
C2 spinous process
Interspinous ligament
Venus plexus
C3 spinous process
C4 spinous process
Spinal cord
C5 spinous process
C6 spinous process
C7 spinous process

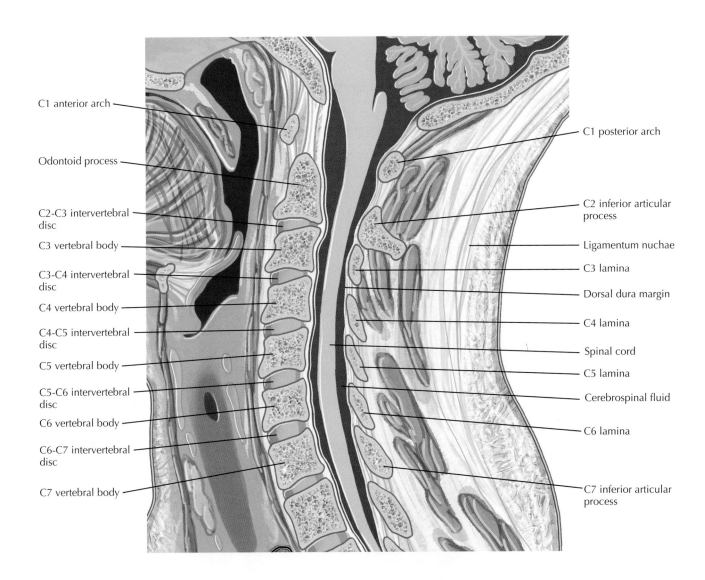

C1 anterior arch

Odontoid process

C2-C3 intervertebral disc

C3 vertebral body

C3-C4 intervertebral disc

C4 vertebral body

C4-C5 intervertebral disc

C5 vertebral body

C5-C6 intervertebral disc

C6 vertebral body

C6-C7 intervertebral disc

C7 vertebral body

C1 posterior arch

C2 inferior articular process

Ligamentum nuchae

C3 lamina

Dorsal dura margin

C4 lamina

Spinal cord

C5 lamina

Cerebrospinal fluid

C6 lamina

C7 inferior articular process

NORMAL ANATOMY

Note the slight spurring of the endplates of the uncovertebral joint at the posterolateral edge of the C2-C3 disc space. This is due to normal aging.

Although generally not present at the level of the foramen magnum, the cerebellar tonsils, if seen, should not protrude more than 5 mm below this foramen best assessed on sagittal images. Tonsils protruding more than 5 mm indicate a Chiari malformation or, more seriously, mass effect in the intracranial vault, causing the cerebellar tonsils to herniate downward.

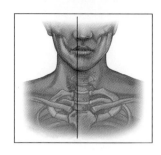

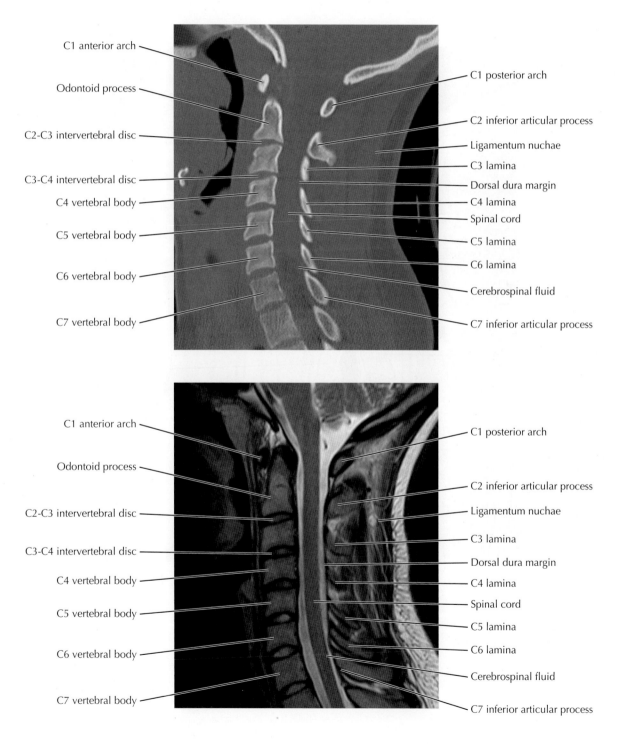

C1 anterior arch

Odontoid process

C2-C3 intervertebral disc

C3-C4 intervertebral disc

C4 vertebral body

C5 vertebral body

C6 vertebral body

C7 vertebral body

C1 posterior arch

C2 inferior articular process

Ligamentum nuchae

C3 lamina

Dorsal dura margin

C4 lamina

Spinal cord

C5 lamina

C6 lamina

Cerebrospinal fluid

C7 inferior articular process

C1 anterior arch

Odontoid process

C2-C3 intervertebral disc

C3-C4 intervertebral disc

C4 vertebral body

C5 vertebral body

C6 vertebral body

C7 vertebral body

C1 posterior arch

C2 inferior articular process

Ligamentum nuchae

C3 lamina

Dorsal dura margin

C4 lamina

Spinal cord

C5 lamina

C6 lamina

Cerebrospinal fluid

C7 inferior articular process

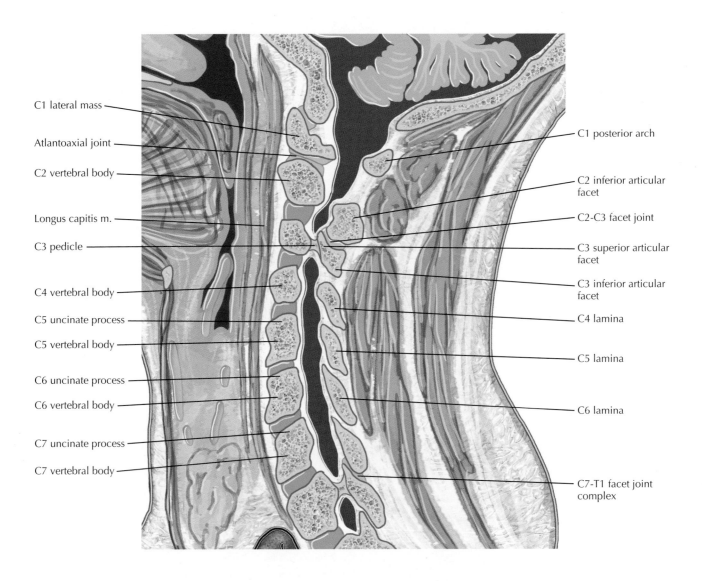

C1 lateral mass

Atlantoaxial joint

C2 vertebral body

Longus capitis m.

C3 pedicle

C4 vertebral body

C5 uncinate process

C5 vertebral body

C6 uncinate process

C6 vertebral body

C7 uncinate process

C7 vertebral body

C1 posterior arch

C2 inferior articular facet

C2-C3 facet joint

C3 superior articular facet

C3 inferior articular facet

C4 lamina

C5 lamina

C6 lamina

C7-T1 facet joint complex

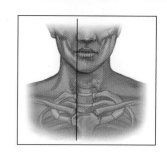

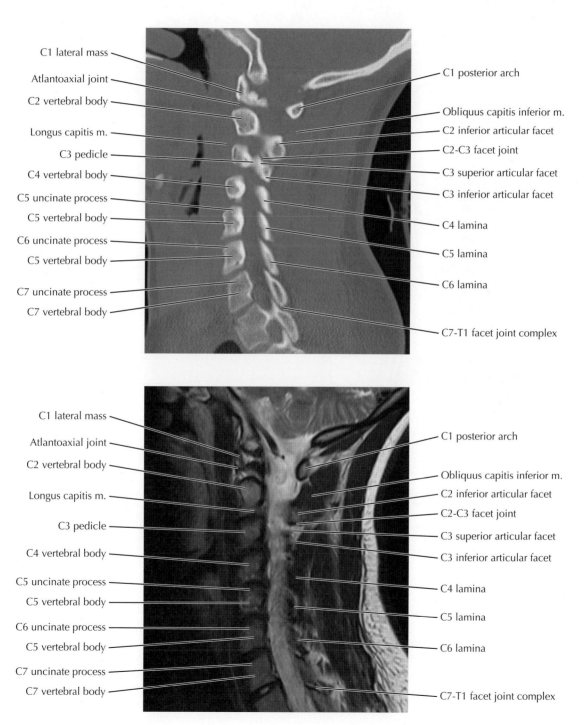

C1 lateral mass — C1 posterior arch

Atlantoaxial joint — Obliquus capitis inferior m.

C2 vertebral body — C2 inferior articular facet

Longus capitis m. — C2-C3 facet joint

C3 pedicle — C3 superior articular facet

C4 vertebral body — C3 inferior articular facet

C5 uncinate process — C4 lamina

C5 vertebral body — C5 lamina

C6 uncinate process — C6 lamina

C5 vertebral body

C7 uncinate process — C7-T1 facet joint complex

C7 vertebral body

C1 lateral mass — C1 posterior arch

Atlantoaxial joint — Obliquus capitis inferior m.

C2 vertebral body — C2 inferior articular facet

Longus capitis m. — C2-C3 facet joint

C3 pedicle — C3 superior articular facet

C4 vertebral body — C3 inferior articular facet

C5 uncinate process — C4 lamina

C5 vertebral body — C5 lamina

C6 uncinate process — C6 lamina

C5 vertebral body

C7 uncinate process

C7 vertebral body — C7-T1 facet joint complex

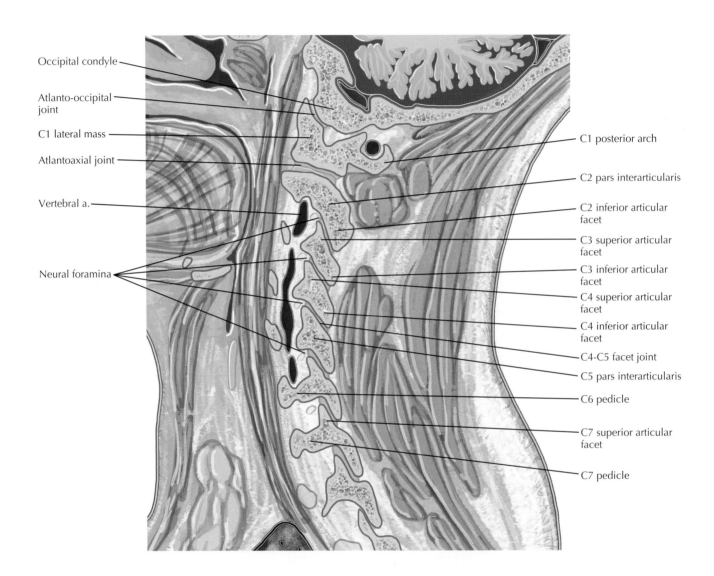

Occipital condyle

Atlanto-occipital joint

C1 lateral mass

Atlantoaxial joint

Vertebral a.

Neural foramina

C1 posterior arch

C2 pars interarticularis

C2 inferior articular facet

C3 superior articular facet

C3 inferior articular facet

C4 superior articular facet

C4 inferior articular facet

C4-C5 facet joint

C5 pars interarticularis

C6 pedicle

C7 superior articular facet

C7 pedicle

NORMAL ANATOMY

The parasagittal CT (top) and MR (bottom) images in Cervical Spine Sagittal 4 demonstrate the normal relationship of the occipital condyle and atlas (C1) arch, as well as the atlantoaxial joint and cervical facet joints. The foramina are somewhat difficult to assess on these images compared with lumbar imaging because of the smaller nature of the cervical vertebra and confounding vertebral artery foramina. Narrowing of the cervical foramina is therefore often better seen on axial imaging.

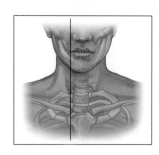

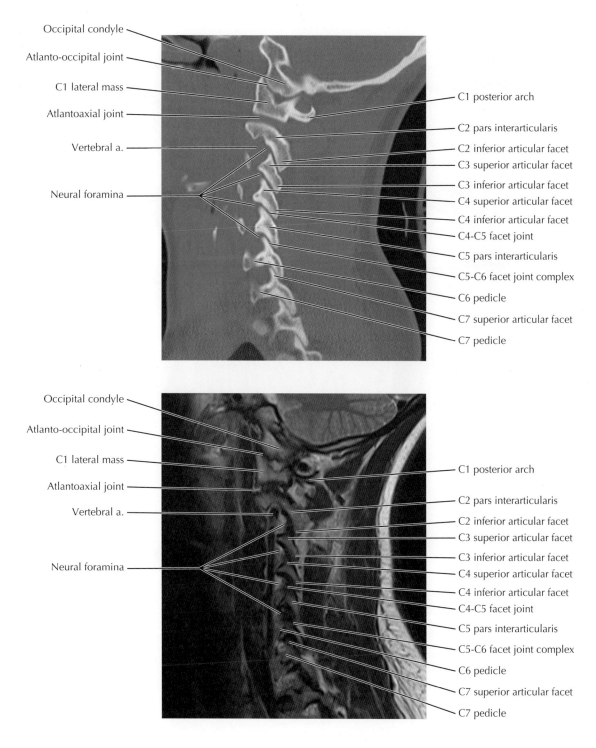

Occipital condyle

Atlanto-occipital joint

C1 lateral mass

Atlantoaxial joint

Vertebral a.

Neural foramina

C1 posterior arch

C2 pars interarticularis

C2 inferior articular facet

C3 superior articular facet

C3 inferior articular facet

C4 superior articular facet

C4 inferior articular facet

C4-C5 facet joint

C5 pars interarticularis

C5-C6 facet joint complex

C6 pedicle

C7 superior articular facet

C7 pedicle

Occipital condyle

Atlanto-occipital joint

C1 lateral mass

Atlantoaxial joint

Vertebral a.

Neural foramina

C1 posterior arch

C2 pars interarticularis

C2 inferior articular facet

C3 superior articular facet

C3 inferior articular facet

C4 superior articular facet

C4 inferior articular facet

C4-C5 facet joint

C5 pars interarticularis

C5-C6 facet joint complex

C6 pedicle

C7 superior articular facet

C7 pedicle

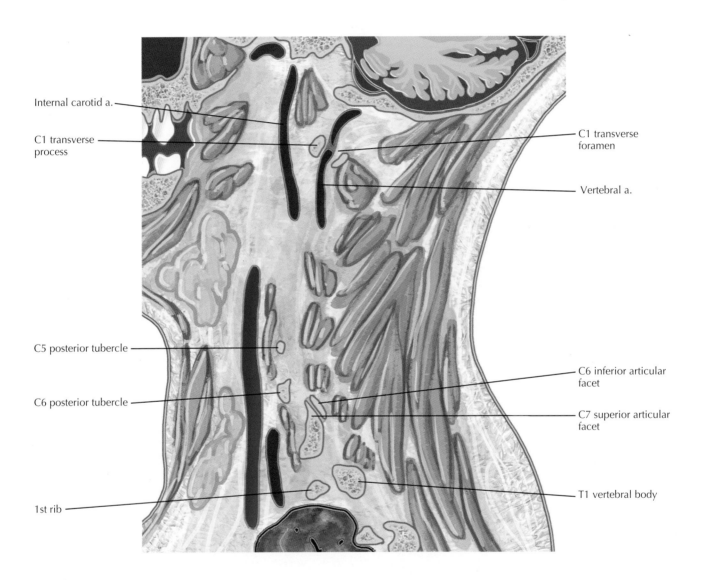

Internal carotid a.

C1 transverse
process

C1 transverse
foramen

Vertebral a.

C5 posterior tubercle

C6 inferior articular
facet

C6 posterior tubercle

C7 superior articular
facet

1st rib

T1 vertebral body

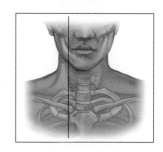

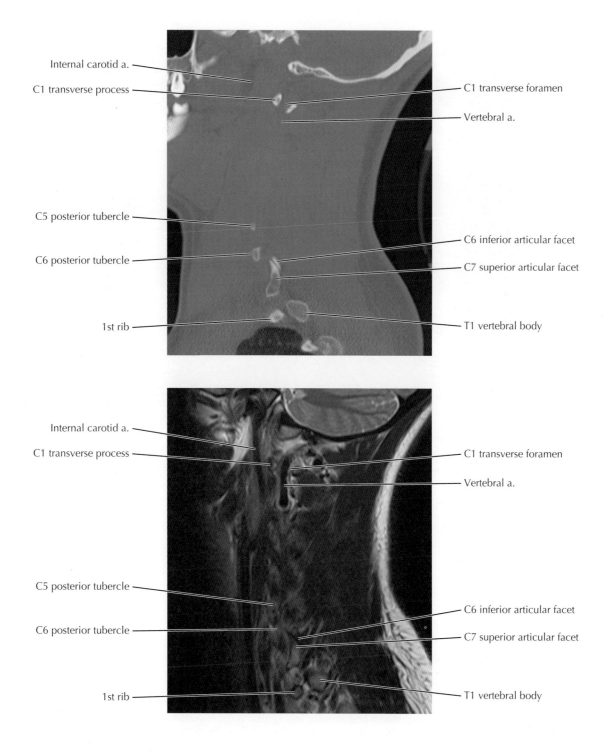

Internal carotid a.

C1 transverse process

C1 transverse foramen

Vertebral a.

C5 posterior tubercle

C6 inferior articular facet

C6 posterior tubercle

C7 superior articular facet

1st rib

T1 vertebral body

Internal carotid a.

C1 transverse process

C1 transverse foramen

Vertebral a.

C5 posterior tubercle

C6 inferior articular facet

C6 posterior tubercle

C7 superior articular facet

1st rib

T1 vertebral body

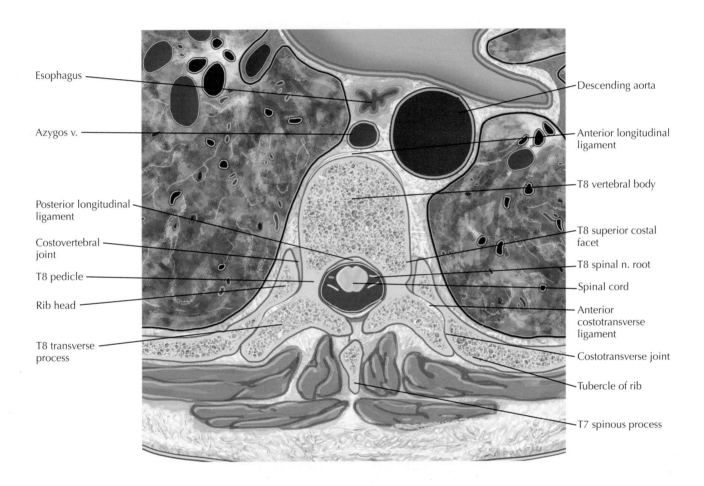

Esophagus

Azygos v.

Posterior longitudinal ligament

Costovertebral joint

T8 pedicle

Rib head

T8 transverse process

Descending aorta

Anterior longitudinal ligament

T8 vertebral body

T8 superior costal facet

T8 spinal n. root

Spinal cord

Anterior costotransverse ligament

Costotransverse joint

Tubercle of rib

T7 spinous process

IMAGING TECHNIQUE CONSIDERATION

Note that the Thoracic Spine Axial 1 MR image (bottom) is a T2-weighted sequence (CSF is bright) with the now-routine "turbo" or fast spin-echo technique (fat is bright). The thoracic vertebrae are larger and require less spatial resolution than in the cervical region. Unlike the cervical region from the third (C3) through seventh (C7) cervical vertebrae, there are no uncovertebral joints in the thoracic region, but instead costovertebral junctions.

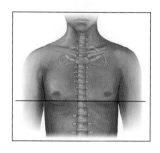

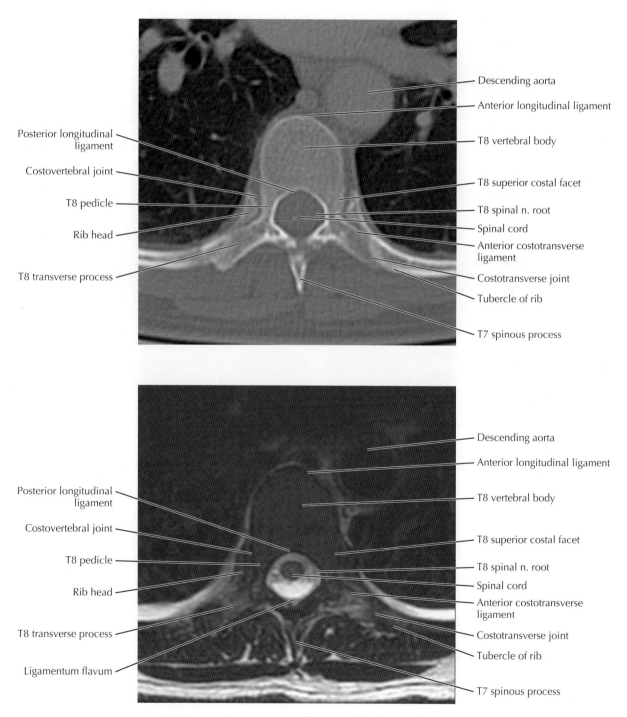

Posterior longitudinal ligament

Costovertebral joint

T8 pedicle

Rib head

T8 transverse process

Descending aorta

Anterior longitudinal ligament

T8 vertebral body

T8 superior costal facet

T8 spinal n. root

Spinal cord

Anterior costotransverse ligament

Costotransverse joint

Tubercle of rib

T7 spinous process

Posterior longitudinal ligament

Costovertebral joint

T8 pedicle

Rib head

T8 transverse process

Ligamentum flavum

Descending aorta

Anterior longitudinal ligament

T8 vertebral body

T8 superior costal facet

T8 spinal n. root

Spinal cord

Anterior costotransverse ligament

Costotransverse joint

Tubercle of rib

T7 spinous process

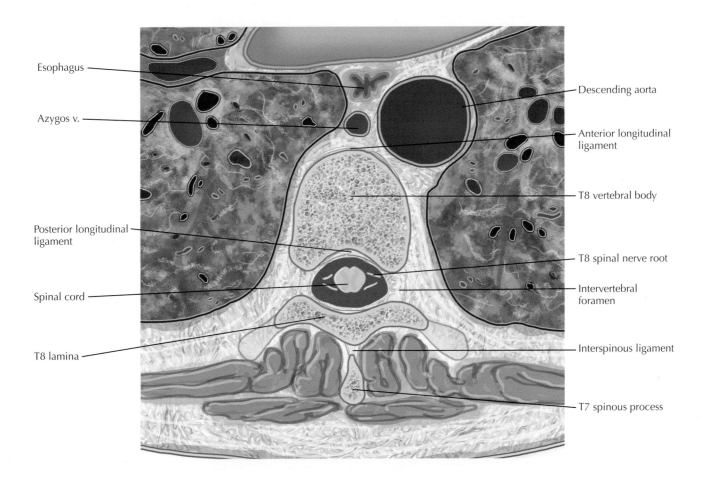

Esophagus

Azygos v.

Posterior longitudinal ligament

Spinal cord

T8 lamina

Descending aorta

Anterior longitudinal ligament

T8 vertebral body

T8 spinal nerve root

Intervertebral foramen

Interspinous ligament

T7 spinous process

NORMAL ANATOMY

The spinal artery of Adamkiewicz, the major blood supply to the thoracic and lumbar portions of the spinal cord, typically arises from the left T10 intercostal artery and enters the left T10-T11 neural foramen before making a hairpin turn on the anterior surface of the cord. In two thirds of cases, the artery will arise from the same side as the descending aorta, and as a variant arise several levels above or below T10 in a bell curve distribution.

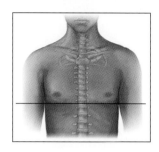

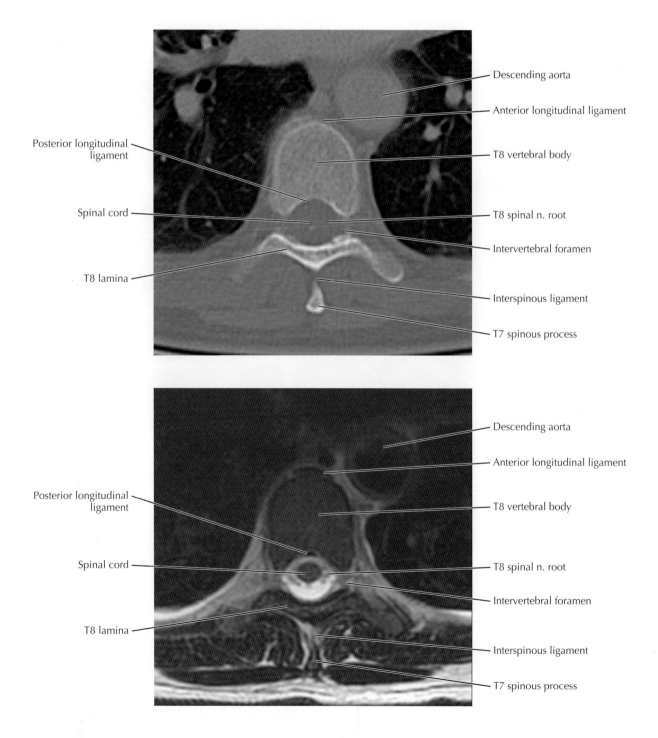

Descending aorta

Anterior longitudinal ligament

Posterior longitudinal ligament

T8 vertebral body

Spinal cord

T8 spinal n. root

Intervertebral foramen

T8 lamina

Interspinous ligament

T7 spinous process

Descending aorta

Anterior longitudinal ligament

Posterior longitudinal ligament

T8 vertebral body

Spinal cord

T8 spinal n. root

Intervertebral foramen

T8 lamina

Interspinous ligament

T7 spinous process

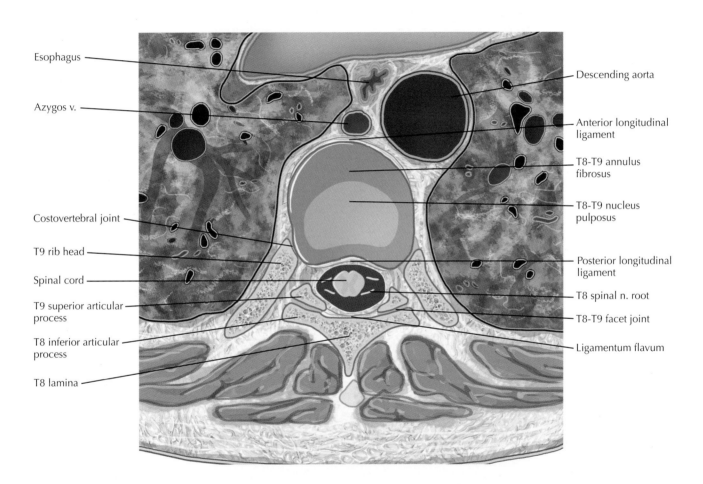

Esophagus

Azygos v.

Costovertebral joint

T9 rib head

Spinal cord

T9 superior articular process

T8 inferior articular process

T8 lamina

Descending aorta

Anterior longitudinal ligament

T8-T9 annulus fibrosus

T8-T9 nucleus pulposus

Posterior longitudinal ligament

T8 spinal n. root

T8-T9 facet joint

Ligamentum flavum

NORMAL ANATOMY

Note the facet joint, which is composed of the superior articular process of the vertebra below, is anterior to the inferior articular process of the vertebra above.

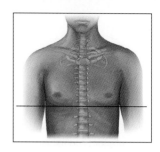

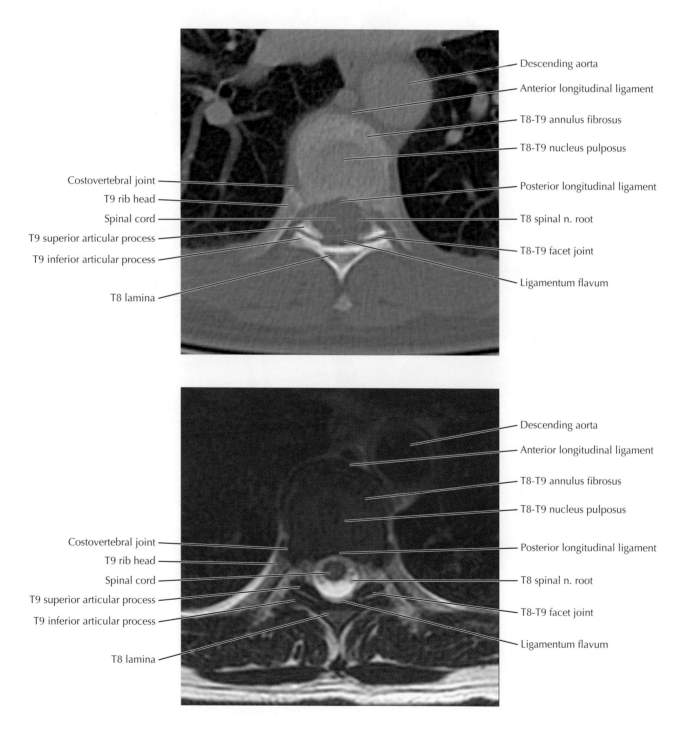

Descending aorta

Anterior longitudinal ligament

T8-T9 annulus fibrosus

T8-T9 nucleus pulposus

Costovertebral joint

T9 rib head

Posterior longitudinal ligament

Spinal cord

T8 spinal n. root

T9 superior articular process

T9 inferior articular process

T8-T9 facet joint

Ligamentum flavum

T8 lamina

Descending aorta

Anterior longitudinal ligament

T8-T9 annulus fibrosus

T8-T9 nucleus pulposus

Costovertebral joint

T9 rib head

Posterior longitudinal ligament

Spinal cord

T8 spinal n. root

T9 superior articular process

T9 inferior articular process

T8-T9 facet joint

Ligamentum flavum

T8 lamina

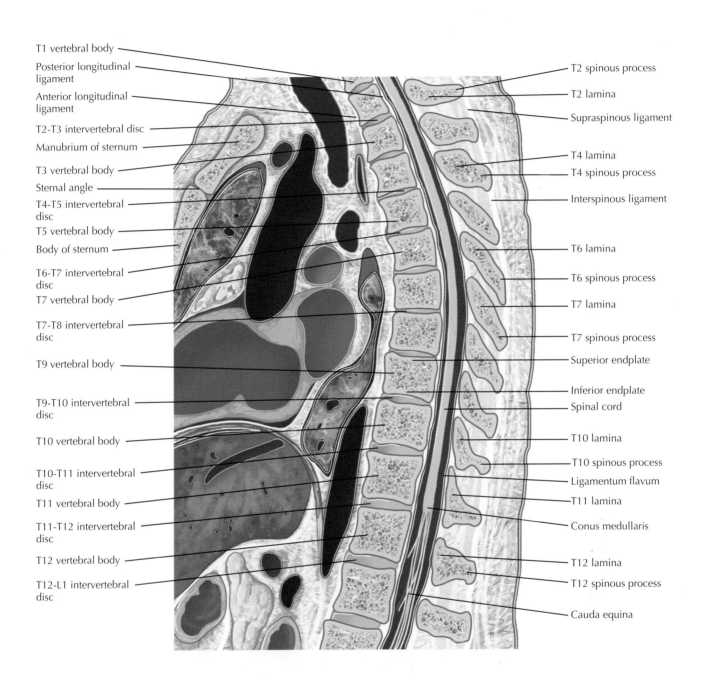

T1 vertebral body

Posterior longitudinal ligament

Anterior longitudinal ligament

T2-T3 intervertebral disc

Manubrium of sternum

T3 vertebral body

Sternal angle

T4-T5 intervertebral disc

T5 vertebral body

Body of sternum

T6-T7 intervertebral disc

T7 vertebral body

T7-T8 intervertebral disc

T9 vertebral body

T9-T10 intervertebral disc

T10 vertebral body

T10-T11 intervertebral disc

T11 vertebral body

T11-T12 intervertebral disc

T12 vertebral body

T12-L1 intervertebral disc

T2 spinous process

T2 lamina

Supraspinous ligament

T4 lamina

T4 spinous process

Interspinous ligament

T6 lamina

T6 spinous process

T7 lamina

T7 spinous process

Superior endplate

Inferior endplate

Spinal cord

T10 lamina

T10 spinous process

Ligamentum flavum

T11 lamina

Conus medullaris

T12 lamina

T12 spinous process

Cauda equina

NORMAL ANATOMY

There is a normal anterior-to-posterior expansion of the spinal cord near the conus, just as there is a normal cervical cord expansion where the brachial plexus nerve roots arise. This should not be confused with expansion from an intramedullary lesion.

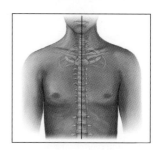

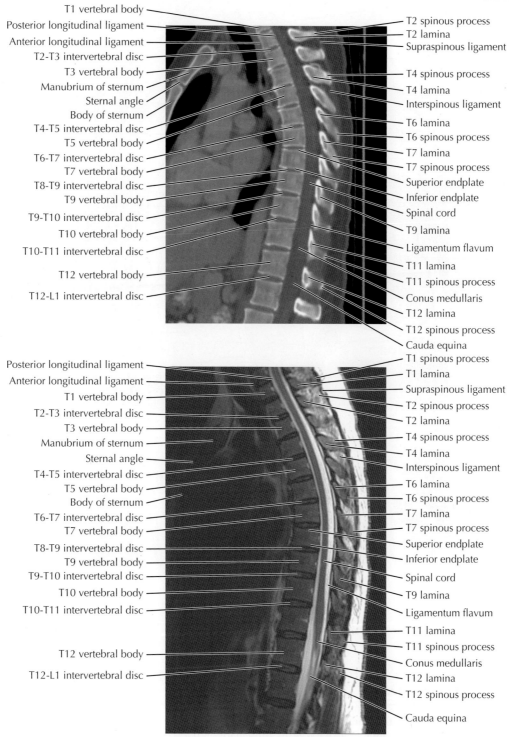

T1 vertebral body

Posterior longitudinal ligament

Anterior longitudinal ligament

T2-T3 intervertebral disc

T3 vertebral body

Manubrium of sternum

Sternal angle

Body of sternum

T4-T5 intervertebral disc

T5 vertebral body

T6-T7 intervertebral disc

T7 vertebral body

T8-T9 intervertebral disc

T9 vertebral body

T9-T10 intervertebral disc

T10 vertebral body

T10-T11 intervertebral disc

T12 vertebral body

T12-L1 intervertebral disc

T2 spinous process

T2 lamina

Supraspinous ligament

T4 spinous process

T4 lamina

Interspinous ligament

T6 lamina

T6 spinous process

T7 lamina

T7 spinous process

Superior endplate

Inferior endplate

Spinal cord

T9 lamina

Ligamentum flavum

T11 lamina

T11 spinous process

Conus medullaris

T12 lamina

T12 spinous process

Cauda equina

Posterior longitudinal ligament

Anterior longitudinal ligament

T1 vertebral body

T2-T3 intervertebral disc

T3 vertebral body

Manubrium of sternum

Sternal angle

T4-T5 intervertebral disc

T5 vertebral body

Body of sternum

T6-T7 intervertebral disc

T7 vertebral body

T8-T9 intervertebral disc

T9 vertebral body

T9-T10 intervertebral disc

T10 vertebral body

T10-T11 intervertebral disc

T12 vertebral body

T12-L1 intervertebral disc

T1 spinous process

T1 lamina

Supraspinous ligament

T2 spinous process

T2 lamina

T4 spinous process

T4 lamina

Interspinous ligament

T6 lamina

T6 spinous process

T7 lamina

T7 spinous process

Superior endplate

Inferior endplate

Spinal cord

T9 lamina

Ligamentum flavum

T11 lamina

T11 spinous process

Conus medullaris

T12 lamina

T12 spinous process

Cauda equina

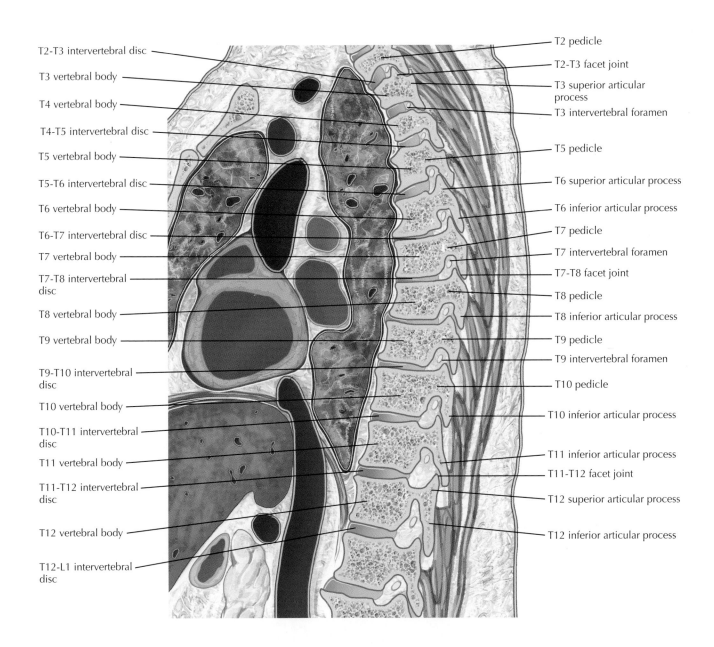

T2-T3 intervertebral disc

T3 vertebral body

T4 vertebral body

T4-T5 intervertebral disc

T5 vertebral body

T5-T6 intervertebral disc

T6 vertebral body

T6-T7 intervertebral disc

T7 vertebral body

T7-T8 intervertebral disc

T8 vertebral body

T9 vertebral body

T9-T10 intervertebral disc

T10 vertebral body

T10-T11 intervertebral disc

T11 vertebral body

T11-T12 intervertebral disc

T12 vertebral body

T12-L1 intervertebral disc

T2 pedicle

T2-T3 facet joint

T3 superior articular process

T3 intervertebral foramen

T5 pedicle

T6 superior articular process

T6 inferior articular process

T7 pedicle

T7 intervertebral foramen

T7-T8 facet joint

T8 pedicle

T8 inferior articular process

T9 pedicle

T9 intervertebral foramen

T10 pedicle

T10 inferior articular process

T11 inferior articular process

T11-T12 facet joint

T12 superior articular process

T12 inferior articular process

NORMAL ANATOMY

Note that the thoracic vertebral anatomy is larger than the cervical vertebral anatomy, making the foramina much easier to appreciate on parasagittal imaging, along with the absence of the confounding vertebral foramina.

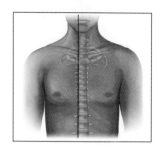

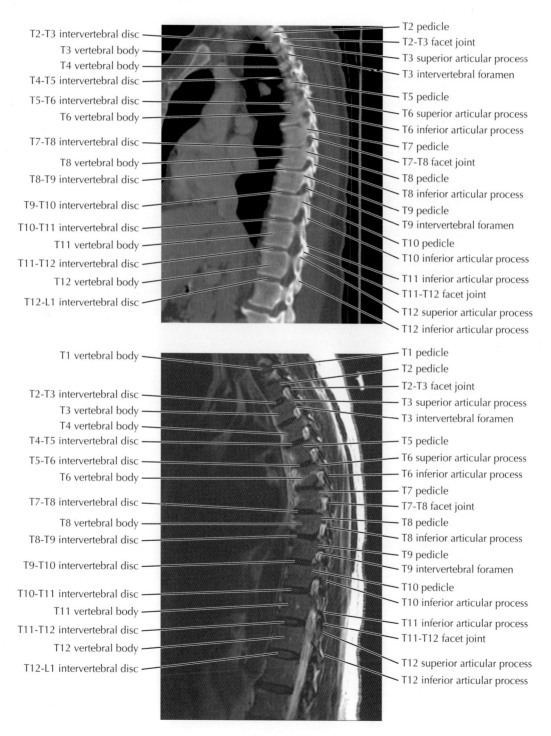

T2-T3 intervertebral disc —
T3 vertebral body —
T4 vertebral body —
T4-T5 intervertebral disc —
T5-T6 intervertebral disc —
T6 vertebral body —
T7-T8 intervertebral disc —
T8 vertebral body —
T8-T9 intervertebral disc —
T9-T10 intervertebral disc —
T10-T11 intervertebral disc —
T11 vertebral body —
T11-T12 intervertebral disc —
T12 vertebral body —
T12-L1 intervertebral disc —

— T2 pedicle
— T2-T3 facet joint
— T3 superior articular process
— T3 intervertebral foramen
— T5 pedicle
— T6 superior articular process
— T6 inferior articular process
— T7 pedicle
— T7-T8 facet joint
— T8 pedicle
— T8 inferior articular process
— T9 pedicle
— T9 intervertebral foramen
— T10 pedicle
— T10 inferior articular process
— T11 inferior articular process
— T11-T12 facet joint
— T12 superior articular process
— T12 inferior articular process

T1 vertebral body —
T2-T3 intervertebral disc —
T3 vertebral body —
T4 vertebral body —
T4-T5 intervertebral disc —
T5-T6 intervertebral disc —
T6 vertebral body —
T7-T8 intervertebral disc —
T8 vertebral body —
T8-T9 intervertebral disc —
T9-T10 intervertebral disc —
T10-T11 intervertebral disc —
T11 vertebral body —
T11-T12 intervertebral disc —
T12 vertebral body —
T12-L1 intervertebral disc —

— T1 pedicle
— T2 pedicle
— T2-T3 facet joint
— T3 superior articular process
— T3 intervertebral foramen
— T5 pedicle
— T6 superior articular process
— T6 inferior articular process
— T7 pedicle
— T7-T8 facet joint
— T8 pedicle
— T8 inferior articular process
— T9 pedicle
— T9 intervertebral foramen
— T10 pedicle
— T10 inferior articular process
— T11 inferior articular process
— T11-T12 facet joint
— T12 superior articular process
— T12 inferior articular process

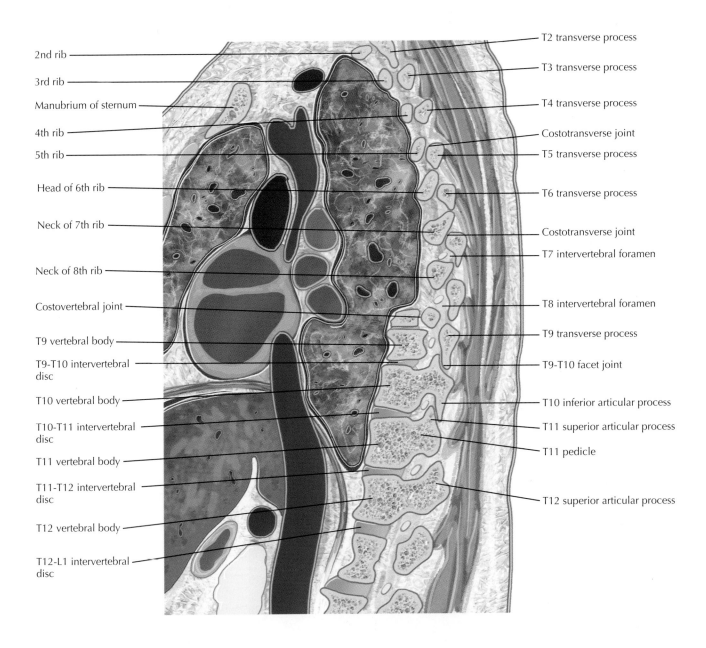

2nd rib

3rd rib

Manubrium of sternum

4th rib

5th rib

Head of 6th rib

Neck of 7th rib

Neck of 8th rib

Costovertebral joint

T9 vertebral body

T9-T10 intervertebral
disc

T10 vertebral body

T10-T11 intervertebral
disc

T11 vertebral body

T11-T12 intervertebral
disc

T12 vertebral body

T12-L1 intervertebral
disc

T2 transverse process

T3 transverse process

T4 transverse process

Costotransverse joint

T5 transverse process

T6 transverse process

Costotransverse joint

T7 intervertebral foramen

T8 intervertebral foramen

T9 transverse process

T9-T10 facet joint

T10 inferior articular process

T11 superior articular process

T11 pedicle

T12 superior articular process

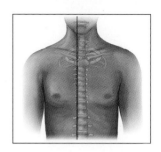

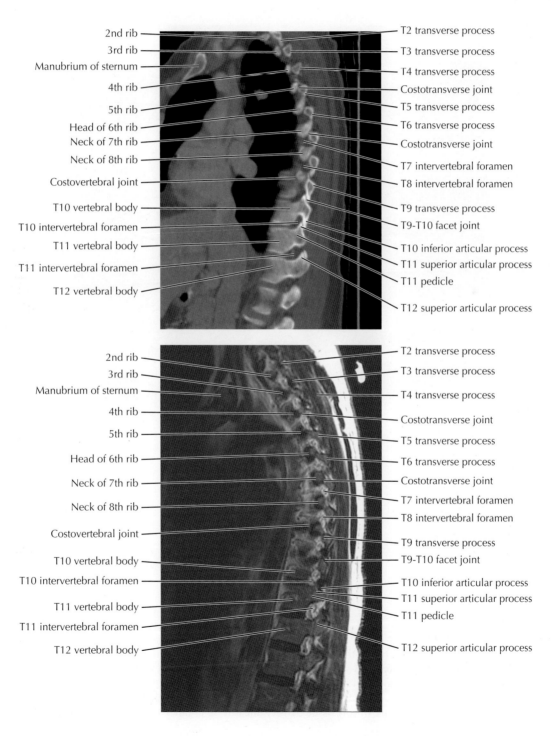

2nd rib — — T2 transverse process
3rd rib — — T3 transverse process
Manubrium of sternum — — T4 transverse process
4th rib — — Costotransverse joint
5th rib — — T5 transverse process
Head of 6th rib — — T6 transverse process
Neck of 7th rib — — Costotransverse joint
Neck of 8th rib — — T7 intervertebral foramen
— T8 intervertebral foramen
Costovertebral joint —
— T9 transverse process
T10 vertebral body — — T9-T10 facet joint
T10 intervertebral foramen —
— T10 inferior articular process
T11 vertebral body — — T11 superior articular process
T11 intervertebral foramen — — T11 pedicle
T12 vertebral body —
— T12 superior articular process

2nd rib — — T2 transverse process
3rd rib — — T3 transverse process
Manubrium of sternum — — T4 transverse process
4th rib — — Costotransverse joint
5th rib — — T5 transverse process
Head of 6th rib — — T6 transverse process
Neck of 7th rib — — Costotransverse joint
Neck of 8th rib — — T7 intervertebral foramen
— T8 intervertebral foramen
Costovertebral joint —
— T9 transverse process
T10 vertebral body — — T9-T10 facet joint
T10 intervertebral foramen — — T10 inferior articular process
— T11 superior articular process
T11 vertebral body — — T11 pedicle
T11 intervertebral foramen —
T12 vertebral body — — T12 superior articular process

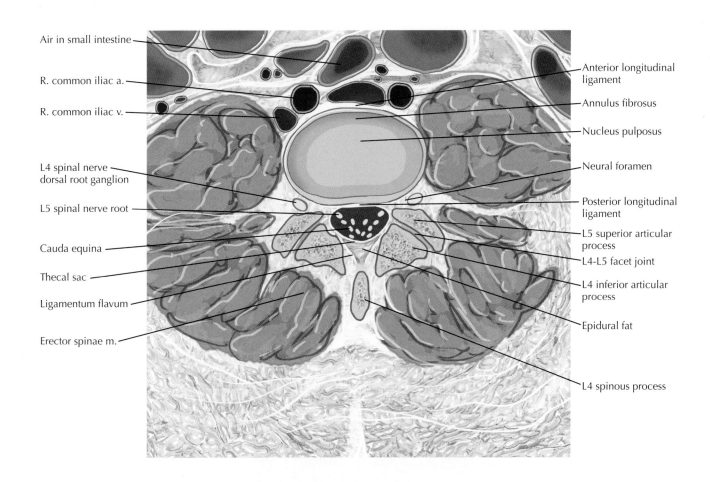

Air in small intestine

R. common iliac a.

R. common iliac v.

L4 spinal nerve dorsal root ganglion

L5 spinal nerve root

Cauda equina

Thecal sac

Ligamentum flavum

Erector spinae m.

Anterior longitudinal ligament

Annulus fibrosus

Nucleus pulposus

Neural foramen

Posterior longitudinal ligament

L5 superior articular process

L4-L5 facet joint

L4 inferior articular process

Epidural fat

L4 spinous process

NORMAL ANATOMY

It is easier to see the triangle of posterior epidural fat on the CT image (top) than on the turbo T2-weighted MR sequence (bottom), where both fluid and fat are bright. Fat has a density of about 10 to −50 Hounsfield units (HU), the scale used to measure density on CT, and appears dark gray, whereas the laterally adjacent right and left ligamentum flavum and spinal canal anteriorly are of soft tissue density, measuring about +40 HU.

This epidural fat is an important target for steroid injection in patients with lumbar degenerative disease and for anesthetic medication injection in pregnant patients during labor and delivery.

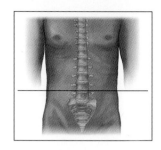

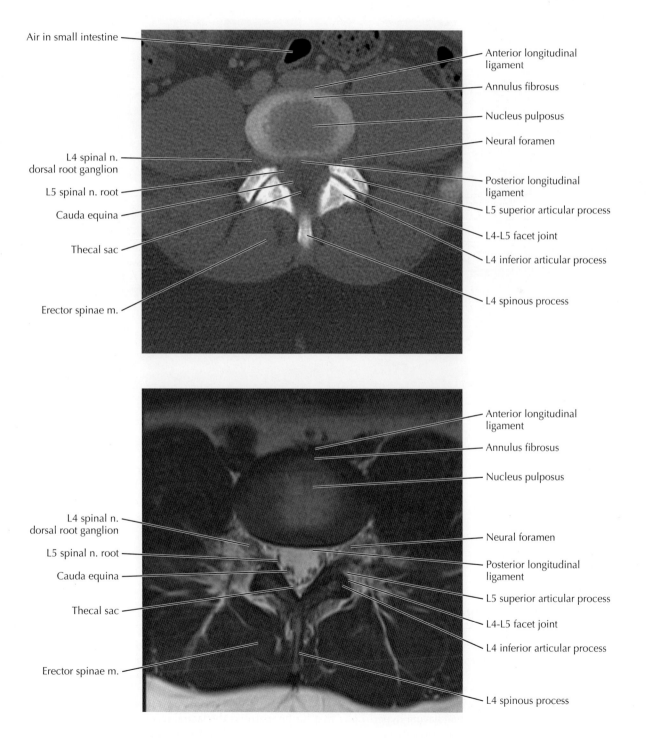

Air in small intestine

Anterior longitudinal ligament

Annulus fibrosus

Nucleus pulposus

Neural foramen

L4 spinal n. dorsal root ganglion

Posterior longitudinal ligament

L5 spinal n. root

L5 superior articular process

Cauda equina

L4-L5 facet joint

Thecal sac

L4 inferior articular process

L4 spinous process

Erector spinae m.

Anterior longitudinal ligament

Annulus fibrosus

Nucleus pulposus

L4 spinal n. dorsal root ganglion

Neural foramen

L5 spinal n. root

Posterior longitudinal ligament

Cauda equina

L5 superior articular process

Thecal sac

L4-L5 facet joint

L4 inferior articular process

Erector spinae m.

L4 spinous process

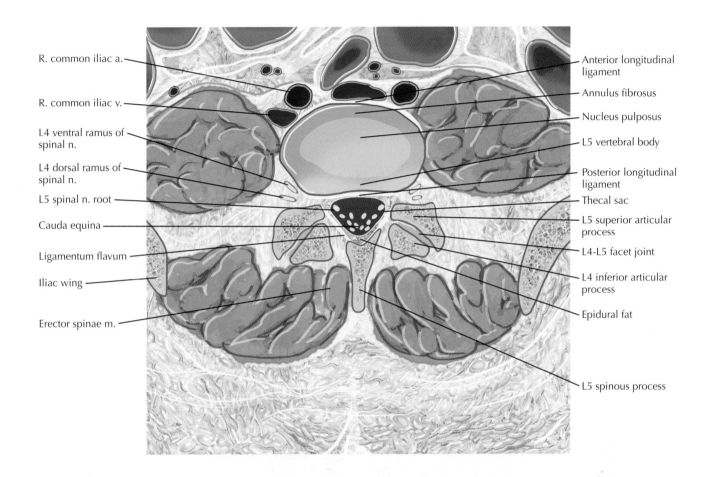

R. common iliac a.

R. common iliac v.

L4 ventral ramus of
spinal n.

L4 dorsal ramus of
spinal n.

L5 spinal n. root

Cauda equina

Ligamentum flavum

Iliac wing

Erector spinae m.

Anterior longitudinal
ligament

Annulus fibrosus

Nucleus pulposus

L5 vertebral body

Posterior longitudinal
ligament

Thecal sac

L5 superior articular
process

L4-L5 facet joint

L4 inferior articular
process

Epidural fat

L5 spinous process

PATHOLOGIC PROCESS

Below the pars of the second lumbar vertebra (L2), the conus gives rise to multiple nerves called the *cauda equina* (Latin, "horse's tail"). A relatively large disc herniation in the lumbar region may not result in significant neural symptoms because these cauda equina nerves may move out of the way, unlike the cord in the thoracic and cervical region. At the lateral aspect of the spinal canal, however, even a small disc protrusion may cause nerve impingement if there is ligamentum flavum hypertrophy that further narrows the lateral recess from posteriorly. With this lateral recess narrowing, the descending L5 nerve that has not yet exited the spinal canal would be impinged, by a lateral L4-5 disc herniation, not the L4 nerve root exiting the neural foramen.

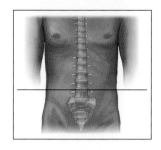

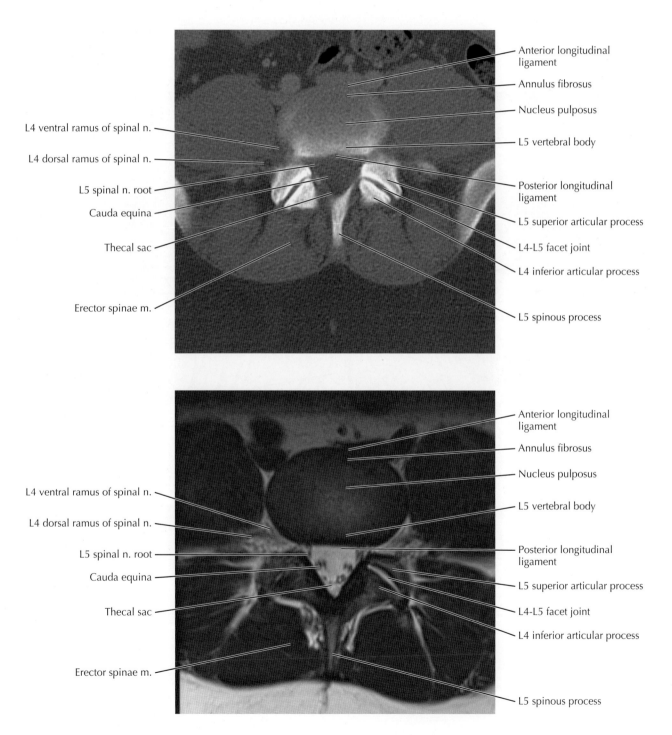

Anterior longitudinal ligament

Annulus fibrosus

Nucleus pulposus

L5 vertebral body

Posterior longitudinal ligament

L5 superior articular process

L4-L5 facet joint

L4 inferior articular process

L5 spinous process

L4 ventral ramus of spinal n.

L4 dorsal ramus of spinal n.

L5 spinal n. root

Cauda equina

Thecal sac

Erector spinae m.

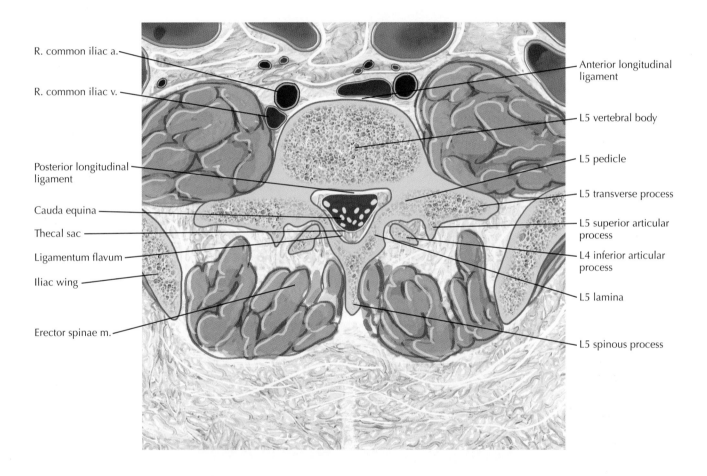

R. common iliac a.

R. common iliac v.

Posterior longitudinal ligament

Cauda equina

Thecal sac

Ligamentum flavum

Iliac wing

Erector spinae m.

Anterior longitudinal ligament

L5 vertebral body

L5 pedicle

L5 transverse process

L5 superior articular process

L4 inferior articular process

L5 lamina

L5 spinous process

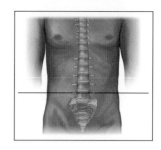

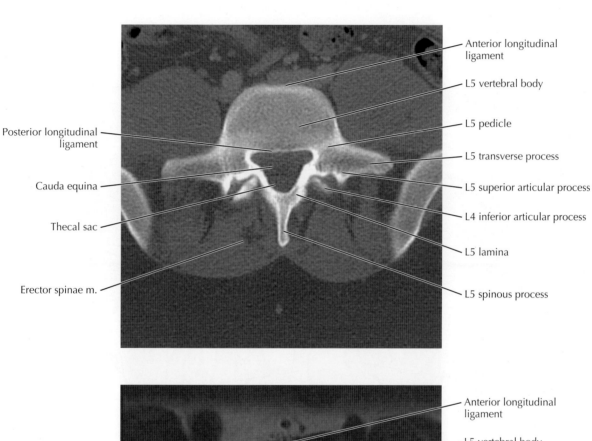

Anterior longitudinal ligament

L5 vertebral body

L5 pedicle

L5 transverse process

L5 superior articular process

L4 inferior articular process

L5 lamina

L5 spinous process

Posterior longitudinal ligament

Cauda equina

Thecal sac

Erector spinae m.

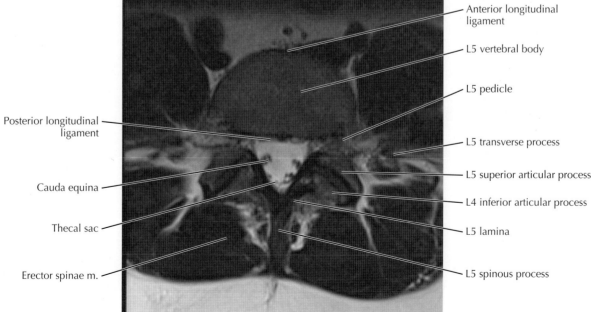

Anterior longitudinal ligament

L5 vertebral body

L5 pedicle

L5 transverse process

L5 superior articular process

L4 inferior articular process

L5 lamina

L5 spinous process

Posterior longitudinal ligament

Cauda equina

Thecal sac

Erector spinae m.

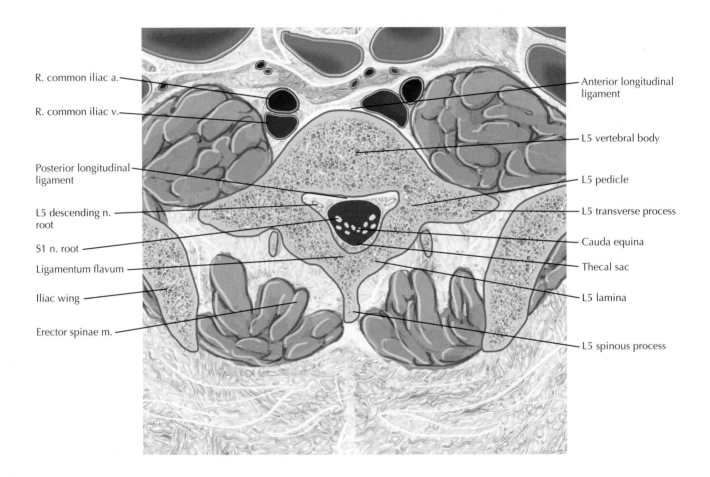

R. common iliac a.

R. common iliac v.

Posterior longitudinal ligament

L5 descending n. root

S1 n. root

Ligamentum flavum

Iliac wing

Erector spinae m.

Anterior longitudinal ligament

L5 vertebral body

L5 pedicle

L5 transverse process

Cauda equina

Thecal sac

L5 lamina

L5 spinous process

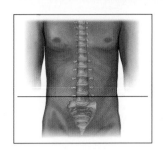

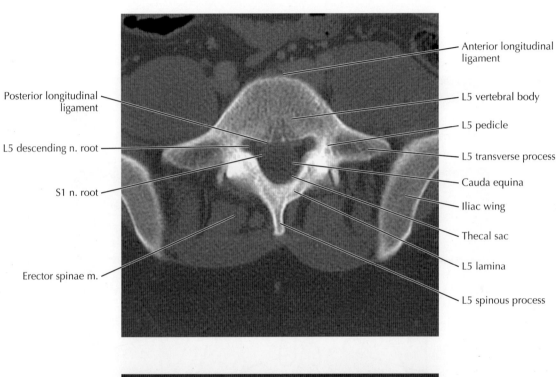

Posterior longitudinal ligament

L5 descending n. root

S1 n. root

Erector spinae m.

Anterior longitudinal ligament

L5 vertebral body

L5 pedicle

L5 transverse process

Cauda equina

Iliac wing

Thecal sac

L5 lamina

L5 spinous process

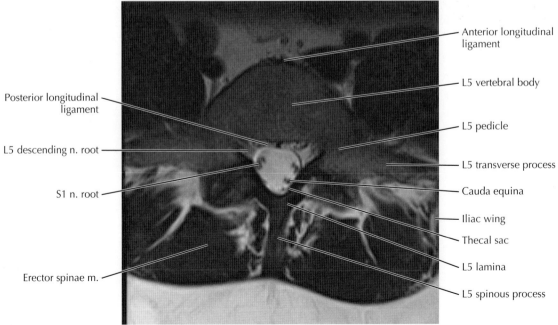

Posterior longitudinal ligament

L5 descending n. root

S1 n. root

Erector spinae m.

Anterior longitudinal ligament

L5 vertebral body

L5 pedicle

L5 transverse process

Cauda equina

Iliac wing

Thecal sac

L5 lamina

L5 spinous process

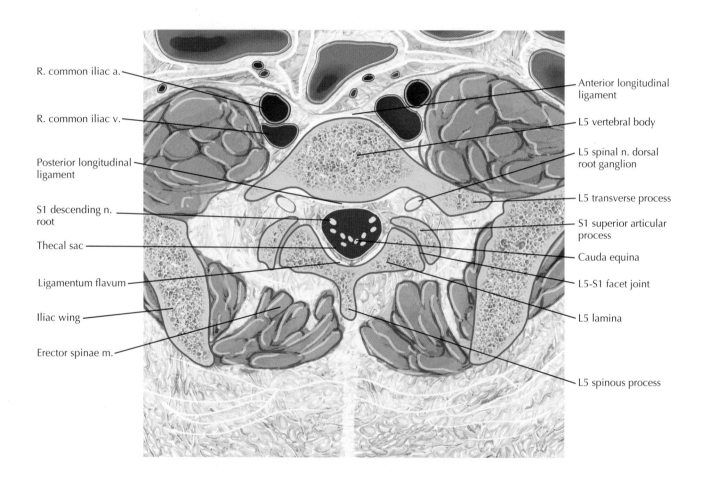

R. common iliac a.

R. common iliac v.

Posterior longitudinal ligament

S1 descending n. root

Thecal sac

Ligamentum flavum

Iliac wing

Erector spinae m.

Anterior longitudinal ligament

L5 vertebral body

L5 spinal n. dorsal root ganglion

L5 transverse process

S1 superior articular process

Cauda equina

L5-S1 facet joint

L5 lamina

L5 spinous process

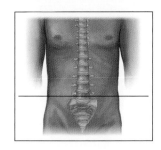

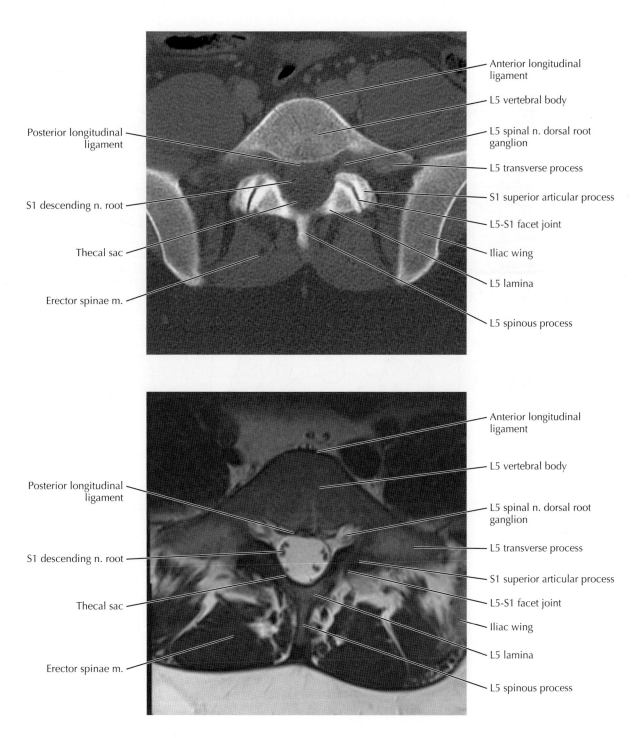

Anterior longitudinal ligament

L5 vertebral body

L5 spinal n. dorsal root ganglion

L5 transverse process

S1 superior articular process

L5-S1 facet joint

Iliac wing

L5 lamina

L5 spinous process

Posterior longitudinal ligament

S1 descending n. root

Thecal sac

Erector spinae m.

Anterior longitudinal ligament

L5 vertebral body

L5 spinal n. dorsal root ganglion

L5 transverse process

S1 superior articular process

L5-S1 facet joint

Iliac wing

L5 lamina

L5 spinous process

Posterior longitudinal ligament

S1 descending n. root

Thecal sac

Erector spinae m.

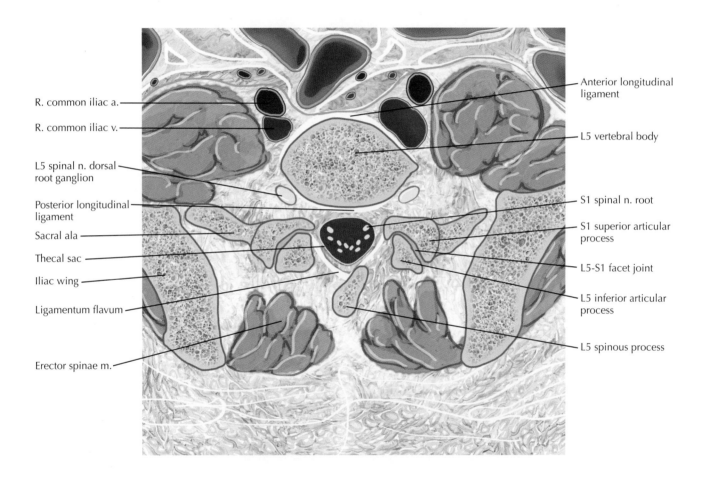

R. common iliac a.

R. common iliac v.

L5 spinal n. dorsal
root ganglion

Posterior longitudinal
ligament

Sacral ala

Thecal sac

Iliac wing

Ligamentum flavum

Erector spinae m.

Anterior longitudinal
ligament

L5 vertebral body

S1 spinal n. root

S1 superior articular
process

L5-S1 facet joint

L5 inferior articular
process

L5 spinous process

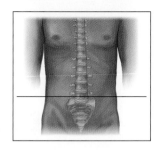

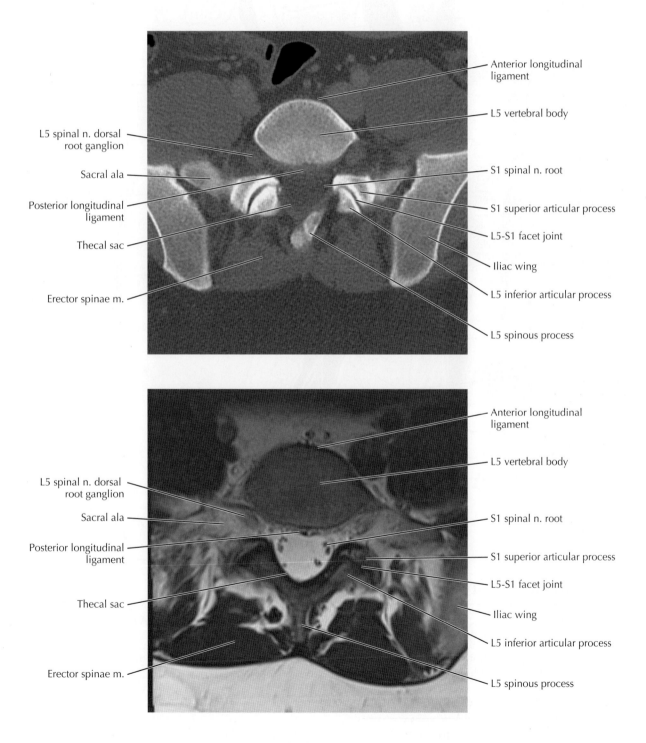

Anterior longitudinal ligament

L5 vertebral body

L5 spinal n. dorsal root ganglion

Sacral ala

Posterior longitudinal ligament

Thecal sac

Erector spinae m.

S1 spinal n. root

S1 superior articular process

L5-S1 facet joint

Iliac wing

L5 inferior articular process

L5 spinous process

Anterior longitudinal ligament

L5 vertebral body

L5 spinal n. dorsal root ganglion

Sacral ala

Posterior longitudinal ligament

Thecal sac

Erector spinae m.

S1 spinal n. root

S1 superior articular process

L5-S1 facet joint

Iliac wing

L5 inferior articular process

L5 spinous process

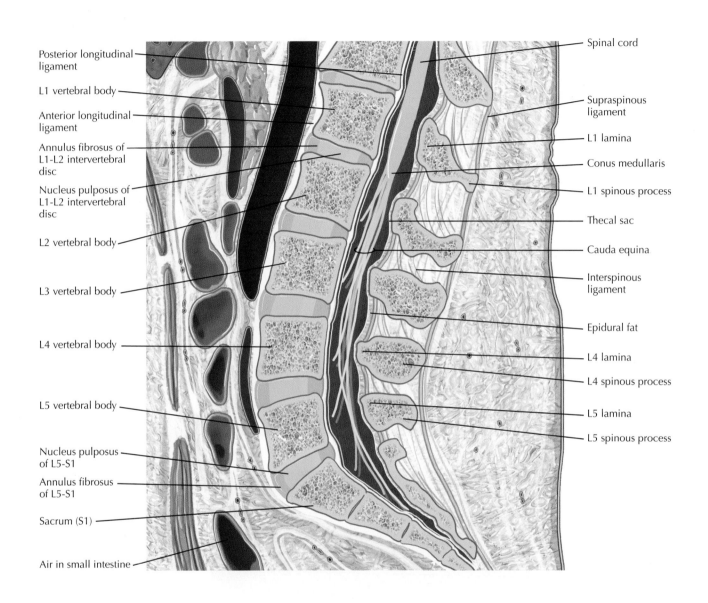

Posterior longitudinal ligament

L1 vertebral body

Anterior longitudinal ligament

Annulus fibrosus of L1-L2 intervertebral disc

Nucleus pulposus of L1-L2 intervertebral disc

L2 vertebral body

L3 vertebral body

L4 vertebral body

L5 vertebral body

Nucleus pulposus of L5-S1

Annulus fibrosus of L5-S1

Sacrum (S1)

Air in small intestine

Spinal cord

Supraspinous ligament

L1 lamina

Conus medullaris

L1 spinous process

Thecal sac

Cauda equina

Interspinous ligament

Epidural fat

L4 lamina

L4 spinous process

L5 lamina

L5 spinous process

NORMAL ANATOMY

The conus of the spinal cord is typically at or above the pars of L2. A lower location can be seen with a tethered cord and spina bifida.

Note that normal, healthy vertebral discs are well hydrated, showing as bright T2 signal, although not as bright as the cerebrospinal fluid.

IMAGING TECHNIQUE CONSIDERATION

Recall that on "turbo" or fast spin-echo T2-weighted imaging, unlike nonturbo T2-weighted imaging, the fat is also bright.

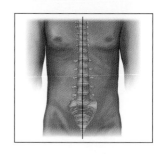

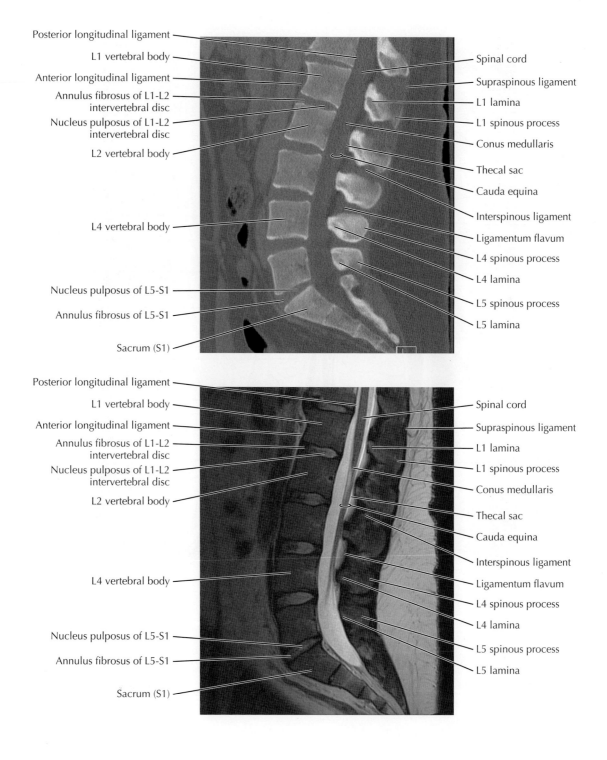

Posterior longitudinal ligament

L1 vertebral body

Anterior longitudinal ligament

Annulus fibrosus of L1-L2 intervertebral disc

Nucleus pulposus of L1-L2 intervertebral disc

L2 vertebral body

L4 vertebral body

Nucleus pulposus of L5-S1

Annulus fibrosus of L5-S1

Sacrum (S1)

Spinal cord

Supraspinous ligament

L1 lamina

L1 spinous process

Conus medullaris

Thecal sac

Cauda equina

Interspinous ligament

Ligamentum flavum

L4 spinous process

L4 lamina

L5 spinous process

L5 lamina

Posterior longitudinal ligament

L1 vertebral body

Anterior longitudinal ligament

Annulus fibrosus of L1-L2 intervertebral disc

Nucleus pulposus of L1-L2 intervertebral disc

L2 vertebral body

L4 vertebral body

Nucleus pulposus of L5-S1

Annulus fibrosus of L5-S1

Sacrum (S1)

Spinal cord

Supraspinous ligament

L1 lamina

L1 spinous process

Conus medullaris

Thecal sac

Cauda equina

Interspinous ligament

Ligamentum flavum

L4 spinous process

L4 lamina

L5 spinous process

L5 lamina

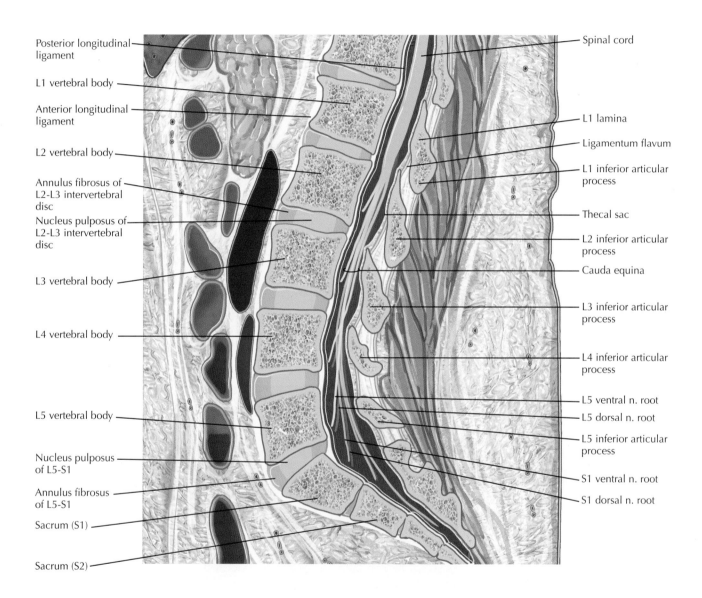

Posterior longitudinal ligament

L1 vertebral body

Anterior longitudinal ligament

L2 vertebral body

Annulus fibrosus of L2-L3 intervertebral disc

Nucleus pulposus of L2-L3 intervertebral disc

L3 vertebral body

L4 vertebral body

L5 vertebral body

Nucleus pulposus of L5-S1

Annulus fibrosus of L5-S1

Sacrum (S1)

Sacrum (S2)

Spinal cord

L1 lamina

Ligamentum flavum

L1 inferior articular process

Thecal sac

L2 inferior articular process

Cauda equina

L3 inferior articular process

L4 inferior articular process

L5 ventral n. root

L5 dorsal n. root

L5 inferior articular process

S1 ventral n. root

S1 dorsal n. root

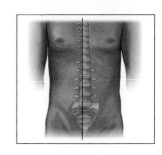

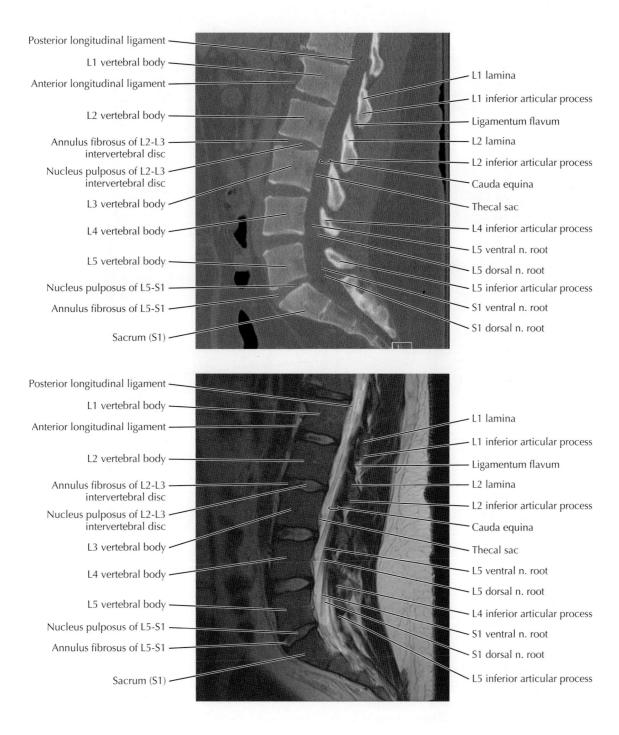

Posterior longitudinal ligament

L1 vertebral body

Anterior longitudinal ligament

L2 vertebral body

Annulus fibrosus of L2-L3 intervertebral disc

Nucleus pulposus of L2-L3 intervertebral disc

L3 vertebral body

L4 vertebral body

L5 vertebral body

Nucleus pulposus of L5-S1

Annulus fibrosus of L5-S1

Sacrum (S1)

L1 lamina

L1 inferior articular process

Ligamentum flavum

L2 lamina

L2 inferior articular process

Cauda equina

Thecal sac

L4 inferior articular process

L5 ventral n. root

L5 dorsal n. root

L5 inferior articular process

S1 ventral n. root

S1 dorsal n. root

Posterior longitudinal ligament

L1 vertebral body

Anterior longitudinal ligament

L2 vertebral body

Annulus fibrosus of L2-L3 intervertebral disc

Nucleus pulposus of L2-L3 intervertebral disc

L3 vertebral body

L4 vertebral body

L5 vertebral body

Nucleus pulposus of L5-S1

Annulus fibrosus of L5-S1

Sacrum (S1)

L1 lamina

L1 inferior articular process

Ligamentum flavum

L2 lamina

L2 inferior articular process

Cauda equina

Thecal sac

L5 ventral n. root

L5 dorsal n. root

L4 inferior articular process

S1 ventral n. root

S1 dorsal n. root

L5 inferior articular process

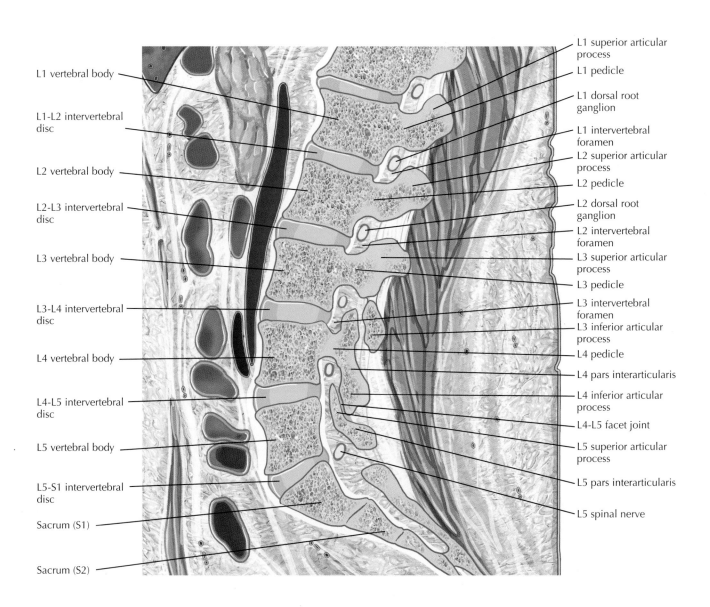

L1 vertebral body

L1-L2 intervertebral disc

L2 vertebral body

L2-L3 intervertebral disc

L3 vertebral body

L3-L4 intervertebral disc

L4 vertebral body

L4-L5 intervertebral disc

L5 vertebral body

L5-S1 intervertebral disc

Sacrum (S1)

Sacrum (S2)

L1 superior articular process

L1 pedicle

L1 dorsal root ganglion

L1 intervertebral foramen

L2 superior articular process

L2 pedicle

L2 dorsal root ganglion

L2 intervertebral foramen

L3 superior articular process

L3 pedicle

L3 intervertebral foramen

L3 inferior articular process

L4 pedicle

L4 pars interarticularis

L4 inferior articular process

L4-L5 facet joint

L5 superior articular process

L5 pars interarticularis

L5 spinal nerve

NORMAL ANATOMY

Note how much better the neural foramina are seen in the lumbar region than in the thoracic or cervical region because of the larger size and absence of confounding vertebral artery foramina. The lumbar foramina are typically keyhole shaped on parasagittal imaging, with the exiting nerve root in the larger upper aspect of the foramen.

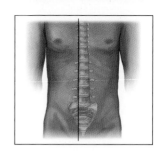

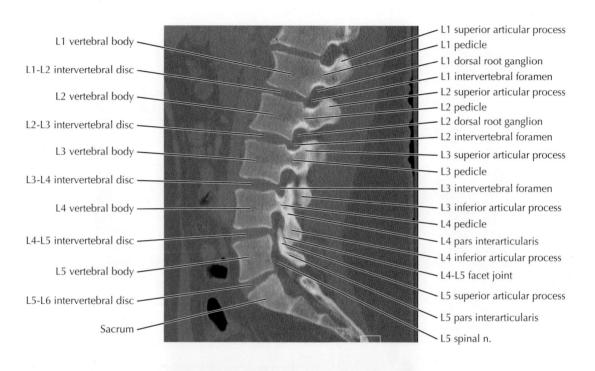

L1 vertebral body

L1-L2 intervertebral disc

L2 vertebral body

L2-L3 intervertebral disc

L3 vertebral body

L3-L4 intervertebral disc

L4 vertebral body

L4-L5 intervertebral disc

L5 vertebral body

L5-L6 intervertebral disc

Sacrum

L1 superior articular process

L1 pedicle

L1 dorsal root ganglion

L1 intervertebral foramen

L2 superior articular process

L2 pedicle

L2 dorsal root ganglion

L2 intervertebral foramen

L3 superior articular process

L3 pedicle

L3 intervertebral foramen

L3 inferior articular process

L4 pedicle

L4 pars interarticularis

L4 inferior articular process

L4-L5 facet joint

L5 superior articular process

L5 pars interarticularis

L5 spinal n.

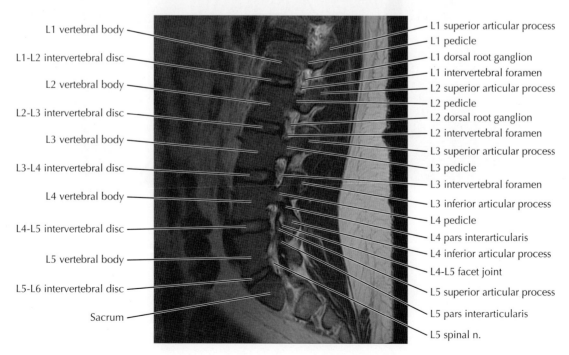

L1 vertebral body

L1-L2 intervertebral disc

L2 vertebral body

L2-L3 intervertebral disc

L3 vertebral body

L3-L4 intervertebral disc

L4 vertebral body

L4-L5 intervertebral disc

L5 vertebral body

L5-L6 intervertebral disc

Sacrum

L1 superior articular process

L1 pedicle

L1 dorsal root ganglion

L1 intervertebral foramen

L2 superior articular process

L2 pedicle

L2 dorsal root ganglion

L2 intervertebral foramen

L3 superior articular process

L3 pedicle

L3 intervertebral foramen

L3 inferior articular process

L4 pedicle

L4 pars interarticularis

L4 inferior articular process

L4-L5 facet joint

L5 superior articular process

L5 pars interarticularis

L5 spinal n.

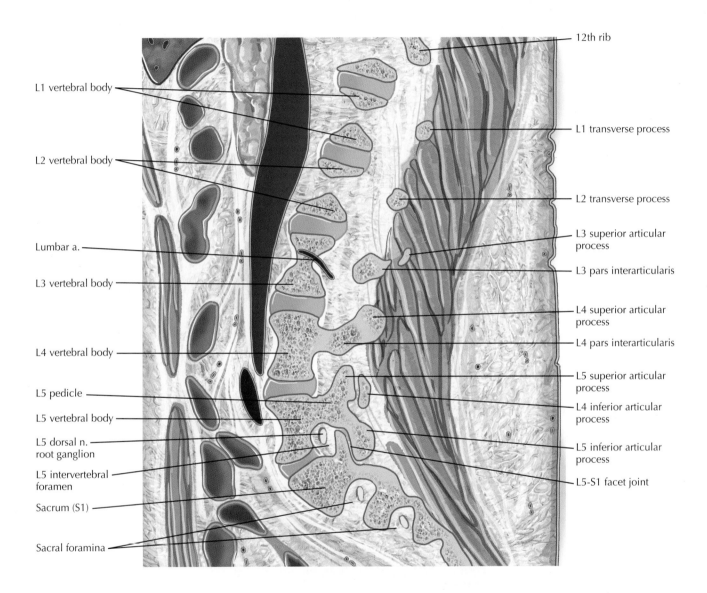

L1 vertebral body

L2 vertebral body

Lumbar a.

L3 vertebral body

L4 vertebral body

L5 pedicle

L5 vertebral body

L5 dorsal n. root ganglion

L5 intervertebral foramen

Sacrum (S1)

Sacral foramina

12th rib

L1 transverse process

L2 transverse process

L3 superior articular process

L3 pars interarticularis

L4 superior articular process

L4 pars interarticularis

L5 superior articular process

L4 inferior articular process

L5 inferior articular process

L5-S1 facet joint

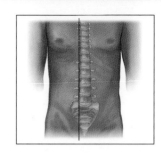

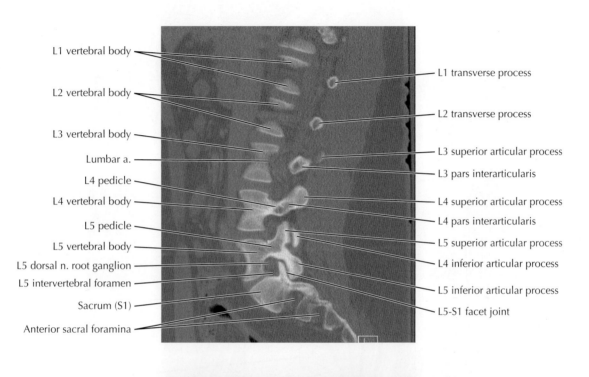

L1 vertebral body

L2 vertebral body

L3 vertebral body

Lumbar a.

L4 pedicle

L4 vertebral body

L5 pedicle

L5 vertebral body

L5 dorsal n. root ganglion

L5 intervertebral foramen

Sacrum (S1)

Anterior sacral foramina

L1 transverse process

L2 transverse process

L3 superior articular process

L3 pars interarticularis

L4 superior articular process

L4 pars interarticularis

L5 superior articular process

L4 inferior articular process

L5 inferior articular process

L5-S1 facet joint

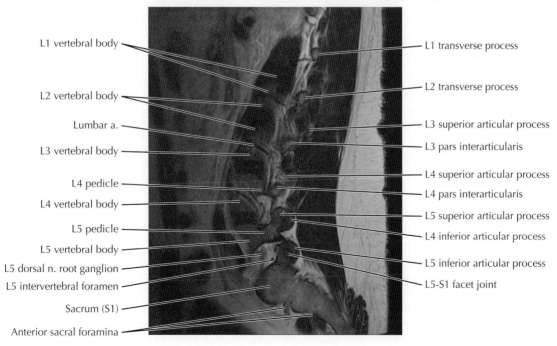

L1 vertebral body

L2 vertebral body

Lumbar a.

L3 vertebral body

L4 pedicle

L4 vertebral body

L5 pedicle

L5 vertebral body

L5 dorsal n. root ganglion

L5 intervertebral foramen

Sacrum (S1)

Anterior sacral foramina

L1 transverse process

L2 transverse process

L3 superior articular process

L3 pars interarticularis

L4 superior articular process

L4 pars interarticularis

L5 superior articular process

L4 inferior articular process

L5 inferior articular process

L5-S1 facet joint

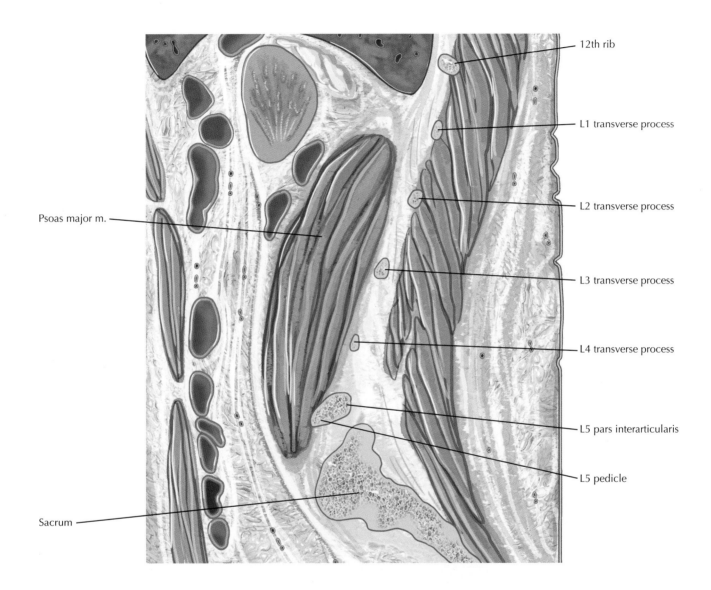

12th rib

L1 transverse process

L2 transverse process

Psoas major m.

L3 transverse process

L4 transverse process

L5 pars interarticularis

L5 pedicle

Sacrum

NORMAL ANATOMY

Lumbosacral Spine Sagittal 5 shows the standard five lumbar transverse processes, although variants can include a missing or accessory rib or a lumbarized S1 vertebral segment. Care must always be taken to declare the numbering of levels used when describing pathology in the spine. The best method is counting down from C1 (atlas), but in the absence of whole-spine imaging, a clearly identifiable landmark should be used.

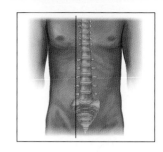

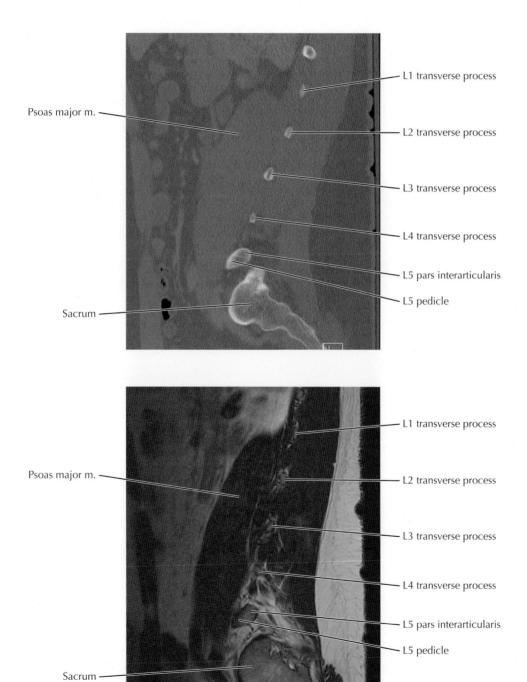

Psoas major m.

L1 transverse process

L2 transverse process

L3 transverse process

L4 transverse process

L5 pars interarticularis

L5 pedicle

Sacrum

Psoas major m.

L1 transverse process

L2 transverse process

L3 transverse process

L4 transverse process

L5 pars interarticularis

L5 pedicle

Sacrum

Index

Note: Page numbers with "*f*" denote figures; "*t*" tables.